英文中醫詞彙入門英文中醫詞彙入門 英文中醫詞
彙入門英文中醫詞彙入門英文中醫詞彙入門英文
中醫詞彙入門英文中醫詞彙入門英文中醫詞彙入
門英文中醫詞彙入門英文中醫詞彙入門英文中醫

英文中医词汇入门

Yīng Wén Zhōng Yī Cí Huì Rù Mén

Introduction to
English Terminology of Chinese Medicine

Nigel Wiseman （魏迺杰）
冯　晔 (Féng Yè)

U.S. Edition

英文中医词汇入门英文中医词汇入门英文中医词
汇入门英文中医词汇入门英文中医词汇入门英文
中医词汇入门英文中医词汇入门英文中医词汇入
门英文中医词汇入门英文中医词汇入门英文中医
词汇入门英文中医词汇入门英文中医词汇入门英

PARADIGM PUBLICATIONS   2002   BROOKLINE, MASSACHUSETTS

CHINESE   MEDICINE   LANGUAGE   SERIES

Introduction to English Terminology of Chinese Medicine
Yīngwén Zhōngyī Cíhuì Rùmén
英文中医词汇入门

Nigel Wiseman （魏迺杰） & 馮曄 (Féng Yè)

Copyright © 2002 Paradigm Publications
44 Linden Street
Brookline, MA 02445 USA
www.paradigm-pubs.com

Library of Congress Cataloging-in-Publication Data

Wiseman, Nigel.
    Introduction to English terminology of Chinese medicine / Nigel Wiseman, Féng Yè =
[Ying wen Zhong yi ci hui ru men / Wei Naijie, Feng Ye].–American ed.
        p. cm.
    Chinese parallel title in Chinese characters.
    Includes index.
    ISBN 0-912111-64-X
    1. Medicine, Chinese–Dictionaries. 2. Chinese language–Dictionaries–English. I. Title:
Ying wen Zhong yi ci hui ru men. II. Feng, Ye, 1967- III. Title.

    R121 .W54 2000
    610'.951'03–dc21

                                                                    00-051045

Council of Oriental Medical Publishers (C.O.M.P.) Designation: Compiled from
primary Chinese sources. English terminology from Wiseman N., 英汉汉英中医
词典 *English-Chinese Chinese-Dictionary of Chinese Medicine*, Húnán Science and
Technology Press, Chángshā, 1995.

Library of Congress Number: 00-051045
International Standard Book Number (ISBN): 0-912111-64-X
Printed in the United States of America

目 录
Contents

自 序
Preface

This book was first published in Táiwān as a text intended to teach Chinese medical English to Chinese students. The present U.S. edition has been prepared in response to demand from English-speaking students who have found the book to be a useful introduction to the concepts of Chinese medicine and to the English terminology described in greater detail in *A Practical Dictionary of Chinese Medicine* (Paradigm Publications, 1998). It is particularly suitable for students who are beginning to learn Chinese medicine after having studied Chinese and for those who wish to master the English terminology for the purposes of translation. Students with a knowledge of Chinese medicine who are new to Chinese might find our *Chinese Medical Chinese: Grammar and Vocabulary* more useful.

The present book covers just over a thousand commonly used Chinese terms in thematic order. Each English term is followed by the corresponding Chinese term in simplified and complex characters, as well as the Pīnyīn transcription. The pronunciation of the English term is given in Kenyon & Knott (KK) transcription for the benefit of non-English speakers. The definitions and clinical significance of terms are written entirely in English. Most of the terms used in the text of each entry are to be found as individual headwords.

At the end of each chapter are exercises. These not only provide activities for students to do in class or at home, but also furnish teachers with examples for examination questions.

The first block of questions tests students on their understanding of the text. Students are encouraged to use the index to find the point in the text where the solution is to be found. The other three blocks of questions ask for English and Pīnyīn equivalents of Chinese terms, Chinese and English equivalents of Pīnyīn terms, and Chinese and Pīnyīn equivalents of English terms, respectively. Questions of this type are of course suitable only for Chinese students learning the English terminology or English-speaking students learning the Chinese terminology.

There are five appendixes. The first appendix explains the Pīnyīn transcription system and the pronunciation of Chinese words.

The second appendix shows the correspondences between the Mandarin phonetic symbols for Chinese characters used in Táiwān and PRC Pīnyīn system that is now used internationally, helping Táiwān students to learn the Pīnyīn.

The third appendix presents the most important characters used in the terminology of Chinese medicine, with examples of their usage. Both single character and example terms are presented in simplified and complex form, so that students can choose which to learn, if not both. This appendix is primarily intended for Western students learning Chinese, but it is also helpful to any student seeking to understand the correspondences between the English and Chinese.

The fourth appendix contains the answers to the questions in the body of the book, so that especially students working on their own have access to the correct answers.

The fifth appendix is a list of entry head terms in the main part of the book. This has been included to help students to memorize terms.

At the end of the bok is a substantial index that includes all English headwords and their corresponding Pīnyīn and Chinese terms as well as English, Pīnyīn/Chinese, and Latin names of medicinals and the English and Pīnyīn/Chinese names of medical formulas. In this way, the index serves the additional function of a Chinese-English English-Chinese dictionary of nearly 70 pages.

The English terminology varies considerably from writer to writer. In this book, most of the terms are rendered in English on the basis of one English word to one Chinese character, discounting grammatical words, e.g., 命门火衰 *mìng mén huǒ shuāi*, debilitation of the life gate fire. The main exceptions are where a multiple-character Chinese term has a single-word English equivalent (e.g., 遗尿 *yí niào*, enuresis; 斜视 *xié shì*, squint) and where two virtually synonymous Chinese characters are used to create a euphonic term (e.g., 舌苔干燥 *shé tāi gān zào*, dry tongue fur; 扬手掷足 *yáng shǒu zhí zú*, flailing of the arms and legs). In translation, we have deliberately avoided rendering traditional Chinese medical concepts with Western medical terms that reflect the Western medical understanding and obscure the Chinese medical understanding. For example, we render 风火眼 *fēng huǒ yǎn* as wind-fire eye rather than as acute conjunctivitis. In this way, it is hoped that we can convey the original concepts of Chinese medicine accurately, without the misleading introduction of the medical ideas of acute and inflammation. Although the correspondences between Chinese medical and Western medical disease names is currently an important issue, discussion of them in translated texts should be reserved for notes and commentaries. In this case, a Western medical term should not be substituted for faithful translation since it deprives the reader of the understanding of the disease in terms of wind and fire.

Many Chinese medical terms have more than one meaning. For example, 滑 *huá* is used in different senses and as different parts of speech: describing the pulse, it refers to the tactile quality of slipperiness; describing the tongue fur, it refers to the visual quality of glossiness (or the tactile quality of slipperiness); and describing loss of semen, it refers to an uncontrolled slipping or flow out of the body. In this text, we have rendered 滑脉 *huá mài* as slippery pulse, 滑苔 *huá tāi* as glossy tongue fur, and 精滑 *jīng huá* as seminal efflux. As a matter of translation principle, we have tried to keep the number of renderings for each character to a minimum so that the correspondences between Chinese terms and English terms can be easily mastered by students and translators.

It should be noted that some of the Latin names of medicinals have been revised to conform to the *Chinese Pharmacopoeia* (2000). As a result of this revision, certain English names of medicinals and formulas have also been changed.

In our view, knowledge of medical Chinese is inestimably valuable for understanding Chinese medicine with clarity and precision. While a good deal of work is required from students to attain perfect comprehension of medical Chinese, each step along the way has its own rewards. Further, a growing body of translated literature that reflects terminology consistent with this text will support students' efforts to learn Chinese. Our aims will have been fulfilled when students can use this knowledge to improve their clinical practice or contribute to the westward transmission of Chinese medicine.

Acknowledgements

Special thanks go to students of China Medical College and Chang Gung University for their suggestions and corrections, and to Thomas Dey for his careful editing of the text.

第一章 基本概念
Basic Concepts

1.1. 阴阳
Yīn-Yáng

1.1.1.

1. 阴〔陰〕*yīn,* **yīn** [jɪn]
2. 阳〔陽〕*yáng,* **yáng** [jæŋ/jɑŋ, jɑŋ]

1. 事物的阴阳属性分类举例表 Yīn-Yáng in General Phenomena					
事物	Phenomenon	阴	Yīn	阳	Yáng
空间	**Space**	地	Earth	天	Heaven
时间	**Time**	黑夜	Night	白天	Day
季节	**Season**	秋 冬	Autumn Winter	春 夏	Spring Summer
性别	**Sex**	女	Female	男	Male
温度	**Temperature**	寒	Cold	热	Hot
重量	**Weight**	重	Heavy	轻	Light
亮度	**Brightness**	晦暗	Dark	光亮	Light
运动	**Motion**	静止	Stasis	运动	Motion
		下降	Downward	上升	Upward
		向内	Inward	向外	Outward

2.　人体部位的阴阳属性分类举例表 Yīn-Yáng in the Human Body			
阴	Yīn	阳	Yáng
里、腹	Interior, abdomen	表、背	Exterior, back
脏	Viscera	腑	Bowels
骨、筋	Bone & sinew	皮毛	Skin & body hair
血、营	Blood and construction	气卫	Qì and defense
抑制	Inhibition	兴奋	Excitation
衰退	Weakness	亢进	Strength

3.　证、脉的阴阳属性分类举例表 Yīn-Yáng in Patterns & Pulses					
		阴	Yīn	阳	Yáng
证	Pattern	里	Interior	表	Exterior
		虚	Vacuity	实	Repletion
		寒	Cold	热	Heat
脉	Pulse	迟	Slow	数	Rapid
		沉	Sunken	浮	Floating
		涩	Rough	滑	Slippery
		虚	Vacuous	实	Replete
		细	Fine	大、洪	Large & surging

1.1.2. 阴阳互动关系 Yīn-Yáng Interaction

3.　阴阳互根〔陰陽互根〕*yīn yáng hù gēn,* **yīn and yáng are rooted in each other** [jɪn ənd jæŋ/jɑŋ ɑr ˈrutɪd ɪn itʃ ˈʌðɚ]: Yīn and yáng are mutually dependent. "Yīn is rooted in yáng and yáng is rooted in yīn." The notion of interdependence means that neither phenomenon of a yīn-yáng pair can exist without the other. Yīn exists by virtue of yáng, and yáng exists by virtue of yīn. Light (yáng) cannot exist without darkness (yīn), and darkness cannot exist without light. Similarly, activity (yáng) cannot exist without rest (yīn). In medicine, the concept of interdependence of yīn and yáng is widely used in physiology, pathology, and treatment. Blood and qì, two fundamental elements of the human body, provide an example: blood is yīn and qì is yáng. It is said that "qì engenders blood," i.e., blood formation relies on the power of qì to move and transform food; "qì moves the blood," meaning that blood circulation relies on the warming and driving power of qì. Furthermore, "qì contains the blood," i.e., it keeps the blood within the vessels. The functions of engendering, moving, and containing the blood are summed up in the phrase, "qì is the commander of the blood." Conversely, qì is dependent on the provision of adequate nutrition by the blood; thus, it is said that "qì has its abode in the blood," and "blood is the mother of qì." Because qì has the power to engender blood, treatment of blood vacuity involves dual supplementation of qì and blood. Massive bleeding, where qì deserts with the blood, is first treated by boosting qì, since blood-nourishing formulas should not be administered until qì is secured. Similarly, formulas used to treat qì vacuity often include blood-nourishing medicinals to enhance qì supplementation. Another example of the interdependence of yīn and yáng, seen in the development of diseases, is the principle that "detriment to yīn affects yáng" and "detriment to yáng affects yīn." Since "without yáng, yīn cannot be born," when yáng vacuity reaches a certain point, the production of yīn humor is affected and yīn also becomes vacuous. Most cases of what Western medicine calls chronic nephritis indicate yáng vacuity and are characterized by water swelling due to the inability of the kidney to transform fluids. However, when the yáng vacuity reaches a certain point, fluid formation is affected and a yīn vacuity pattern evolves. This demonstrates the principle that "detriment to yáng affects yīn." Similarly, yīn vacuity, when reaching a certain peak, leads to simultaneous yáng vacuity, since "without yīn, yáng cannot arise." What is termed hypertension in Western medicine usually corresponds to hyperactivity of yáng caused by vacuity of yīn. In severe cases, this condition may develop into a dual yīn-yáng vacuity, illustrating the principle that "detriment to yīn affects yáng."

4. 阴阳制约〔陰陽制約〕*yīn yáng zhì yuē,* **yīn and yáng counterbalance each other** [jɪn ənd jæŋ/jɑŋ ˌkɑʊntəˈbæləns itʃ ˈʌðɚ]: Yīn and yáng both prevent their complement from becoming disproportionately strong. When either pole weakens, the other may grow stronger. Thus, in the body, when yīn humor is depleted, yáng qì appears relatively stronger and manifests in the form of heat (vacuity heat). In the body, yīn and yáng counterbalance each other. A deficit of one naturally leads to a surfeit of the other, while a surfeit of one will weaken the other. In both cases, yīn and yáng no longer counterbalance each other, and disease arises as a result. In medicine, the notion of counterbalancing is widely applied in physiology, pathology, and therapy. In physiology, for example, liver yīn counterbalances liver yáng, preventing it from becoming too strong. If liver yīn becomes insufficient and fails to counter-

balance its complement, ascendant hyperactivity of liver yáng develops. In the relationship of evils and the human body, yáng evils invading the body will cause a surfeit of yáng, which may result in damage to yīn humor and the emergence of a heat pattern. Conversely, a yīn evil entering the body will lead to a surfeit of yīn and cause damage to the body's yáng qì and the emergence of a cold pattern. These processes are described in *Elementary Questions (Sù Wèn)* in the following way: "If yáng abounds, yīn ails, and if yīn abounds, yang ails; when yáng prevails there is heat, and when yīn prevails there is cold." In therapy, if a disease is caused by heat evil, it is treated with cool or cold medicinals according to the principle that "cold can counteract heat," meaning yīn medicinals combat yáng evils. Similarly, diseases caused by cold evil are treated with warm or hot medicinals, since "heat can overcome cold," i.e., yáng medicinals can combat yīn evils. This is summed up in a guiding principle of therapy, "heat is treated with cold; cold is treated with heat." It is most often applied in patterns of repletion characterized by a surfeit of either yīn or yáng. In conditions caused by a deficit of yīn or yáng, the opposing complement is no longer kept in check and becomes disproportionately strong. If yīn is vacuous, yáng is no longer kept in check and its strength will grow out of proportion to that of yīn. Such a condition is at root a yīn vacuity that manifests as vacuity heat. For this reason, treatment by draining fire and clearing heat alone is not only ineffective but also detrimental to the patient's health. It is replaced by a method such as enriching yin and downbearing fire, or fostering yīn and subduing yáng, whereby clearing heat and draining fire are secondary to enriching yīn. By supplementing yīn, the yáng surfeit will naturally diminish. This explains the principle "invigorate the governor of water to restrain the brilliance of yáng." In the reverse situation, where yáng is vacuous and fails to keep yīn in check, there is exuberant internal yīn cold that can manifest as clear-food diarrhea, fifth-watch diarrhea, or water swelling. Here, treatment should aim not simply at dissipating cold evil, but also at supplementing the yáng vacuity through such methods as assisting yáng, boosting fire, and supplementing qì. This demonstrates the principle that "where warming is to no avail, fire is lacking" and "boost the source of fire to disperse the shroud of yīn." It is important to note the difference between the natural ebb and flow of yīn and yáng and a surfeit of one or the other complement. **Waxing and waning of yīn and yáng** refers to their normal relationship in the human body, which is one of constant fluctuation, rather than a rigid, immutable balance. "When yīn rises, yáng ebbs," and "when yáng swells, yīn subsides." This constant fluctuation is apparent in all the body's functions, such as fluid production and metabolism, the role of the five viscera in storing essential qì, and the role of the six bowels in conveyance and transformation of food. By contrast, "deficit" and "surfeit" denote the disturbance of the normal relative balance and failure to rectify the imbalance immediately. This is known as imbalance of yīn and yáng, which is the underlying cause of all disease.

5. 阴阳消长〔陰陽消長〕*yīn yáng xiāo zhǎng*, **waxing and waning of yīn and yáng** ['wæksɪŋ ənd wenɪŋ əf jɪn ənd jæŋ/jɑŋ]: See yīn and yáng counterbalance each other.

6. 阴阳转化〔陰陽轉化〕*yīn yáng zhuǎn huà*, **yīn and yáng convert into each other** [jɪn ənd jæŋ/jɑŋ kənˈvɜɻt ɪntu itʃ ˈʌðɚ]: Yáng can change into or give way to yīn, and vice versa. When an exuberant heat evil creates a severe yīn-yáng imbalance by damaging the blood fluids of the body, it "burns itself out" and has nothing left to thrive on. As a result, the original pattern of repletion heat converts into vacuity cold. Conversely, when yáng qì becomes so insufficient that it can no longer transform the fluids of the body, the fluids become a secondary evil that causes further disturbance in the body by accumulating in the abdomen in the form of drum distention (ascites). The original vacuity pattern turns into a repletion pattern. This form of conversion is due to failure of the mutual counterbalancing relationship of yīn and yáng.

7. 阳胜则热〔陽勝則熱〕*yáng shèng zé rè*, **when yáng prevails, there is heat** [wɛn jæŋ/jɑŋ prɪˈvelz, ðɛr ɪz hit]: When yáng qì is especially strong, febrile conditions develop.

8. 阴胜则寒〔陰勝則寒〕*yīn shèng zé hán*, **when yīn prevails, there is cold** [wɛn jɪn prɪˈvelz, ðɛr ɪz kold]: When yīn qì prevails, yáng qì is debilitated; hence, cold signs appear.

1.2. 五行
Five Phases

1.2.1.

9. 木〔木〕*mù*, **wood** [wʊd]

10. 火〔火〕*huǒ*, **fire** [fɑɪr]

11. 土〔土〕*tǔ*, **earth (soil)** [ɜˈθ(sɔɪl)]

12. 金〔金〕*jīn*, **metal** [mɛtl]

13. 水〔水〕*shuǐ,* **water** ['wɔtɚ]

事物的五行属性分类举例表 Five Phases in Nature				
木 Wood	火 Fire	土　Earth (Soil)	金 Metal	水 Water
酸 Sour	苦 Bitter	甘　Sweet	辛 Acrid	咸 Salty
青 Green-blue	赤 Red	黄　Yellow	白 White	黑 Black
生 Birth	长 Growth	化　Trans-formation	收 Withdrawal	藏 Storage
风 Wind	暑 Summerheat	湿　Dampness	燥 Dryness	寒 Cold
东 East	南 South	中　Center	西 West	北 North
春 Spring	夏 Summer	长夏 Long summer	秋 Autumn	冬 Winter

1.2.2. 五行互动关系 Five-Phase Interactions

14. **相生**〔相生〕*xiāng shēng,* **engendering** [ɪn'gɛndərɪŋ]: The nurturing effect that the five phases and their corresponding phenomena have on each other. Wood (liver) engenders fire; fire (heart) engenders earth; earth (spleen) engenders metal; metal (lung) engenders water; water (kidney) engenders wood. Engendering thus follows the sequence wood → fire → earth → metal → water → wood. It reflects the way in which spring gives way to summer, summer gives way to long summer, etc.

15. **相克**〔相剋〕*xiāng kè,* **restraining** [rɪ'strenɪŋ]: The action of the five phases and their corresponding phenomena of keeping each other in check. Wood (liver) restrains earth; earth (spleen) restrains water; water (kidney) restrains fire; fire (heart) restrains metal; metal (lung) restrains wood. Restraining thus follows the sequence wood → earth → water → fire → metal → wood. When the restraining cycle breaks down, the resulting disharmonies are called rebellion or overwhelming.

16. **相侮**〔相侮〕*xiāng wǔ,* **rebellion** [rɪ'bɛlɪən]: In the doctrine of the five phases, a reversal of the restraining relationship, where one of the five phases is disproportionately strong and rebels against the phase that should normally restrain it. For example, wood is normally restrained by metal, but if wood becomes too strong it will rebel against metal.

Powerless to withstand the attack, metal will succumb. In terms of the bowels and viscera, this means that when the liver, normally restrained by the lung, becomes too strong, it will rebel against the lung and overcome it.

17. 相乘〔相乘〕*xiāng chéng,* **overwhelming** [ˌovəʳˈ(h)wɛlmɪŋ]: In the doctrine of the five phases, an abnormal exaggeration of restraining where one of the phases is weakened and causes the phase that under normal circumstances would overcome it to invade and weaken it further. For example, wood normally restrains earth, but if earth is weak, then wood overwhelms it, rendering earth even weaker. In terms of the viscera, this means that the spleen, which the liver normally restrains, will, if weak, be completely overwhelmed by the liver and become even weaker.

1.2.3. 五行说明五脏之间的关系 Five-Phase Explanations of Relationships Between Viscera

18. 木火刑金〔木火刑金〕*mù huǒ xíng jīn,* **wood fire tormenting metal** [wud fɑɪr tɔrˈmɛntɪŋ ˈmɛtl̩]: Liver fire affecting the lung. Wood in the five phases is the liver, and metal is the lung. When liver fire becomes excessively effulgent, it can scorch lung yīn and cause dry cough, chest and rib-side pain, heart vexation, bitter taste in the heart, red eyes, and, in severe cases, expectoration of blood. This is the manifestation of wood fire tormenting metal.

19. 火盛刑金〔火盛刑金〕*huǒ shèng xíng jīn,* **exuberant fire tormenting metal** [ɪˈgzubərənt fɑɪr tɔrˈmɛntɪŋ ˈmɛtl̩]: See wood fire tormenting metal.

20. 木郁化火〔木鬱化火〕*mù yù huà huǒ,* **depressed wood transforming into fire** [dɪˈprɛst wud trænsˈfɔrmɪŋ ˈɪntə fɑɪr]: Depressed liver qì that gives rise to fire signs such as red face, red eyes, headache, dizziness, vomiting and retching, coughing of blood, and, in severe cases, mania. "Wood" in this context means the liver according to the five-phase understanding that the liver belongs to wood. However, "fire" means fire as an evil, not the viscus that belongs to fire, which is the heart. See liver depression transforming into fire.

21. 水火相济〔水火相濟〕*shuǐ huǒ xiāng jì,* **fire and water help each other** [fɑɪr ənd ˈwɔtəʳ hɛlp itʃ ˈʌðəʳ]: Heart fire and kidney water balance each other. In the doctrine of the five phases, the heart belongs to fire and the kidney belongs to water, and each restrains the other.

22. 水亏火旺〔水虧火旺〕*shuǐ kuī huǒ wàng,* **depleted water and effulgent fire** [dɪˈplitɪd ˈwɔtəʳ ənd ɪˈfʌldʒənt fɑɪr]: **1.** Insufficiency of kidney-

water that causes effulgent heart fire, characterized by heart vexation, dizziness, insomnia or unquiet sleep, red-tipped tongue, and a rapid fine pulse. **2.** A yīn-yáng imbalance of the kidney characterized by yīn vacuity and yáng hyperactivity. **3.** Kidney yīn depletion with hyperactivity of the life gate fire, characterized by loosening of and pain in the teeth, excessive libido, and seminal emission.

23. 火不生土〔火不生土〕 *huǒ bù shēng tǔ,* **fire failing to engender earth** [fɑɪr ˈfelɪŋ tu mˈdʒɛndɚ ɝθ]: Kidney yáng failing to warm the spleen. Earth represents the spleen, whereas fire represents kidney yáng (not the heart). In kidney yáng vacuity (insufficiency of the life gate fire), the spleen is deprived of warmth and its ability to transform food and water-damp is affected. Hence, there are signs of spleen-kidney yáng vacuity such as cold limp lumbus and knees, nontransformation of food, inhibited urination, swelling, and fifth-watch diarrhea.

24. 母病及子〔母病及子〕 *mǔ bìng jí zǐ,* **disease of the mother affects the child** [dɪˈziz əf ðə mʌðɚ əˈfɛkts ðə tʃaɪld]: The five-phase law that disease can spread from one bowel or viscus to the other according to the engendering sequence. For example, liver-wood is the mother of heart-fire, and ascendant liver yáng that causes exuberant heart fire is a disease of the mother affecting the child. Spleen-earth is the mother of lung-metal, and spleen-stomach vacuity giving rise to insufficiency of lung qì is another example.

1.2.4. 五脏 Five Viscera

25. 肝〔肝〕 *gān,* **liver** [ˈlɪvɚ]: Belongs to wood.
26. 心〔心〕 *xīn,* **heart** [hɑrt]: Belongs to fire.
27. 脾〔脾〕 *pí,* **spleen** [splin]: Belongs to earth (soil).
28. 肺〔肺〕 *fèi,* **lung** [lʌŋ]: Belongs to metal.
29. 肾〔肾〕 *shèn,* **kidney** [ˈkɪdnɪ]: Belongs to water.

1.2.5. 五脏所主 Governings of the Five Viscera

30. 筋〔筋〕 *jīn,* **sinew** [ˈsɪnju]: Tough, stringy, elastic parts of the body (tendon, muscle). Governed by liver.
31. 脉〔脉〕 *mài,* **vessel** [ˈvɛsl̩]: Governed by the heart.
32. 肌肉〔肌肉〕 *jī ròu,* **flesh** [flɛʃ]: Governed by the spleen.
33. 皮毛〔皮毛〕 *pí máo,* **skin and [body] hair** [skɪn, ˈbɑdɪ–hɛr]: Governed by the lung.
34. 骨〔骨〕 *gǔ,* **bone** [bon]: Governed by the kidney.

1.2.6. 五官 Five Offices

35. 目〔目〕*mù,* **eye** [ɑɪ]: Governed by the liver.

36. 舌〔舌〕*shé,* **tongue** [tʌŋ]: Governed by the heart.

37. 唇〔唇〕*chún,* **lips** [lɪps]: Governed by the spleen.

38. 鼻〔鼻〕*bí,* **nose** [noz]: Governed by the lung.

39. 耳〔耳〕*ěr,* **ear** [ir]: Governed by the kidney.

5. 人体的五行属性分类举例表 Five Phases in Man				
木 Wood	火 Fire	土 Earth (Soil)	金 Metal	水 Water
肝 Liver	心 Heart	脾 Spleen	肺 Lung	肾 Kidney
胆 Gall-bladder	小肠 Small intestine	胃 Stomach	大肠 Large intestine	膀胱 Bladder
目 Eyes	舌 Tongue	口 Mouth	鼻 Nose	耳 Ears
筋 Sinew	脉 Vessels	肉 Flesh	皮毛 Skin & body hair	骨 Bone
怒 Anger	喜 Joy	思 Thought	悲 Sorrow	恐 Fear
呼 Shouting	笑 Laughing	歌 Singing	哭 Wailing	呻 Moaning
泪 Tears	汗 Sweat	涎 Drool	涕 Snivel	唾 Spittle
弦 Stringlike	洪 Surging	缓 Moderate	毛 Downy	石 Stone-like

1.2.7. 五色 Five Colors

40. 青〔青〕*qīng,* **green-blue** [grin blu]: Color associated with wood.

41. 赤〔赤〕*chì,* **red** [rɛd]: Color associated with fire.

42. 黄〔黄〕*huáng,* **yellow** ['jɛlo]: Color associated with earth (soil).

43. 白〔白〕*bái,* **white** [wɑɪt, hwɑɪt]: Color associated with metal.

44. 黑〔黑〕*hēi,* **black** [blæk]: Color associated with water.

1.2.8. 五液 Five Humors

45. 泪〔淚〕*lèi,* **tears** [tirz]: Humor of the liver.

46. 汗〔汗〕*hàn,* **sweat** [swɛt]: Humor of the heart.

47. 涎〔涎〕*xián,* **drool** [drul]: Humor of the spleen. Drool is said to spring from the cheeks and to flow out from the corners of the mouth during sleep.

48. 涕〔涕〕*tì,* **snivel; nasal mucus** [ˈsnɪvl̩, ˈnezl̩ ˈmjukəs]: Humor of the lung.

49. 唾〔唾〕*tuò,* **spittle** [ˈspɪtl̩]: Humor of the kidney. Spittle is said to spring from under the tongue and to be spat out of the mouth.

1.2.9. 五味 Five Flavors

50. 酸〔酸〕*suān,* **sour, sourness** [saʊr, ˈsaʊrnɪs]: Flavor associated with wood.

51. 苦〔苦〕*kǔ,* **bitter, bitterness** [ˈbɪtɚ, ˈbɪtɚnɪs]: Flavor associated with fire.

52. 甘〔甘〕*gān,* **sweet, sweetness** [swit, ˈswitnɪs]: Flavor associated with earth (soil).

53. 辛〔辛〕*xīn,* **acrid, acridity** [ˈækrɪd, əˈkrɪdɪtɪ]: Flavor associated with metal.

54. 咸〔鹹〕*xián,* **salty, saltiness** [ˈsɔltɪ, ˈsɔltɪnɪs]: Flavor associated with water.

1.2.10. 五志 Five Minds

55. 怒〔怒〕*nù,* **anger** [æŋgɚ]: Mind associated with liver-wood.

56. 喜〔喜〕*xǐ,* **joy** [dʒɔɪ]: Mind associated with heart-fire.

57. 思〔思〕*sī,* **thought** [θɔt]: Mind associated with spleen-earth.

58. 忧〔憂〕*yōu,* **anxiety** [æŋgˈzaɪətɪ]: Mind associated with lung-metal.

59. 恐〔恐〕*kǒng,* **fear** [fir]: Mind associated with kidney-water.

60. 七情〔七情〕*qī qíng,* **seven affects** [ˈsɛvən ˈæfɛkts]: The seven affects are an alternative classification of mental states. They comprise the five minds given above, sorrow, and fright. Note that the affects and minds are often referred to generically as "affect-mind" (情志 *qíng zhì*).

61. 情志〔情志〕*qíng zhì,* **affect-mind** [ˈæfɛkt–ˌmaɪnd]: See seven affects.

62. 悲〔悲〕*bēi,* **sorrow** [ˈsɔro]: One of the seven affects.

63. 惊〔驚〕*jīng,* **fright** [fraɪt]: One of the seven affects.

1.3. 脏腑、人体部位及基本物质
Bowels & Viscera, Body Parts, and Basic Substances

1.3.1. 五脏 Five Viscera

The liver, heart, spleen, lung, and kidney (introduced in the first chapter). In acupuncture theory, the pericardiac network vessel is taken as a sixth viscus so that the viscera match the bowels in number.

64. 心包络〔心包絡〕*xīn bāo luò*, **pericardiac network** [ˌpɛrɪˈkɑrdɪæk ˈnɛtwɝk]

1.3.2. 六腑 Six Bowels

65. 胃〔胃〕*wèi*, **stomach** [ˈstʌmək]
66. 小肠〔小腸〕*xiǎo cháng*, **small intestine** [smɔl inˈtɛstɪn]
67. 大肠〔大腸〕*dà cháng*, **large intestine** [lɑrdʒ inˈtɛstɪn]
68. 胆〔膽〕*dǎn*, **gallbladder** [ˈgɔlblædɚ]
69. 膀胱〔膀胱〕*páng guāng*, **bladder** [ˈblædɚ]
70. 三焦〔三焦〕*sān jiāo*, **triple burner** [ˈtrɪpl̩ ˈbɝnɚ]

1.3.3. 人体部位 Body Parts

71. 身〔身〕*shēn*, **body** [ˈbɑdɪ]
72. 形〔形〕*xíng*, **body** [ˈbɑdɪ]
73. 体〔體〕*tǐ*, **body; constitution** [ˈbɑdɪ, ˌkɑnstɪˈt(j)uʃən]
74. 头〔頭〕*tóu*, **head** [hɛd]
75. 额〔額〕*é*, **forehead** [ˈfɔrɪd]
76. 面〔面〕*miàn*, **face (*n.*); facial (*adj.*)** [fes, ˈfeʃl̩]
77. 囟〔囟〕*xìn*, **fontanel** [ˈfɑntəˌnɛl]: Either of two gaps between the bones of the skull that close between the age of six months and two years, especially the larger one. The larger fontanel, the "fontanel gate" or "forehead fontanel" (额囟 *é xìn*, called anterior fontanel in Western medicine), is located just in front of the vertex; the smaller one, the "pillow fontanel" (枕囟 *zhěn xìn*, called the posterior fontanel in Western medicine), is on the back of the head.
78. 囟门〔囟門〕*xìn mén*, **fontanel gate, anterior fontanel** [ˈfɑntəˌnɛl get, ænˈtɪrɪɚ ˈfɑntəˌnɛl] See fontanel.
79. 口〔口〕*kǒu*, **mouth (*n.*); oral (*adj.*)** [mɑʊθ, ˈɔrəl]

80. 齿〔齒〕*chǐ,* **tooth** (*n.*); **dental** (*adj.*) [tuθ, ˈdɛntl̩]: The teeth are said to be the surplus of the bone (齿为骨之余 *chǐ wéi gǔ zhī yú*).

81. 牙〔牙〕*yá,* **tooth** (*n.*); **dental** (*adj.*) [tuθ, ˈdɛntl̩]

82. 牙齿〔牙齒〕*yá chǐ,* **tooth** (*n.*); **dental** (*adj.*) [tuθ, ˈdɛntl̩]

83. 齿牙〔齒牙〕*chǐ yá,* **tooth** (*n.*); **dental** (*adj.*) [tuθ, ˈdɛntl̩]

84. 龈〔齦〕*yín,* **gum** [gʌm]

85. 齿龈〔齒齦〕*chǐ yín,* **gum** [gʌm]

86. 颈〔頸〕*jǐng,* **neck** [nɛk]

87. 项〔項〕*xiàng,* **nape** [nep]

88. 咽〔咽〕*yān,* **pharynx** (*n.*), **pharyngeal** (*adj.*); **throat** (*n.*) [ˈfærɪŋks, fəˈrɪndʒɪəl, θrot]

89. 喉〔喉〕*hóu,* **throat, larynx** [θrot, ˈlærɪŋks]

90. 喉核〔喉核〕*hóu hé,* **throat node** [θrot nod]: Either of two slight protrusions on each side of the throat. The throat nodes correspond to the tonsils in Western medicine.

91. 喉关〔喉關〕*hóu guān,* **throat pass** [θrot pæs]: The isthmus faucium (咽峡 *yān xiá*).

92. 悬雍垂〔懸雍垂〕*xuán yōng chuí,* **uvula** [ˈjuvjələ]: The fleshy protuberance hanging down at the back of the palate.

93. 会厌〔會厭〕*huì yàn,* **epiglottis** [ˌɛpɪˈglɑtɪs]

94. 结喉〔結喉〕*jié hóu,* **laryngeal prominence** [ləˈrɪndʒɪəl ˈprɑmɪnəns]: The Adam's apple.

95. 胸〔胸〕*xiōng,* **chest** [tʃɛst, θəˈræsɪk]

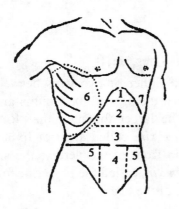

1. [Region] below the heart

2. Stomach duct

1, 2, and 3. Greater abdomen

4. Smaller abdomen

5. Lesser abdomen

6. Rib-side

7. Vacuous lǐ

96. 胁〔脅〕 *xié*, **rib-side** [ˌrɪbsɑɪd]: The area from the armpit down to the bottom of the ribs (i.e., to the lowest of the 12 ribs). The rib-side is traversed by the foot reverting yīn (*jué yīn*) liver and foot lesser yáng (*shào yáng*) gallbladder channels; hence, pain in this area is associated with diseases of the liver and gallbladder.

97. 乳〔乳〕 *rǔ*, **breast** [brɛst]: Either of two fleshy protruberances of the female chest each headed by a nipple and whose function is to produce milk for breast-feeding. The breasts lie on the foot yáng brightness (*yáng míng*) channel. See nipple.

98. 乳头〔乳頭〕 *rǔ tóu*, **nipple** [nɪpl̩]: The dark-colored protruding head of the breast in the female, and in males in the corresponding position. The nipples belong to the liver and diseases of them are often treated through the liver channel.

99. 虚里〔虛里〕 *xū lǐ*, **vacuous lǐ** [ˈvæk(j)uəs li]: The place below the nipple at which a throbbing can be felt and that is said to be the collecting place of ancestral qì. Vacuous lǐ corresponds in channel theory to the great network vessel of the stomach, and since stomach qì is the foundation of human life and is the source of ancestral qì in the chest, vacuous lǐ reflects the state of ancestral qì and stomach qì. Vacuous lǐ corresponds to the apical pulse in Western medicine.

100. 心下〔心下〕 *xīn xià*, **[region] below the heart** [ˈridʒən bɪˈlo ðə hɑrt]: The part of the abdomen located just below the breast bone; the pit of the stomach (胸口 *xiōng kǒu*).

101. 胃脘〔胃脘〕 *wèi wǎn*, **stomach duct** [ˈstʌmək-dʌkt]: The stomach cavity and adjoining sections of the small intestine and gullet. The stomach duct is divided into the upper, center, and lower stomach ducts.

102. 脘〔脘〕 *wǎn*, **stomach duct** [ˈstʌmək-dʌkt]: See preceding item.

103. 腹〔腹〕 *fù*, **abdomen** (*n.*); **abdominal** (*adj.*) [ˈæbdəmən, əbˈdamɪnl̩]: The anterior aspect of the body from the ribs down to the genitals, considered yīn in relationship to the back, which is yáng.

104. 脐〔臍〕 *qí*, **umbilicus** (*n.*); **umbilical** (*adj.*) [ˌʌmbəˈlaɪkəs, ʌmˈbɪlɪkl̩]: The rounded, knotty depression in the center of the abdomen, caused by the detachment of the umbilical cord after birth. Also called navel.

105. 大腹〔大腹〕 *dà fù*, **greater abdomen** [ˈgretɚ ˈæbdəmən]: The part of the abdomen above the umbilicus. Corresponds to "epigastrium" in Western medical terminology.

106. 小腹〔小腹〕 *xiǎo fù*, **smaller abdomen** [ˈsmɔlɚ ˈæbdəmən]: The part of the abdomen below the umbilicus.

107. 少腹〔少腹〕*shào fù,* **lesser abdomen** [ˈlɛsɚ ˈæbdəmən]: The smaller abdomen or the lateral parts of it.

108. 肩〔肩〕*jiān,* **shoulder** [ˈʃoldɚ]: The upper part of the trunk below the neck.

109. 背〔背〕*bèi,* **back** [bæk]: The posterior aspect of the trunk, from the shoulder to lumbus.

110. 膈〔膈〕*gé,* **diaphragm (*n.*); diaphragmatic (*adj.*)** [ˈdɑɪəˌfræm, ˌdɑɪəfræˈm ætɪk]

111. 腰〔腰〕*yāo,* **lumbus (*n.*); lumbar (*adj.*)** [ˈlʌmbəs, ˈlʌmbɚ]: The lower part of the back. "The lumbus is the house of the kidney" (腰为肾之府 *yāo wéi shèn zhī fǔ*). This reflects the observation that lumbar pain is often a manifestation of kidney qì vacuity.

112. 肢〔肢〕*zhī,* **limb** [lɪm]

113. 手〔手〕*shǒu,* **hand** [hænd]: See next item.

114. 手（臂）〔手（臂）〕*shǒu (bèi),* **arm** [ɑrm]: In Chinese "arm" and "hand" are not distinguished as clearly as in English: 手 means "hand" or "arm and hand"; 手臂 means "arm."

115. 足〔足〕*zú,* **foot** [fʊt]

116. 足〔足〕*zú,* **leg** [lɛg]

117. 手足〔手足〕*shǒu zú,* **extremities** [ɪksˈtrɛmɪtɪz]: Arms/hands and legs/feet.

118. 腿〔腿〕*tuǐ,* **leg** [lɛg]

119. 膝〔膝〕*xī,* **knee** [ni]

120. 肘〔肘〕*zhǒu,* **elbow** [ˈɛlbo]

121. 踝〔踝〕*huái,* **ankle** [ˈæŋkl]

122. 腕〔腕〕*wàn,* **wrist** [rɪst]

123. 腠理〔腠理〕*còu lǐ,* **interstices** [ˈɪntɚˌstɪsɪz]: An anatomical entity of unclear identity, explained in modern dictionaries as being the "grain" of the skin, flesh, and organs or the connective tissue in the skin and flesh. *Elementary Questions (Sù Wèn)* states, "Clear yáng effuses through the interstices." Modern usage of the term suggests that the interstices correspond to the sweat ducts in Western medicine.

124. 窍〔竅〕*qiào,* **orifice** [ˈɔrəfɪs]: Any one of the openings of the body. The *upper orifices* (上窍 *shàng qiào*) or *clear orifices* (清窍 *qīng qiào*) are the eyes, ears, nostrils, and mouth, whereas the *lower orifices* (下窍 *xià qiào*) or *turbid orifices* (浊窍 *zhuó qiào*) are the anal and genital orifices. These are collectively known as the *nine orifices* (九窍 *jiǔ qiào*).

125. 命门〔命門〕 *mìng mén,* **life gate** [lɑɪf get]: A physiological entity of disputed morphological identity. The term "life gate" first appears in *The Inner Canon (Nèi Jīng),* where it refers to the eyes. Reference to a "life gate" as an internal organ first appears in *The Classic of Difficult Issues (Nàn Jīng, 36),* which states, "The two kidneys are not both kidneys. The left one is the kidney, and the right is the life gate." The question of the life gate invited little discussion until the Míng and the Qīng, when various theories were put forward: a) both kidneys contain the life gate; b) the space between the kidneys is the life gate; c) the life gate is the stirring qì between the kidneys; d) the life gate is the root of original qì and the house of fire and water; e) the life gate is the fire of earlier heaven or the true yáng of the whole body; and f) the life gate is the gate of birth, i.e., in women the "birth gate" (产门 *chǎn mén*) and in men the "essence gate" (精室 *jīng shì*). Nowadays, the life gate is usually understood as the fire of earlier heaven or the true yáng of the whole body.

126. 精关〔精關〕 *jīng guān,* **essence gate** [ˈɛsəns get]: The barrier that regulates the discharge of semen. The Chinese term *jīng* means essence and, its physical manifestation, semen. The "essence gate" is not clearly defined as an anatomical structure. Zhāng Jiè-Bīn (Míng, 1563–1640) described a "gate that is felt to open on ejaculation," which is now often called the essence gate. Signs such as seminal efflux, seminal emission, and premature ejaculation are attributed to "insecurity of the essence gate" due to kidney disease.

127. 真元〔眞元〕 *zhēn yuán,* **true origin** [tru ˈɔrədʒɪn]: Original qì in its relationship to the kidney.

128. 膏肓〔膏肓〕 *gāo huāng,* **gāo-huāng** [gɑʊ-hwaŋ]: The region below the heart and above the diaphragm. When a disease is said to have entered the gāo-huāng, it is difficult to cure.

129. 膜原〔膜原〕 *mó yuán,* **membrane source** [ˈmɛmbren–ˌsɔrs]: A membrane of the chest or diaphragm that is not clearly defined. In the warm disease doctrine concerning externally contracted heat (febrile) disease, the term membrane source denotes a location between the exterior and interior; hence "evil in the membrane source" corresponds to midstage patterns in the cold damage doctrine.

130. 丹田〔丹田〕 *dān tián,* **cinnabar field** [ˈsɪnəbɑr fild]: **1.** An area three body-inches (*cùn*) below the umbilicus, believed by Daoists to be the chamber of essence (semen) in males and the uterus in females. **2.** Any of three mustering positions in qi-gong, including the lower cinnabar field (*xià dān tián*) located below the umbilicus, the middle cinnabar

field (*zhōng dān tián*) located in the pit of the stomach (scrobiculus cordis), and the upper cinnabar field (*shàng dān tián*) located in the center of the brow.

131. 血室〔血室〕*xuè shì,* **blood chamber** [ˈblʌd–ˌtʃembɚ]: A place where blood is stored, variously defined as the uterus, the liver, or the thoroughfare vessel.

132. 气海〔氣海〕*qì hǎi,* **sea of qì** [si əv tʃi]: **1.** The center of the chest. **2.** Cinnabar field.

1.3.4. 基本物质 Basic Substances

133. 气〔氣〕*qì,* **qì** [tʃi]: The Chinese term qì has the following meanings: **1.** Air, gas, vapor, flatus (e.g., belching of putrid qì). **2.** Smell, odor (as in 气味 *qì wèi,* smell, odor), usually translated as such rather than as qì. **3.** Environmental forces (e.g., cold; dampness; dryness). **4.** Nature (e.g., the four qì of medicinals—cool, cold, warm, hot). **5.** Anything of a particular nature (e.g., yīn qì, the yīn forces of the body). **6.** Breath; breathing (see rough breathing). **7.** Any of various dynamic phenomena of the body (e.g., source qì; construction qì; defense qì; bowel and visceral qì; channel qì) understood to have the functions of: powering bodily activity; transforming qì, blood, fluids, and essence; keeping the body warm; defending the body against evils invading it from outside; containing fluids (keeping blood flowing in the vessels and containing sweat and urine). **8.** Strength. **9.** Anger. **10.** Disease (e.g., leg qì, mounting qì, plum-pit qì). **11.** An abbreviation for diseases of qì (qì vacuity, qì stagnation), as appearing in the terms qì constipation (气秘 *qì bì*) and qì tumor (气瘤 *qì liú*), etc.

134. 阳气〔陽氣〕*yáng qì,* **yáng qì** [jæŋ/jɑŋ tʃi]: **1.** Anything yáng in nature, in complementary opposition to yīn qì. **2.** The active or functional aspect of the body, in complementary opposition to yīn-blood or yīn humor.

135. 阴气〔陰氣〕*yīn qì,* **yīn qì** [jɪn tʃi]: Anything yīn in nature, in complementary opposition to yáng qī.

136. 原气〔原氣〕*yuán qì,* **source qì** [ˈsɔrs–tʃi]: The basic form of qì in the body, which is made up of a combination of three other forms: the essential qì of the kidney; qì of grain and water, derived through the transformative function of the spleen; and air (great qì) drawn in through the lung. Source qì springs from the kidney (or life gate) and is stored in the cinnabar field (丹田 *dān tián*), the area three body-inches (寸 *cùn*) below the umbilicus; it reaches all parts of the body through the pathways of the triple burner, activating all the bowels and viscera. It is

the basis of all physiological activity. All other forms of qì inherent in the body are considered to be manifestations or derivatives of source qì.

137. 营气 〔 營氣 〕 *yíng qì,* **construction qì** [kən'strʌkʃən–tʃi]: The qì that forms the blood and flows with it in the vessels, helping to nourish the entire body.

138. 卫气 〔 衛氣 〕 *wèi qì,* **defense qì** [dɪ'fɛns–tʃi]: A qì described as being "fierce, bold, and uninhibited" and unable to be contained by the vessels and therefore flowing outside them. In the chest and abdomen it warms the bowels and viscera, whereas in the exterior it flows through the skin and flesh, regulates the opening and closing of the interstices (i.e., the sweat glands/ducts), and keeps the skin lustrous and healthy, thereby protecting the fleshy exterior (肌表 *jī biǎo*) and preventing the invasion of external evils.

139. 正气 〔 正氣 〕 *zhèng qì,* **right qì** ['rɑɪt–tʃi]: True qì, especially in opposition to disease. Right qì is the active aspect of all components including the bowels and viscera, blood, fluids, and essence and the abovementioned forms of qì in maintaining health and resisting disease. Right qì stands in opposition to evil qì, which is any entity in its active aspect of harming the body.

140. 邪气 〔 邪氣 〕 *xié qì,* **evil qì** ['ivl̩–tʃi]: An evil or evils as an active force.

141. 元气 〔 元氣 〕 *yuán qì,* **original qì** [ə'rɪdʒɪnl̩–tʃi]: **1.** Source qì. **2.** Right qì.

142. 宗气 〔 宗氣 〕 *zōng qì,* **ancestral qì** [æn'sɛstrəl–tʃi]: The qì that converges or concentrates in the chest (or the "sea of qì," as it is often called in this context), pervades the respiratory tract and controls breathing, and penetrates the heart and vessels. Ancestral qì drives the heart and regulates the pulses; its health is reflected in the strength of breathing and in the voice.

143. 脏腑之气 〔 臟腑之氣 〕 *zàng fǔ zhī qì,* **bowel and visceral qì** ['bɑʊəl ənd 'vɪsərəl tʃi]: The qì of the bowels and viscera. Each bowel and viscus has its own qì, which is the basis of its physiological activity and manifests as a major aspect of its physiological function. The heartbeat is the manifestation of heart qì, and bowel movements are a manifestation of large intestine qì.

144. 经络之气 〔 經絡之氣 〕 *jīng luò zhī qì,* **channel and network vessel qì** ['tʃænl̩ ənd 'nɛtwɝk–ˌvɛsl̩ tʃi]: The qì that flows through the channels and network vessels. Its movement is seen in the channels' function of transmission and conveyance. The sensation produced by needling an

acupuncture point, known as "obtaining qì" (得气 *dé qì*), demonstrates the presence of channel qì.

145. 气化〔氣化〕*qì huà,* **qì transformation** [tʃi ˌtrænsfɚˈmeʃən]: The movement, mutation, and conversion of qì. In ancient Chinese thought, qì is considered to be a material entity having yīn and yáng aspects that are interdependent and opposing. Yáng qì is formless and intangible (无形 *wú xíng*), yet can evolve to assume tangible forms, which are yīn qì. Yīn qì and yáng qì form a unity of opposites and undergo constant mutation from which the material world springs. This constant mutation is called "qì transformation." In the human body, qì in a wider sense denotes essence, qì (yáng qì), liquid, humor, and blood, as well as disease-causing entities, or so-called "evils," such as wind, cold, summerheat, etc. (see **six qì**). The term "qì transformation" refers to the processes by which these qì produce each other and convert from one to another. Qì transformation is therefore life activity. The five viscera and six bowels, the limbs and bones, etc., are all involved in the process of qì transformation. The movement of blood and essential qì, the distribution of fluids, the digestion and assimilation of food, the discharge of waste, the moistening of the sinews and bones, the warming of the skin, the maintenance of the sheen of the hair of the head and body, and the regulation of the bowels and viscera all rely upon qì transformation. For this reason, some writers have said that qì transformation is roughly equivalent to the Western medical concept of metabolism. Growth and development of the body, and defense against external evils, are similarly dependent upon qì transformation. Cessation of qì transformation is the cessation of life. This is the broadest meaning of "qì transformation." In a narrower meaning, the term denotes the qì transformation of the triple burner, especially in the context of fluid metabolism.

146. 血〔血〕*xuè,* **blood** [blʌd]: The red fluid of the body that flows through blood vessels. Blood is traditionally said to be created from the essential qì derived from food by the stomach and spleen, which becomes red blood after being transformed by construction qì and the lung. It flows to all parts of the body and is governed by the heart. By the action of the heart and lung, it flows through the vessels, carrying nourishment to the whole of the body. All the bowels and viscera and all parts of the body rely on the blood for nourishment. The heart and liver are said to have their own blood, the terms "heart blood" and "liver blood" meaning blood in relation to the functions of those two viscera.

147. 阴血〔陰血〕*yīn xuè,* **yīn-blood** [jɪn blʌd]: Blood as a yīn substance.

148. 精〔精〕*jīng,* **essence** ['ɛsəns]: That which is responsible for growth, development, and reproduction, which determines the strength of the constitution, and which, in the male, is manifest physically in the form of semen. Essence is stored by the kidney. It is composed of earlier heaven essence and later heaven essence. Earlier heaven essence (先天之精 *xiān tiān zhī jīng,* also called congenital essence) is the essence present from birth that is inherited from the parents and that is constantly supplemented by later heaven essence (后天之精 *hòu tiān zhī jīng,* also called acquired essence), which is the essence acquired after birth that is produced from food by the stomach and spleen.

149. 津液〔津液〕*jīn yè,* **liquid and humor (fluids)** ['lɪkwɪd ənd 'hjumɚ ('fluɪdz)]: All the fluids of the human body, comprising "liquid" (津 *jīn*), thinner fluids, and "humor" (液 *yè*), thicker turbid ones. The term "fluids" embraces all the normal fluid substances of the human body. The term refers to fluids actually flowing within the human body and to sweat, saliva, stomach juices, urine, and other fluids secreted by or discharged from the body. The main functions of fluids are to moisten the bowels and viscera, the flesh, the skin, the hair, and the orifices, to lubricate the joints, and to nourish the brain, marrow, and bones.

150. 神〔神〕*shén,* **spirit** ['spɪrɪt]: **1.** (In the narrow sense) that which is said to be stored by the heart and to return to the abode of the heart during sleep. Spirit is what normally makes us conscious and alert during the day, what becomes inactive during sleep. When there are heart palpitations, susceptibility to fright, heart vexation, or insomnia, the heart-spirit is said to be disquieted. In wind stroke or when evils enter the pericardium, loss of consciousness is described as "clouded spirit." **2.** (In the broad sense) the vitality manifest in a healthy complexion, bright eyes, erect bearing, physical agility, and clear coherent speech. It is said, "If the patient is spirited, he lives; if he is spiritless, he dies."

151. 君火〔君火〕*jūn huǒ,* **sovereign fire** ['savrɪn–,faɪr]: The heart fire. The name "sovereign fire" derives from the statement contained in *The Inner Canon* (*Nèi Jīng*) that the "heart holds the office of sovereign." The sovereign fire stands in complementary opposition to the ministerial fire.

152. 相火〔相火〕*xiàng huǒ,* **ministerial fire** [,mɪnɪ'stɪrɪəl–,faɪr]: A fire in the body inhabiting the life gate, liver, gallbladder, and triple burner and thought to come essentially from the life gate (to which extent it is indissociable from kidney yáng). It stands in complementary opposition to the sovereign fire, which is the heart fire. The sovereign and minis-

terial fires together warm the bowels and viscera and power activity in the body.

1.3.5. 残物 Waste Substances

153. 大便〔大便〕*dà biàn,* **stool** (*n.*); **fecal** (*adj.*); **defecation** (*n.*) [stul, ˈfik!, ˌdɛfiˈkeʃən]: Stool is the waste matter discharged from the anus. The English term "stool" also means defecation, the act of emptying the bowels.

154. 小便〔小便〕*xiǎo biàn,* **urine** (*n.*), **urinary** (*adj.*); **urination, voiding** (*n.*) [ˈjurɪn, ˈjurɪˌnɛrɪ, ˌjurɪˈneʃən, ˈvɔɪdɪŋ]: The English "urine" denotes the fluid discharged from the bladder. "Urination" and "voiding" both refer to the act or an instance of discharging urine.

155. 尿〔尿〕*niào,* **urine** (*n.*), **urinary** (*adj.*); **urination** (*n.*) [ˈjurɪn, ˈjurɪˌnɛrɪ, ˌjurɪˈneʃən]: See preceding item.

1.4. 病因
Causes of Disease

156. 三因〔三因〕*sān yīn,* **three causes (of disease)** [θri ˈkɔzɪz (əv dɪˈziz)]: Three categories of disease causes: external causes, internal causes, and neutral causes, reflecting the notions of heaven, humankind, and earth, respectively.

157. 内因〔內因〕*nèi yīn,* **internal cause** [ɪnˈtɝn! kɔz]: One of the three causes (of disease); the seven affects—joy, anger, anxiety, thought, grief, fear, and fright—as causes of disease. The seven affects are normal responses of the individual, but when excessively intense or persistent, they can disturb the yīn-yáng and qì-blood balance and cause diseases of the bowels and viscera. This is known as internal damage by the seven affects or affect damage (see next item). Internal causes are not to be confused with evils that arise internally. (Internal fire and internal wind, for example, may be the result of affect damage, but they can also develop from insufficiency or from transformation of external evils, which are not internal causes.)

158. 内伤七情〔內傷七情〕*nèi shāng qī qíng,* **internal damage by the seven affects; affect damage** [ɪnˈtɝn! ˈdæmɪdʒ baɪ ðə ˈsɛvən ˈæfɛkts; ˈæfɛkt-ˌdæmɪdʒ]: Any detrimental effect on bowel and visceral qì produced by intemperance of the seven affects (mental and emotional problems); any disease pattern resulting from such causes.

159. 外因〔外因〕*wài yīn,* **external cause** [ɪksʼtɜ̃nḷ ʼkɔz]: One of the three causes (of disease). External causes are the six excesses and warm evil.

160. 不内外因〔內因外因〕*bù nèi wài yīn,* **neutral cause** [n(j)utrəl ʼkɔz]: One of the three causes (of disease). Dietary irregularities, taxation fatigue, knocks and falls, and animal and insect wounds.

161. 六淫〔六淫〕*liù yín,* **six excesses** [sɪks ɛkʼsɛsɪz]: The six qì—wind, cold, summerheat, dampness, dryness, and fire—as causes of disease. Wind diseases are most common in spring, summerheat diseases in summer, damp diseases in long summer (长夏 *cháng xià*), dryness diseases in autumn, and cold diseases in winter. *The Inner Canon (Nèi Jīng)* referred to the six excesses as the "six qì" (the six kinds of weather), but recognized them as causes of diseases. Each of the six excesses is associated with a season. Fire and summerheat are both forms of heat. Heat in the summer (from the Summer Solstice, 夏至 *xià zhì,* to Beginning of Autumn, 立秋 *lì qiū*) is generally called summerheat, whereas heat that occurs untimely in other seasons is called fire (or heat). Fire in other contexts denotes an intense form of heat and is contrasted with a milder form, warmth.

1.4.1. 六淫 Six Excesses

162. 风〔風〕*fēng,* **wind** [wɪnd]: **1.** Environmental wind as a cause of disease; a yáng evil. The nature of wind as an evil and its clinical manifestations are similar to those of the meteorological phenomenon from which its name derives: it comes and goes quickly, moves swiftly, blows intermittently, and sways the branches of the trees. "Wind is swift and changeable," and its clinical manifestations as an evil have the following characteristics: (1) rapid onset and swift changes in condition; (2) convulsions, tremor, shaking of the head, dizziness, and wandering pain and itching; (3) invasion of the upper part of the body and the exterior, e.g., the head (the uppermost part of the body), the lung (the uppermost of the bowels and viscera), and the skin and [body] hair; and (4) facial paralysis and hemiplegia. Note that although wind is associated with movement, by causing stiffness and clenched jaw, it can also be seen to have the power to check normal movement, as in facial paralysis. **2.** Internal wind, i.e., wind arising within the body by the following pathomechanisms: liver yáng transforming into wind, which occurs when liver yáng and liver fire transform into wind, that manifests in dizziness, tremor, and convulsions; extreme heat engendering wind, which occurs in externally contracted diseases such as fright wind and manifests in convulsions, stiffness of the neck, arched-back rigidity, etc.; blood

vacuity engendering wind, which occur when great sweating, great vomiting, great diarrhea, major loss of blood, damage to yīn in enduring illness (久病 jiǔ bìng), or kidney-water failing to moisten liver-wood causes (a) desiccation of the blood that deprives the sinews of nourishment and (b) insufficiency of liver yīn that leaves yáng unsubdued and allows liver wind to scurry around internally. It is marked by dizziness, tremor, worm-like movement in the extremities, or clouding collapse.

163. 寒〔寒〕 *hán*, **cold** [kold]: Cold weather as a cause of disease. Cold in the body causes disease and is classified as "cold" among the eight principles. The nature of cold as an evil and its clinical manifestations are similar to those of cold in the natural environment, e.g., low temperature, deceleration of activity, and congealing. Diseases caused by cold evil result from severe or sudden exposure to cold, excessive consumption of cold fluids, or exposure to frost. They bear the following features: (1) Generalized or local signs of cold, such as aversion to cold, desire for warmth, pronounced lack of warmth in the extremities, and cold and pain in the lower abdomen. (2) Cold, thin, clear excreta; for example, a runny nose with clear mucus, clear phlegm, watery vomitus, long voidings of clear urine, or clear watery diarrhea. *Elementary Questions* (*Sù Wèn, zhì zhēn yào dà lùn*) states, "All disease with water humors that are clear, pure, and cold is ascribed to cold" (诸病水液澄澈清冷，皆属于寒 *zhū bìng shuǐ yè shéng chè qīng lěng, jiē shǔ yú hán*).

164. 暑〔暑〕 *shǔ*, **summerheat** [ˈsʌmərhit]: Hot summer weather as a cause of disease, or the disease caused by it. Distinction is made between summerheat-heat and summerheat-damp. Summerheat-heat is exposure to the heat of summer; this is called "summerheat stroke," and is what English speakers normally refer to as sunstroke or heatstroke. Summerheat-damp refers to certain externally-contracted diseases occurring in hot weather that in China used to be loosely called "summerheat disease," and that include "summerheat warmth," which is equivalent to infectious encephalitis B. Summerheat-heat is associated with torrid summer weather, whereas summerheat-damp is associated with hot humid weather. This difference is reflected in signs: summerheat-heat is marked by high fever, thirst, heart vexation, absence of sweating, and a surging pulse. High fever can easily damage qì and fluids, causing lack of strength, short hasty breathing, and dry tongue fur. Summerheat-damp, by contrast, is marked by fluctuating generalized heat [effusion], fatigued limbs, poor appetite, oppression in the chest, nausea and vomiting, abnormal stool, short voidings of reddish urine, soggy pulse, and thick slimy tongue fur.

165. 湿〔濕〕*shī,* **damp, dampness** [ˈdæmp(nɪs)]: **1.** Dampness in the environment as a cause of disease. Dampness in the body is qualitatively analogous and causally related to dampness in the natural environment. It is associated with damp weather or damp climates and with stagnant water in places where ground drainage is poor. To some extent, it is seasonal in nature, tending to occur when the weather is wet or damp. Sitting and lying in wet places, living in damp conditions, working in a damp or wet environment, or wearing sweat-soaked clothing can also cause dampness diseases. Dampness has a number of characteristics: (1) It is clammy, viscous, and lingering. Dampness diseases are persistent and difficult to cure. (2) Dampness tends to stagnate. When dampness evil invades the exterior, the patient may complain of physical fatigue, heavy cumbersome limbs, and heavy-headedness. If it invades the channels and the joints, the patient may complain of aching joints and inhibited bending and stretching. Dampness can also trap and dampen the effect of heat by causing an unsurfaced heat, one that can be felt only by prolonged palpation. (3) The spleen is particularly vulnerable to dampness evil; signs of dampness encumbering the spleen include poor appetite, glomus and oppression in the chest and stomach duct, upflow nausea, abdominal distention, sloppy stool, short voidings of scant urine, thick and slimy tongue fur, and a soggy moderate pulse. The lack of desire for fluids—though especially in the case of damp-heat there may be thirst—is a sign of the "clogging" or "encumbering" effect of dampness. (4) There may be generalized or local stagnation or accumulation of water-damp that manifests in water swelling, leg qì, vaginal discharge, or exudating sores such as eczema. Dampness in the body is often referred to as damp turbidity to highlight it as the antithesis of clear yáng qì. (5) Over time, dampness can gather to form phlegm.

166. 燥〔燥〕*zào,* **dryness** [ˈdraɪnɪs]: **1.** Dryness as an environmental qì that causes disease. In China, dryness is associated with autumn. Signs include dry nostrils, nosebleed, dry mouth, dry cracked lips, dry "tickly" or sore throat, dry cough with little or no phlegm, rough dry skin, and dry tongue with relatively little liquid. **2.** A state of the body caused by depletion of yīn-humor and presenting signs similar to those created by the environmental qì dryness.

167. 火〔火〕*huǒ,* **fire** [faɪr]: **1.** Heat in the environment as a cause of disease. Fire is characterized by the following signs: (1) Pronounced generalized or local signs of heat, such as high fever, aversion to heat, desire for coolness, red facial complexion, red eyes, reddish urine, red tongue, yellow fur, rapid pulse, or, in sore patterns, redness, heat, pain, and swelling. (2) Thick, sticky excreta, such as thick snivel (nasal mucus),

thick yellow phlegm, sour watery vomitus, murky urine, blood and pus in the stool, acute diarrhea, or foul-smelling stools, often with a burning sensation on discharge. For this reason *Elementary Questions (Sù Wèn)* states, "Turbid water is associated with heat" (水液混浊，皆属于热 *shuǐ yè hùn zhuó, jiē shǔ yú rè*) and "all sour retching and vomiting, fulminant downpour, and lower body distress are ascribed to heat" (诸呕吐酸，暴注下迫，皆属于热 *zhū ǒu tù suān, bào zhù xià pò, jiē shǔ yú rè*). (3) Damage to the fluids characterized by a dry tongue with little liquid, thirst with desire for cold fluids, and dry hard stool. (4) Bleeding and maculopapular eruptions that occur when the fire evil scorches the blood and causes frenetic movement of hot blood. (5) Disturbances of the spirit and vision; as *Elementary Questions (Sù Wèn)* states, "All heat with visual distortion is ascribed to fire" (诸热瞀瘛，皆属于火 *zhū rè mào qì, jiē shǔ yú huǒ*) and "excessive agitation and mania are ascribed to fire" (诸躁狂越，皆属于火 *zhū zào kuáng yuè, jiē shǔ yú huǒ*). **2.** A pathological state that is either caused by fire as one of the six excesses, and classified as heat among the eight principles, or any similar pathological state stemming from the transformation of other evils, from the transformation of yáng qì, or from yīn vacuity. **2a.** The transformation of yáng qì due to affect damage (emotional disturbance) and the transformation of exterior evils as they enter the interior cause repletion fire. This condition is characterized by high fever, headache, red eyes, bitter taste in the mouth, dry mouth, thirst with desire for cold drinks, vexation and agitation, rib-side pain, abdominal pain that refuses pressure, constipation, red tongue with dry yellow fur and sometimes prickles, and a rapid replete pulse. In severe cases, there is blood ejection, spontaneous external bleeding, or maculopapular eruptions. The most common repletion fire patterns are gastrointestinal repletion fire or liver-gallbladder repletion fire. **2b.** Depletion of yīn humor and yīn-yáng imbalance among the bowels and viscera causes vacuity fire, which is characterized by mild heat signs, tidal reddening of the face, vexing heat in the five hearts, steaming bone taxation heat [effusion], vexation and insomnia, night sweating, short voidings of reddish urine, dry mouth and throat, red tongue with scant fur or a smooth bare red tongue without fur, and a forceless rapid fine pulse.

168. 温邪〔溫邪〕*wēn xié,* **warm evil** [wɔrm ˈivl]: Any evil causing warm heat disease, including spring warmth, wind warmth, and summerheat warmth. *On Warm Heat (Wēn Rè Lùn)* states, "Warm evil contracted in the upper body first invades the lung."

1.4.2. 其他 Miscellaneous

169. 疠气〔癘氣〕*lì qì,* **pestilential qì** [ˌpɛstɪˈlɛnʃ(ɪ)əl tʃi]: Any disease evil that is highly contagious.

170. 毒〔毒〕*dú,* **toxin** [ˈtɑxɪn]: **1.** Any substance that is harmful to the body when eaten or when entering the body through a wound or through the skin, such as lacquer toxin (漆毒 *qī dú*) or pitch toxin (沥青毒 *lì qīng dú*). The toxin of animals is called venom. **2.** Any virulent evil qì, e.g., toxic qì, which denotes scourge epidemic qì; occasionally, a disease caused by this, e.g., seasonal toxin.

171. 瘀血〔瘀血〕*yū xuè,* **static blood** [ˈstætɪk blʌd]: Blood affected by stasis, i.e., blood that does not move freely, stagnates in the vessels, or accumulates outside the vessels. Static blood and the morbid changes to which it gives rise are identified by localized pain, stasis macules, and masses; these changes indicate the presence of concretions, conglomerations, and accumulations and gatherings. When blood vessels are blocked by static blood and can no longer withstand the pressure, bleeding may occur. This is most commonly seen in gynecological diseases. Generalized signs of blood stasis include a dull complexion, blue-green or purple lips and tongue, and stasis macules on the edge of the tongue. The pulse is fine or rough.

172. 血瘀〔血瘀〕*xuè yū,* **blood stasis** [ˈblʌd ˈstesɪs]: The formation or presence of static blood.

173. 痰〔痰〕*tán,* **phlegm** [flɛm]: A viscid substance traditionally understood to be a product and a cause of disease. Phlegm may gather in the lung, from where it can be expelled by coughing. However, phlegm as referred to in Chinese medicine is wider in meaning than sputum spoken of in Western medicine. It is understood as a viscous fluid that can accumulate anywhere in the body causing a variety of diseases such as wind stroke, epilepsy, scrofula, etc., but which in the absence of expectoration is usually characterized by a slimy tongue fur and a slippery or slippery stringlike pulse. Phlegm is a thick turbid substance that is distinguished from a thinner, clearer form of accumulated fluid, rheum (饮 *yǐn*), although the term "phlegm" is sometimes used to cover both. Phlegm and rheum may be the result of the impaired movement and transformation of fluids that is associated with morbidity of the lung, spleen, and kidney. Phlegm—but not rheum—may also result from the "boiling" of the fluids by depressed fire. Invasion of the six excesses, affect damage, and damage by food and drink may all affect the dynamic of bowel and visceral qì and cause water humor to gather and form phlegm. The two most important viscera in the formation of phlegm are

the spleen and the lung. Phlegm is the product of a transformation of fluids; most commonly it is the product of congealing water-damp. The spleen normally moves and transforms water-damp, but when its qì is weak or dampness evil is exuberant (邪气盛 xié qì shèng), the normal movement and transformation of water-damp is impaired, and dampness gathers to form phlegm. For this reason it is said that the "spleen is the source of phlegm formation" (脾为生痰之源 pí wéi shēng tán zhī yuán). It is said that "obese people tend to have copious phlegm" (肥人多痰 féi rén duō tán). This saying can be explained by the observation that excessive consumption of sweet or fatty rich foods causes spleen dampness to gather. The lung is the upper source of water; it governs depurative downbearing and regulation of the waterways. When dampness and phlegm accumulate, these functions can be overloaded, so that phlegm collects in the lung; hence it is said that the "lung is the receptacle that holds phlegm" (肺为贮痰之器 fèi wéi zhù tán zhī qì). Phlegm may also form in the lung when heat scorches lung liquid. Phlegm, however, appears not only in the lung; it can follow the upbearing and downbearing of qì and arrive at all places, so it is not just expectorated, but can, depending on the organ or channel affected, cause vomiting of phlegm-drool, clouded spirit, mania and withdrawal, phlegm rale in the throat, numbness of the limbs, hemiplegia, scrofula, goiter, phlegm nodes, plum-pit qì, or dizziness.

174. 饮〔飲〕 yǐn, **rheum** [rum]: See phlegm.

175. 水湿〔水濕〕 shuǐ shī, **water-damp** [ˈwɔtɚ–dæmp]: Any water or dampness as an actual or potential cause of disease. The term "water-damp" is commonly used in the context of the spleen, especially regarding its function of governing the movement and transformation of fluids and its intolerance of dampness.

176. 饮食不节〔飲食不節〕 yǐn shí bù jié, **dietary irregularities** [ˈdaɪəˌtɛrɪˌɾɛgjəˈlærɪtɪz]: A neutral cause [of disease]; any excess in the consumption of food, including: ingestion of raw, cold, or unclean foodstuffs; voracious eating and drinking; predilection for sweet fatty foods; habitual consumption of liquor or hot-spicy foods. Dietary irregularities may not only affect the spleen and stomach, causing digestive disturbances, food accumulation, stomach pain, diarrhea, etc., but in cases of excessive liquor consumption and excessive consumption of sweet and fatty foods, they may create heat, phlegm, and dampness. In addition, dietary irregularities may combine with the six excesses to cause disease, e.g., ingestion of raw or cold foodstuffs in summer.

177. 暴饮暴食〔暴飲暴食〕*bào yǐn bào shí*, **voracious eating and drinking** [vəˈreʃəs itɪŋ ənd ˈdrɪŋkɪŋ]: Eating and drinking large quantities in a short space of time.

178. 过食生冷〔過食生冷〕*guò shí shēng lěng*, **excessive consumption of raw and cold foods** [ɪkˈsɛsɪv kənˈsʌmpʃən əv rɔ ənd kold fudz]: See dietary irregularities.

179. 过食肥甘〔過食肥甘〕*guò shí féi gān*, **excessive consumption of sweet and fatty foods** [ɪkˈsɛsɪv kənˈsʌmpʃən əv swit ənd ˈfætɪ fudz]: See dietary irregularities.

180. 偏嗜油腻厚味〔偏嗜油膩厚味〕*piān shì yóu nì hòu wèi*, **predilection for greasy and rich foods** [ˌprɛdɪˈlɛkʃən fɚ ˈgrisɪ ənd rɪtʃ fudz]: See dietary irregularities.

181. 过食辛辣〔過食辛辣〕*guò shí xīn là*, **excessive consumption of hot-spicy acrid foods** [ɪkˈsɛsɪv kənˈsʌmpʃən əv hɑt ˈspaɪsɪ ˈækrɪd fudz]: See dietary irregularities.

182. 跌打〔跌打〕*diē dǎ*, **knocks and falls** [nɑks ənd fɔlz]: Blows, collisions, collapses, or falls from heights, especially when resulting in injuries that cause stasis swelling (bruises), cuts and grazes, sprains, bone fractures, dislocations, and damage to the bowels and viscera.

183. 虫兽伤〔蟲獸傷〕*chóng shòu shāng*, **animal and insect wounds** [ˈænɪml ənd ˈɪnsɛkt wundz] Wounds inflicted by animals and bites and stings from insects.

184. 房室不节〔房室不節〕*fáng shì bù jié*, **sexual intemperance** [ˈsɛksjuəl ɪnˈtɛmpərəns]: Excessive sexual activity and in women excessive childbirth. Sexual intemperance damages kidney essence and causes signs of kidney vacuity such as aching lumbus, seminal emission, lassitude of spirit and lack of strength, and dizziness. Excessive childbirth in women can cause menstrual irregularities, menstrual block, and vaginal discharge.

185. 劳倦〔勞倦〕*láo juàn*, **taxation fatigue** [tækˈseʃən-fəˌtig]: Overexertion, intemperate living (including dietary irregularities and sexual intemperance), or the seven affects (emotional imbalance) as a cause of disease.

习题
Questions

Answer the following questions in English:

1. Name the five viscera and six bowels. ....

2. To what Western anatomical category/categories do the sinews belong? ....

3. What is the difference between drool and spittle?
....

4. What flavor is associated with metal? ....

5. What is the difference between the upper abdomen and the lower abdomen? ....

6. What is the modern understanding of life gate? ....

7. Name the nine orifices. ....

8. Which viscus stores essence? ....

9. What are the interstices? ....

10. What is said of diseases that have entered the gāo-huāng?
....

11. Where does ancestral qì concentrate? ....

12. What phase does anger correspond to? ....

13. What color is associated with the spleen? ....

14. In simple terms, what is the difference between fire and summer-heat among the six excesses? ....

15. What is rheum? ....

16. Which of the six excesses is associated with disease of rapid onset and swift changes? ....

17. By which viscus are the vessels governed? ....

18. Which disease evil may be characterized by unsurfaced heat?
....

19. What is the yīn counterpart of defense qì? ....

20. To what qì is right qì opposed? ....

21. What substance is expelled from the lung by coughing and is considered to be the cause of a wide range of morbid conditions?

22. What is the name of the lower part of the back? ....

23. What is stored by the heart? ....

24. What is the difference between liquid and humor?
....

25. Where is the membrane source? ....

26. From which of the six bowels is urine discharged? ....

27. Which of the five viscera governs the eyes? ....

28. What is the "fontanel gate" called in Western medicine?
....

29. Which of the five viscera governs the flesh?
....

30. With which phase is saltiness associated? ....

Give the Pīnyīn and English for the following Chinese terms:

31. 膀胱 ....

32. 命门 ....

33. 元气 ....

34. 胸 ....

35. 喉关 ....

36. 结喉 ....

37. 悬雍垂 ....

38. 龈 ....

39. 小肠 ....

40. 胆 ....

41. 膈 ....

42. 囟 ....

43. 胁 ....

44. 内伤七情 ....

45. 不内外因 ....

46. 脏腑之气 ....

47. 膜原 ....

48. 膝 ....

49. 腹 ....

50. 肩 ....

Supply the Chinese and English for the following:

51. *Nù.* ....

52. *Tóu.* ....

53. *Huì yàn.* ....

54. *Xié.* ....

55. *Xū lǐ.* ....

56. *Wèi wǎn.* ....

57. *Huái.* ....

58. *Zhǒu.* ....

59. *Còu lǐ.* ....

60. *Jīng luò zhī qì.* ....

61. *Dà biàn.* ....

62. *Fēng.* ....

63. *Qì huà.* ....

64. *Yá chǐ.* ....

65. *Xīn bāo luò.* ....

66. *Dà fù.* ....

67. *Hóu hé.* ....

68. *Zhèng qì.* ....

69. *Jīn yè.* ....

70. *Shén.* ....

Give the Chinese and Pīnyīn for the following:

71. Source qì. ....

72. Urine. ....

73. Limb. ....

74. Hand. ....
75. [Region] below the heart. ....
76. Large intestine. ....
77. Fear. ....
78. Triple burner. ....
79. Snivel. ....
80. Bitter. ....
81. Sweat. ....
82. Lip. ....
83. Fontanel. ....
84. Lesser abdomen. ....
85. Orifice. ....
86. Original qì. ....
87. Construction qì. ....
88. Defecation. ....
89. Rib-side. ....
90. Diaphragm. ....

第二章　经络
The Channels and Network Vessels

186. 经络〔經絡〕*jīng luò,* **channels and network vessels** [ˈtʃænlz ənd ˈnɛtwɜ·k–ˌvɛslz]: The pathways of blood and qì pervading the whole body, connecting the bowels and viscera, the limbs and joints. The channels are the main pathways of qì and blood, whereas the network vessels are smaller branches ensuring supply of qì and blood to all localities. Disturbances in the channels are reflected in abnormalities along their course. Acupuncture (针灸 *zhēn jiǔ*), acupressure (指压 *zhǐ yā*), and fire cupping (拔火罐 *bá huǒ guàn*) are largely based on the theory of the channels and network vessels.

187. 十二经〔十二經〕*shí èr jīng,* **twelve channels** [twɛlv ˈtʃænlz]: The channels that form the basic structure of the channel system. The twelve channels comprise six channels of the hand and six channels of the foot, each channel duplicated on both sides of the body. Each channel "homes" and "nets" (属、络 *shǔ、 luò*) to bowels and viscera that stand in interior-exterior relationship.

188. 十二经筋〔十二經筋〕*shí èr jīng jīn,* **twelve channel sinews** [twɛlv ˈtʃænl ˈsɪnjuz]: Sinews following the path of the channels, together filling the entire surface of the body. They are named after the channels (e.g., hand yáng brightness channel sinews). Morbidity of the channel sinews manifests as hypertonicity, slackening, cramps, rigidity, and convulsions.

189. 络脉〔絡脈〕*luò mài,* **network vessel** [ˈnɛtwɜ·k–ˌvɛsl]: Any branch of the channels that enmesh the body. (1) In a broader sense, "network vessel" denotes any of the fifteen network vessels, the network vessels (in the narrower sense), and grandchild network vessels. Fourteen vessels connect the twelve regular channels, and the governing (*dū*) and controlling (*rèn*) vessels. These together with the great network vessel of the spleen constitute the fifteen network vessels (also called *diverging network vessels*). (2) In the narrow sense, "network vessel" denotes the branches of the fifteen network vessels, which enmesh the whole body, the smaller branches of which are known as the grandchild network vessels. (3) "Network vessel" also denotes any of the

small branches of the network vessels in the surface of the body, which are more precisely rendered as superficial network vessels.

190. 十五络〔十五絡〕*shí wǔ luò,* **fifteen network vessels** [ˈfɪftin ˈnɛt-wɝk–ˌvɛsl̩z]: See network vessel.

191. 浮络〔浮絡〕*fú luò,* **superficial network vessel** [ˌsupɚˈfɪʃl̩ ˈnɛtwɝk–ˌvɛsl̩]: See network vessel.

192. 孙络〔孫絡〕*sūn luò,* **grandchild network vessel** [ˈgrændtʃaɪld ˈnɛt-wɝk–ˌvɛsl̩]: See network vessel.

193. 脾之大络〔脾之大絡〕*pí zhī dà luò,* **great network vessel of the spleen** [gret ˈnɛtwɝk–ˌvɛsl̩ əv ðə splin]: A large network vessel that branches off directly from the spleen, issues at SP-21 (*dà bāo,* Great Embracement), and disperses over the chest and rib-side.

194. 胃之大络〔胃之大絡〕*wèi zhī dà luò,* **great network vessel of the stomach** [gret ˈnɛtwɝk–ˌvɛsl̩ əv ðə ˈstʌmək]: A large network vessel that branches directly from the stomach, passes up the stomach, traverses the diaphragm, and after connecting with the lung, turns outward to exit below the left breast, at the Vacuous lǐ (*xū lǐ*), roughly corresponding to ST-18 (*rǔ gēn,* Breast Root).

2.1. 六经
The Six Channels

195. 太阳〔太陽〕*tài yáng,* **greater yáng** [ˈgretɚ jæŋ/jɑŋ]: The hand greater yáng (*tài yáng*) small intestine (abbreviation: SI) and foot greater yáng bladder (BL) channels. Greater yáng is the exuberance of yáng qì. The greater yáng channels are the most exterior of all the yáng channels and are most susceptible to contraction of external evils; hence it is said that "greater yáng governs openness." It has copious blood and scant qì.

196. 阳明〔陽明〕*yáng míng,* **yáng brightness** [jæŋ/jɑŋ ˈbraɪtnɪs]: The hand yáng brightness (*yáng míng*) large intestine (LI) and foot yáng brightness stomach (ST) channels. The yáng brightness is the last stage in the development of yáng qì. It is the innermost of the three yáng channels, hence it is said that "yáng brightness is the closedness." Yáng brightness has copious qì and copious blood.

197. 少阳〔少陽〕*shào yáng*, **lesser yáng** [ˈlɛsɚ jæŋ/jɑŋ]: The hand lesser yáng (*shào yáng*) triple burner (TB) and foot lesser yáng gallbladder (GB) channels. "Lesser" implies the waning of yáng. The lesser yáng is between the greater yáng (*tài yáng*) and yáng brightness (*yáng míng*); hence it is said that "the lesser yáng is the pivot." The lesser yáng has copious qì and scant blood.

198. 太阴〔太陰〕*tài yīn*, **greater yīn** [ˈgretɚ jɪn]: The hand greater yīn (*tài yīn*) lung (LU) and foot greater yīn spleen (SP) channels. Greater yīn is characterized by an exuberance of yīn qì. Among the yīn channels, the greater yīn is the most closely associated with the exterior; hence it is said that "greater yīn governs opening." Greater yīn has copious blood and scant qì.

199. 少阴〔少陰〕*shào yīn*, **lesser yīn** [ˈlɛsɚ jɪn]: The hand lesser yīn (*shào yīn*) heart (HT) and foot lesser yīn kidney (KI) channels. "Lesser" implies a waning of yīn qì. The lesser yīn is said to have copious qì and scant blood. The lesser yīn is located between the greater yīn (*tài yīn*) and reverting yīn (*jué yīn*); hence it is said "lesser yīn is the pivot." It has copious qì and scant blood.

200. 厥阴〔厥陰〕*jué yīn*, **reverting yīn** [rɪˈvɝtɪŋ jɪn]: The hand reverting yīn (*jué yīn*) pericardium (PC) and foot reverting yīn liver (LR) channels. The name reverting yīn indicates yīn qì developing to its final stage and then reverting toward yáng. The reverting yīn is located within the greater yīn (*tài yīn*) and lesser yīn (*shào yīn*), and hence it is said that "reverting yīn is the closedness." It has copious blood and scant qì.

2.2. 奇经八脉
The Eight Extraordinary Vessels

201. 任脉〔任脈〕*rèn mài*, **controlling vessel** [kənˈtrolɪŋ–ˌvɛsl̩]: *Abbreviation:* CV. The vessel whose principal course ascends from the pelvis along the midline of the abdomen and chest, and splits to skirt around the mouth and nose, and which is the sea of the yīn channels; it regulates menstruation and matures the fetus.

202. 督脉〔督脈〕*dū mài*, **governing vessel** [ˈgʌvɚnɪŋ–ˌvɛsl̩]: *Abbreviation:* GV. The vessel whose main pathway ascends the spine and whose main function is to regulate the yáng channels.

203. **冲脉**〔衝脈〕*chōng mài*, **thoroughfare vessel** [ˈθəro(ə)fɛr–ˌvɛsl̩]]: *Abbreviation:* TV. The vessel whose main pathway starts from near the point ST-30 (*qì chōng*, Qì Thoroughfare), rising parallel with the lesser yīn kidney channel, passing either side of the umbilicus, and ascending to the chest, where it disperses. Disease indicators of this vessel include qì surging up into the heart, menstrual irregularities, flooding and spotting, and infertility.

204. **带脉**〔帶脈〕*dài mài*, **girdling vessel** [ˈgɝdlɪŋ–ˌvɛsl̩]: *Abbreviation:* GIV. The vessel that encircles the body at the waist. This channel serves to bind up all the channels running up and down the trunk, thus regulating the balance between upward and downward flow of qì in the body. Signs associated with disease of this vessel include vaginal discharge, prolapse of the uterus, abdominal distention and fullness, and limp lumbus.

205. **阴跷（蹻）脉**〔陰蹻（蹻）脈〕*yīn qiāo mài*, **yīn springing vessel** [jɪn ˈsprɪŋɪŋ–ˌvɛsl̩]: *Abbreviation:* YIS. The vessel whose pathway branches off from the foot lesser yīn channel, starting just behind KI-2 (*rán gǔ*, Blazing Valley), and passes up the ankle and inside of the leg, enters the genitals, proceeds up the chest to the empty basin (缺盆 *quē pén*, supraclavicular fossa). It issues in front of ST-9 (*rén yíng*, Man's Prognosis), proceeds to the cheek to home to the inner canthus, where it unites with the foot greater yáng (*tài yáng*) and yáng springing vessel. The main disease indicators are inhibited bending and stretching, and abnormalities of the opening and closing of the eye.

206. **阳跷（蹻）脉**〔陽蹻（蹻）脈〕*yáng qiāo mài*, **yáng springing vessel** [jæŋ/jɑŋ ˈsprɪŋɪŋ–ˌvɛsl̩]]: *Abbreviation:* YAS. A vessel that starts from the heal, passes over the outer ankle, up the leg, over the hip and rib-side, to the lateral margin of the shoulder blade. It then proceeds up the face, passing over the cheek to reach the inner canthus. From there, it runs over the head, entering the brain at GB-20 (*fēng chí*, Wind Pool). As with the yīn springing vessel, the main disease indicators are inhibited bending and stretching, and abnormalities of the opening and closing of the eye.

207. **阴维脉**〔陰維脈〕*yīn wéi mài*, **yīn linking vessel** [jɪn ˈlɪŋkɪŋ–ˌvɛsl̩]: *Abbreviation:* YIL. A vessel whose pathway starts from KI-9 (*zhú bīn*, Guest House), ascends the medial aspect of the lower limb, enters the smaller abdomen, and ascends through the rib-side and chest to the throat. Its disease indicators are yīn channel interior signs such as heart pain and stomach pain.

208. 阳维脉〔陽維脈〕*yáng wéi mài,* **yáng linking vessel** [jæŋ/jɑŋ ˈlɪŋkɪŋ‑ˌvɛsl]: *Abbreviation:* YAL. A vessel that starts from BL-63 (*jīn mén,* Metal Gate), ascends the lateral aspect of the lower limb, and passes over the rib-side to the shoulder blade, from where it ascends to behind the ear and the side of the head. The disease indicators are greater yáng channel signs such as aversion to cold and heat effusion.

2.3. 穴道
Acupuncture Points

209. 穴道〔穴道〕*xué dào,* **acupuncture point** [ˈækjəˌpʌnktʃɚ pɔɪnt]: A place on the surface of the body where qì and blood of the channels and network vessels gather or pass.

210. 同身寸〔同身寸〕*tóng shēn cùn,* **body inch** [ˈbɑdɪ ɪntʃ]: A proportional unit of measurement used to determine the location of acupuncture points on the body, calculated from the length of specific body parts according to the *finger standard* (指寸法 *zhǐ cùn fǎ*) and *bone standard* (骨度 *gǔ dù*).

211. 属络〔屬絡〕*shǔ luò,* **homing and netting** [ˈhomɪŋ ənd ˈnɛtɪŋ]: Each of the six channels "homes" to the bowel or viscus to which it belongs, and "nets" the bowel or viscus standing in exterior-interior relationship. For example, the greater yīn (*tài yīn*) lung channel "homes" to the lung, and "nets" the large intestine.

212. 交会穴〔交會穴〕*jiāo huì xué,* **intersection point** [ˌɪntɚˈsɛkʃən pɔɪnt]: Any point at which two or more channels intersect. Intersection points have the ability to transmit a stimulus through both or all channels that intersect at the point. Intersection points are used to treat disease affecting two or more of the intersecting channels.

213. 背俞〔背兪〕*bèi shū,* **back transport [point]** [bæk ˈtrænspɔrt]: Any of a group of points on the bladder channel, 1.5 body-inches either side of the spinal column, each associated with, and named after, an organ whose qì is said to pass through its location. Back transport points are used to diagnose and treat the bowels and viscera with which they are associated.

214. 募穴〔募穴〕*mù xué,* **alarm point; mustering point** [əˈlɑrm pɔɪnt; ˈmʌstərɪŋ pɔɪnt]: Any of a group of points on the abdomen or chest, each of which is the collecting point of the qì of a bowel or viscus in whose

vicinity it lies. Disease in a given bowel or viscus may be reflected in tenderness, lumps, gatherings, depressions, or other aberrant signs at its alarm point, and can be treated by applying a stimulus at the point.

215. 原穴〔原穴〕 *yuán xué,* **source point** [sɔrs pɔɪnt]: Any of the points that lie on the twelve channels and at which the source qì of the bowels or viscus related to that channel collects. The source points of the six yīn channels are the same as the *stream points* on the six yīn channels. Those of the six yáng channels are located one point proximal to the stream points. Source points can be palpated to identify repletion or vacuity of source qì in the channel's associated bowel or viscus (repletion being characterized by swelling or distention, and vacuity by a depression at the point). These points are primarily used for the treatment of diseases affecting the bowels and viscera. They can be drained or supplemented to treat vacuity or repletion in the channel or its associated organ.

216. 络穴〔絡穴〕 *luò xué,* **network point; connecting point** [ˈnɛtwɚk pɔɪnt, kəˈnɛktɪŋ pɔɪnt]: The point at which a network vessel separates from its main channel is the network point of that channel. For example, the network vessel of the hand reverting yīn (*jué yīn*) pericardium channel splits from the main channel at PC-6 (*nèi guān,* Inner Pass), thus PC-6 is the network point of the pericardium channel. Each channel that possesses its own points has a network point; thus each of the twelve regular channels and the governing (*dū*) and controlling (*rèn*) vessels have network points. Two network vessels are associated with the spleen: the spleen network vessel and the great network vessel of the spleen. Each of these has a network point. Hence there are in total fifteen network points. The network points are used to treat a) internally-externally coupled organs; and b) signs specifically associated with the network vessels.

217. 下合穴〔下合穴〕 *xià hé xué,* **lower uniting point** [ˈloɚ juˈnaɪtɪŋ pɔɪnt]: Any of a group of points located on the lower limbs, used to treat disease of the six bowels. Each organ has a uniting point located on its associated channel in the vicinity of the elbows or knees (LU-5, LI-11, ST-36, SP-9, HT-3, SI-8, BL-40, KI-10, PC-3, TB-10, GB-34, LR-8; see transport point). In addition to these, the three bowels associated with the yáng channels of the arm each have a uniting point located on one of the yáng channels of the foot. The lower uniting points of the small and large intestines are located on the stomach channel at ST-37 (*shàng jù xū,* Upper Great Hollow) and ST-39 (*xià jù xū,* Lower Great Hollow), respectively, whereas that of the triple burner is on the bladder

channel at BL-39 (*wěi yáng,* Bend Yáng). Each point is used to treat disease of its respective bowel.

218. 五俞穴〔五俞穴〕*wǔ shū xué,* **five transport points** [faɪv ˈtrænspɔrt pɔɪnt]: Any of a series of five points below the elbows or knees on each of the twelve channels. The five points are the well (井穴 *jǐng xué*), brook (spring) (荥穴 *yíng xué*), stream (俞穴 *shū xué*), channel (river) (经穴 *jīng xué*), and uniting points (合穴 *hé xué*), which each have five-phase correspondences that differ from the yáng to the yīn channels. On the lung channel, for example, LU-11 (*shào shāng,* Lesser Shang) is the well point corresponding to wood; LU-10 (*yú jì,* Fish Border) is the brook point corresponding to fire; LU-9 (*tài yuān,* Great Abyss) is the stream point corresponding to earth (soil); LU-8 (*jīng qú,* Channel Ditch) is the channel point corresponding to metal; LU-5 (*chǐ zé,* Cubit Marsh) is the uniting point corresponding to water.

219. 四总穴〔四總穴〕*sì zǒng xué,* **four command points** [fɔr kəˈmænd pɔɪnts]: Points ST-36 (*zú sān lǐ,* Leg Three Li), BL-40 (*wěi zhōng,* Bend Center), LU-7 (*liè quē,* Broken Sequence), and LI-4 (*hé gǔ,* Union Valley), which "command" the body and are used to treat disease in specific areas of the body. ST-36 is the command point of the abdomen, and treats diarrhea, constipation, and abdominal pain and distention. BL-40 is the command point of the back and lumbus, and treats pain in those parts. LU-7 is the command point of the head and nape, and treats headache and stiffness of the nape. LI-4 is the command point of the face and mouth and is useful for treating such diseases as toothache, swollen cheeks, nosebleed, and headache. Command points are often combined with points more specific to the disease being treated. For example, treatment of lumbar pain might pair BL-40, the command point of the back, with local points such as BL-23 and BL-30.

习题
Questions

Answer the following questions in English:

91. What term refers to the branches of the channels that enmesh the body? ....

92. Name the twelve regular channels. ....

93. Name the eight extraordinary vessels. ....

94. What does the abbreviation HT refer to? ....

95. Name the four command points. ....

96. What does the abbreviation TB refer to? ....

97. The yáng brightness (*yáng míng*) channels are associated with which bowels?

....

98. The lesser yáng (*shào yáng*) channels are associated with which bowels? ....

99. With which viscus and which bowel is the hand greater yáng (*tài yáng*) small intestine channel associated? ....

100. Which of the eight extraordinary vessels is considered the sea of the yīn channels? ....

101. Which of the eight extraordinary vessels starts from the pelvis and ascends the anterior aspect of the body? ....

102. What does YAS mean? ....

103. Which of the eight extraordinary vessels starts at KI-9?

....

104. What does the abbreviation KI refer to? ....

105. Which of the eight extraordinary vessels encircles the body at the waist? ....

106. Name the five transport points. ....

107. What does the abbreviation BL refer to? ....

108. What is the network point of the pericardium channel?

....

109. What point is the lower uniting point of the hand yáng brightness (*yáng míng*) large intestine channel? ....

110. What does the abbreviation GV stand for? ....

Give the Pīnyīn and English for the following Chinese terms:

111. 原穴 ....

112. 同身寸 ....

113. 交会穴 ....

114. 络穴 ....

115. 太阴 ....

116. 属络 ....

117. 募穴 ....

118. 四总穴 ....

119. 十二经筋 ....

120. 经络 ....

121. 胃之大络 ....

122. 阳明 ....

123. 穴道 ....

124. 阳跷（蹻）脉 ....

125. 输穴 ....

126. 下合穴 ....

127. 厥阴 ....

128. 任脉 ....

129. 阴维脉 ....

130. 带脉 ....

Supply the Chinese and English for the following:

131. *Shí èr jīng.* ....

132. *Shí wǔ luò.* ....

133. *Fú luò.* ....

134. *Shào yīn.* ....

135. *Yīn qiāo mài.* ....

136. *Bèi shū.* ....

137. *Xià hé xué.* ....

138. *Wǔ shū xué.* ....

139. *Sūn luò.* ....

140. *Jīng xué.* ....

141. *Jǐng xué.* ....

142. *Shí èr jīng jīn.* ....

143. *Yíng xuè.* ....

144. *Pí zhī dà luò.* ....

145. *Luò mài.* ....

146. *Tài yáng.* ....

147. *Luò xué.* ....

148. *Tóng shēn cùn.* ....

149. *Jiāo huì xué.* ....

150. *Chōng mài.* ....

Give the Chinese and Pīnyīn for the following:

151. Yīn linking vessel. ....

152. Controlling vessel. ....

153. Thoroughfare vessel. ....

154. Yáng linking vessel. ....

155. Alarm point. ....

156. Body inch. ....

157. Great network vessel of the spleen. ....

158. Fifteen network vessels. ....

159. Governing vessel. ....

160. Stream point. ....

161. Uniting point. ....

162. Reverting yīn. ....

163. Yáng brightness. ....

164. The twelve channel sinews. ....

165. The eight extraordinary vessels. ....

166. The five transport points. ....

167. The four command points. ....

168. Yīn springing vessel. ....

169. Superficial network vessel. ....

170. Fire cupping. ....

第三章　五脏六腑
Five Viscera and Six Bowels

3.1. 心
The Heart

220. 心属火〔心屬火〕*xīn shǔ huǒ,* **heart belongs to fire** [hɑrt bɪˈlɔŋz tə faɪr]: The heart is associated with fire among the five phases.

221. 心与小肠相表里〔心與小腸相表裡〕*xīn yǔ xiǎo cháng xiāng biǎo lǐ,* **heart and small intestine stand in interior-exterior relationship** [hɑrt ənd smɔl ɪnˈtɛstɪn stænd ɪn ɪnˈtɪrɪə ɪksˈtɪrɪə rɛˈleʃənʃɪp]: The heart is in the interior and the small intestine is its corresponding bowel in the exterior. This relationship is manifest in heart heat spreading to the small intestine, which is characterized by bloody urine.

222. 心主血脉〔心主血脈〕*xīn zhǔ xuè mài,* **heart governs the blood and vessels** [hɑrt ˈgʌvənz ðə blʌd ənd ˈvɛsl̩z]: The heart is responsible for moving the blood around the body.

223. 心藏神〔心藏神〕*xīn cáng shén,* **heart stores the spirit** [hɑrt stɔrz ðə ˈspɪrɪt]: The heart is the seat of consciousness and mental vitality. Insomnia is a sign of disquieted heart-spirit.

224. 心开窍于舌〔心開竅於舌〕*xīn kāi qiào yú shé,* **heart opens at the tongue** [hɑrt ˈopənz ət ðə tʌŋ]: Heart disease is sometimes reflected in stiffness of the tongue or erosion of the mouth and tongue.

3.2. 肺
The Lung

225. **肺属金**〔肺屬金〕 *fèi shǔ jīn*, **lung belongs to metal** [lʌŋ bɪˈlɔŋz tə ˈmɛtl̩]: The lung is associated with metal among the five phases.

226. **肺与大肠相表里**〔肺與大腸相表裡〕 *fèi yǔ dà cháng xiāng biǎo lǐ*, **lung and large intestine stand in interior-exterior relationship** [lʌŋ ənd lɑrdʒ ɪnˈtɛstɪn stænd ɪn ɪnˈtɪrɪɚ ɪksˈtɪrɪɚ rɛˈleʃənʃɪp]: The lung stands in interior-exterior relationship with the large intestine. The lung channel "nets" (connects with) the large intestine, and the large intestine channel "nets" the lung. The lung's depurative downbearing helps the large intestine's function of conveying and transforming waste, and vice versa. Panting due to phlegm congestion can be treated with draining precipitants (泻下药 *xiè xià yào*, i.e., laxatives) to free lung qì, whereas some types of constipation are best treated by opening the lung. Medicinals that transform phlegm and suppress cough, such as apricot kernel (*xìng rén*) and trichosanthes (*guā lóu*), also have the effect of moistening the intestines.

227. **肺主气**〔肺主氣〕 *fèi zhǔ qì*, **lung governs qì** [lʌŋ ˈgʌvɚnz tʃi]: The lung takes in clear, natural qì and expels turbid qì. "The lung governs qì" denotes the respiratory function and role played by the lung in the production of true qì. *Qì*, in Chinese, means breath and breathing as well as qì.

228. **肺主肃降**〔肺主肅降〕 *fèi zhǔ sù jiàng*, **lung governs depurative downbearing** [lʌŋ ˈgʌvɚnz dɪˈpjurətɪv ˈdɑʊnˌbɛrɪŋ]: Under normal circumstances, lung qì bears downward, drawing breath down the windpipe into the lung and keeping the lung clean of phlegm. The compound term "depurative downbearing" reflects the downward movement of qì and its action of maintaining a clean lung.

229. **肺主通调水道**〔肺主通調水道〕 *fèi zhǔ tōng tiáo shuǐ dào*, **lung governs regulation of the waterways** [lʌŋ ˈgʌvɚnz ˌrɛgjəˈleʃən əv ðə ˈwɔtɚˌwez]: The spleen, lung, kidney, intestines, and bladder are jointly responsible for regulating water metabolism. The specific role of the lung is called "governing regulation of the waterways," and represents a combination of the two functions of diffusion and depurative downbearing.

230. **肺主皮毛**〔肺主皮毛〕 *fèi zhǔ pí máo*, **lung governs the skin and [body] hair** [lʌŋ ˈgʌvɚnz ðə skɪn ənd ˈbɑdɪ–hɛr]: The skin and [body] hair are dependent on the essential qì supplied by the lung. Certain

forms of lung vacuity such as lung wilting may be reflected in dry lusterless skin. In a broader sense, the skin and [body] hair represent the exterior of the body as a defense against external evils. Invasion of external evils is associated with disturbance of normal sweating (absence of sweating or profuse sweating).

231. 肺开窍于鼻〔肺開竅於鼻〕*fèi kāi qiào yú bí,* **lung opens at the nose** [lʌŋ ˈopəns ət ðə noz]: The nose is the outer opening of the respiratory tract, through which air enters the lung. *Elementary Questions (Sù Wèn, yīn yáng yìng xiàng dà lùn)* states, "The lung governs the nose." The sense of smell can function normally only if lung qì is in harmony and breathing is smooth. Thus, *The Magic Pivot (Líng Shū)* states, "Lung qì flows to the nose; when the lung is in harmony, the nose can perceive fragrance and malodor." In addition, snivel (nasal mucus) is the humor of the lung. Many lung diseases are the result of the contraction of external evils through the nose and mouth, and are reflected in the condition of the nose. For example, colds may be characterized by nasal congestion and a runny nose, attributable to nondiffusion of lung qì. Also, lung qì ascending counterflow, caused by evil heat congestion in the lung, frequently leads to rapid breathing and flaring nostrils.

3.3. 脾、胃、肠
The Spleen, Stomach, and Intestines

232. 脾属土〔脾屬土〕*pí shǔ tǔ,* **spleen belongs to earth (soil)** [splin bɪˈlɔŋz tu ɝθ(sɔɪl)]: The spleen is associated with earth (soil) among the five phases.

233. 脾与胃相表里〔脾與胃相表裡〕*pí yǔ wèi xiāng biǎo lǐ,* **spleen and stomach stand in interior-exterior relationship** [splin ənd ˈstʌmək stænd ɪn ɪnˈtɪriɚ ɪksˈtɪriɚ rɛˈleʃənʃɪp]: The spleen is in the interior; its corresponding bowel in the exterior is the stomach, to which it is connected by channels. The spleen and stomach are complementary in their functions: the spleen governs movement and transformation, while the stomach governs intake; the spleen governs upbearing of the clear, while the stomach governs downbearing of the turbid; the spleen is averse to dampness, while the stomach likes moisture. Furthermore, the stomach's governing decomposition of grain and water is to some extent attributable to the spleen because the spleen "moves the fluids of the stomach."

234. **脾主运化**〔脾主運化〕*pí zhǔ yùn huà*, **spleen governs movement and transformation** [splin ˈgʌvɚnz ˈmuvmənt ənd ˌtrænsfɚˈmeʃən]: The spleen is in charge of digestion. Food enters the stomach where it is decomposed. The spleen "moves the fluids of the stomach," extracts the essence of grain and water (nutrients in food), and dispatches it to the other organs, so that the essence is ultimately carried to all parts of the body. Modern writers explain this function as comprising digestion, assimilation, and distribution of nutrients. *Elementary Questions* (*Sù Wèn*) explains it in the following terms: "Drink (饮 *yǐn*, imbibed fluid) enters the stomach, where it is churned and its essential qì is strained off. The essential qì is then carried to the spleen and further distributed by spleen qì. It passes up to the lung, which ensures regular flow through the waterways down to the bladder. In this way, water essence is distributed throughout the five channels and the four parts of the body." Because of its importance in providing nutrients for the production of blood and qì that maintain the life and health of the organism, the spleen is described as the *source of engendering transformation* (生化之源 *shēng huà zhī yuán*, i.e., the basis of qì and blood production) and the root of later heaven (后天之本 *hòu tiān zhī běn*, i.e., the chief factor in the acquired constitution). This productive aspect of the spleen explains the five-phase association with earth (soil). Abnormality of the spleen's governing of movement and transformation is called the spleen failing to move and transform.

235. **脾主升清**〔脾主升清〕*pí zhǔ shēng qīng*, **spleen governs upbearing of the clear** [splin ˈgʌvɚnz ˈʌpbɛrɪŋ əv ðə klɪr]: Upbearing of the clear refers to the spleen's governing of movement and transformation. The clear refers to essence of grain and water (nutrients absorbed from food), which by the action of spleen qì is carried upward and outward around the whole body.

236. **脾主肌肉、四肢**〔脾主肌肉、四肢〕*pí zhǔ jī ròu, sì zhī*, **spleen governs the flesh and limbs** [splin ˈgʌvɚnz ðə flɛʃ ənd lɪmz]: The fullness of the flesh and the strength of the limbs are dependent upon the spleen's movement and transformation function. Because the spleen is the source of blood and qì formation, all the muscles of the body rely for their nourishment on the capacity of the stomach and spleen to move and transform the essence of grain and water. Only when the stomach and spleen are functioning properly are the muscles full and sound and the limbs powerful. Impairment of spleen function may therefore lead to emaciation, loss of limb power, and, in severe cases, wilting of the flesh and paralysis.

237. 脾，其华在唇四白〔脾，其華在唇四白〕*pí, qí huá zài chún sì bái,* **spleen... its bloom is in the four whites of the lips** [splin, ɪts blʌm ɪz ɪn ðə fɔr waɪts əv ðəlɪps]: The health of the spleen is reflected in the lips and surrounding area, which is generally slightly paler than other parts of the face. Strong movement of spleen qì is also reflected in red, moist, and lustrous lips. The "four whites of the lips" (唇四白 *chún sì bái*) is understood to mean the pale flesh above, below, and on either side of the mouth.

238. 脾开窍于口〔脾開竅於口〕*pí kāi qiào yú kǒu,* **spleen opens at the mouth** [splin ˈopənz ət ðə mɑʊθ]: The mouth is the outer orifice of the spleen. This phrase refers to the relationship of the spleen's movement and transformation to appetite and taste in the mouth. If stomach and spleen function is normal, the individual has a good appetite and normal taste in the mouth.

239. 胃主受纳〔胃主受納〕*wèi zhǔ shòu nà,* **stomach governs intake** [ˈstʌmək ˈgʌvənz ˈɪntek]: The function of the stomach is to receive ingested foods and perform the initial stage of digestion. Normal performance of this function is dependent on the downward passage of food to the small intestine. It is less important than the spleen, and to some extent dominated by it, since "the spleen moves the fluids of the stomach." Impairment of stomach function may take the form of stomach qì disharmony, characterized by distention and fullness in the stomach duct and abdomen, torpid stomach intake (presenting signs such as sluggishness of the intake function such as poor appetite and indigestion), stomach pain, or stomach qì ascending counterflow (nausea, vomiting, belching, or hiccup).

240. 胃主腐熟〔胃主腐熟〕*wèi zhǔ fǔ shú,* **stomach governs decomposition; stomach governs rotting and ripening** [ˈstʌmək ˈgʌvənz diˌkɑmpəˈzɪʃən (ˈratɪŋ ənd ˈraɪpənɪŋ)]: The stomach is responsible for "rotting and ripening" grain and water (food) so that its essence can be extracted by the spleen. See stomach governs intake.

241. 胃主降浊〔胃主降濁〕*wèi zhǔ jiàng zhuó,* **stomach governs downbearing of the turbid** [ˈstʌmək ˈgʌvənz ˈdaʊnˌbɛrɪŋ əv ðə ˈtɝbɪd]: The stomach sends food down to the small intestine. The spleen removes essence of grain and water, which is the "clear" part of the food. What remains is the "turbid" part, which after further transformation is discharged from the anus.

242. 小肠主分别清浊〔小腸主分別清濁〕*xiǎo cháng zhǔ fēn bié qīng zhuó,* **small intestine governs separation of the clear and turbid** [smɔl ɪnˈtɛstɪn ˈgʌvənz ˌsɛpəˈreʃən əv ðə klɪr ənd ˈtɝbɪd]: The small

intestine further transforms food already decomposed by the stomach. The clear refers to what is useful to the body, while the turbid denotes waste. In the small intestine, the essence of grain and water is assimilated into the body by the action of the spleen. Waste water is absorbed and, by kidney qì transformation, is conveyed to the bladder. Hence, "The small intestine governs humor."

243. 小肠主液〔小腸主液〕*xiǎo cháng zhǔ yè*, **small intestine governs humor** ['smɔl-ɪn'tɛstɪn 'ɡʌvɚnz 'hjumɚ]: See small intestine governs separation of the clear and the turbid.

244. 大肠主传化糟粕〔大腸主傳化糟粕〕*dà cháng zhǔ chuán huà zāo pò*, **large intestine governs the conveyance and transformation of waste** [lɑrdʒ ɪn'tɛstɪn 'ɡʌvɚnz ðə kən'veəns ənd ‚trænsfɚ'meʃən əv west]: The large intestine conveys waste downward and out of the body, transforming it into stool as it does so.

245. 大肠主津〔大腸主津〕*dà cháng zhǔ jīn*, **large intestine governs liquid** [lɑrdʒ ɪn'tɛstɪn 'ɡʌvɚnz 'lɪkwɪd]: The large intestine is said to govern liquid because it absorbs fluid from the food waste so that it forms into firm stool.

3.4. 肝
The Liver

246. 肝属木〔肝屬木〕*gān shǔ mù*, **liver belongs to wood** [lɪvɚ bɪ'lɔŋz tə wʊd]: The liver is associated with wood among the five phases.

247. 肝与胆相表里〔肝與膽相表裡〕*gān yǔ dǎn xiāng biǎo lǐ*, **liver and gallbladder stand in interior-exterior relationship** ['lɪvɚ ənd 'ɡɔlblædɚ stænd ɪn ɪn'tɪrɪɚ ɪks'tɪrɪɚ rɛ'leʃənʃɪp]: The liver stands in interior-exterior relationship with the gallbladder. The liver channel nets the gallbladder, and the gallbladder channel nets the liver. Effulgent gallbladder heat and ascendant liver yáng can both manifest in rashness, impatience, and tendency to anger. Liver-calming medicinals can also drain gallbladder fire, and medicinals that drain gallbladder fire can also calm the liver.

248. 肝主疏泄〔肝主疏泄〕*gān zhǔ shū xiè*, **liver governs free coursing** ['lɪvɚ 'ɡʌvɚnz 'fri kɔrsɪŋ]: In the five phases, wood is said to "like orderly reaching." Accordingly, the liver maintains the normal flow of qì throughout the whole body. The liver's governing of free coursing is reflected in the regularity and smoothness of qì dynamic. When this function is normal, qì dynamic is smooth and regular, so that qì and

blood remain in harmony, the channels are kept free, and the bowels and viscera all function normally. When it is impaired, qì dynamic is disturbed and a whole variety of diseases may arise as a result. If liver qì is depressed in the liver itself and its associated channel, distending pain develops in the chest and rib-side or in the lesser abdomen, or the breasts become painfully swollen. If liver qì invades the stomach, there are signs such as attacks of pain (阵痛 *zhèn tòng*) in the stomach duct and abdomen, and nausea, vomiting, and belching; if liver qì invades the spleen, there is distending pain in the chest, rib-side, and abdomen, with rumbling intestines and diarrhea. The free coursing function is easily upset by emotional factors.

249. 肝藏血〔肝藏血〕 *gān cáng xuè,* **liver stores blood** [ˈlɪvɚ stɔrz blʌd]: The liver is capable of retaining blood and regulating the amount of blood in the body. The amount of blood in the various parts of the body varies in accordance with physiological needs. During physical exertion, blood is distributed throughout the body, meeting the increased need for nutrients. When the body is at rest or asleep, blood flows back to the liver to be stored. Therefore it is said, "When the body moves, blood flows through the channels, and when the body is at rest, the blood flows back to the liver where it is stored"; and "the legs receive blood and walk, the hands receive blood and grip." When the liver's blood-storing function is disturbed, two possible conditions may arise. In the first case, the storage capacity of the liver is reduced so that there is not enough blood in the body to supply all needs; if the blood does not nourish the eyes, such diseases as flowery vision (blurred or mottled vision), dry eyes, and night blindness may occur; if the blood fails to nourish the sinews, hypertonicity (tension, stiffness) of the sinews gives rise to inhibited bending and stretching; in women, blood may fail to flow into the thoroughfare (*chōng*) and controlling (*rèn*) vessels, causing scant menstruation or menstrual block. In the second case, the blood-storing function of the liver is impaired, causing a tendency toward bleeding, such as profuse menstruation, flooding and spotting, and other forms of bleeding; such conditions are known as the liver failing to store blood (肝不藏血 *gān bù cáng xuè*).

250. 肝主筋〔肝主筋〕 *gān zhǔ jīn,* **liver governs the sinews** [ˈlɪvɚ ˈgʌvɚnz ðə ˈsɪnjuz]: The sinews (tendons, muscles; see sinew) are dependent on the liver. Only when liver blood is abundant can its nourishing influence reach the sinews and enable them to move normally. If liver blood is insufficient, the resulting failure of the blood to nourish the sinews adequately brings on hypertonicity (tension and stiffness) or numbness in the limbs, with difficulty in bending and stretching. When

liver wind stirs internally, tremors, convulsions, and arched-back rigidity are observed.

251. 肝，其华在爪〔肝，其華在爪〕 *gān, qí huá zài zhǎo,* **liver... its bloom is in the nails** [ˈlɪvɚ, ɪts blum ɪz ɪn ðə nelz]: Bloom means the outward manifestation of health. This phrase reflects the observation that when liver blood is abundant, the nails are red, lustrous, and healthy. When liver blood is insufficient, the nails are pale in color and brittle.

252. 肝开窍于目〔肝開竅於目〕 *gān kāi qiào yú mù,* **liver opens at the eyes** [ˈlɪvɚ ˈopənz ət ðə ɑɪz]: The liver and the eyes are intimately related. The phrase "the liver opens at the eyes" appears in an enumeration of five phase correspondences in *Essential Prescriptions of the Golden Coffer (Jīn Guì Yào Lüè). The Magic Pivot (Líng Shū, mài dù piān)* states, "Liver qì flows to the eyes; when the liver is in harmony, the eyes can identify the five colors," and *Elementary Questions (Sù Wèn, wǔ zàng shēng chéng piān)* states, "The liver receives blood, so there is sight." These lines emphasize that the eyes are dependent on the nourishing action of liver blood. Insufficiency of liver blood may provoke such conditions as night blindness, dry eyes, and blurred vision; liver fire flaming upward can cause reddening and painful swelling of the eyes; ascendant liver yáng can manifest as dizzy vision; and internal liver wind may cause a sideways or upward squint.

253. 肝为刚脏〔肝爲剛臟〕 *gān wéi gāng zàng,* **liver is the unyielding viscus** [ˈlɪvɚ ɪz ði ʌnˈjildɪŋ ˈvɪskəs]: The liver likes orderly reaching, and is averse to being repressed or constrained and to hyperactivity [of its yáng aspect]. The unyielding nature of the liver is mainly seen in liver qì: mental stimulus gives rise to rashness, impatience, and anger. Conversely, insufficiency of liver qì gives rise to susceptibility to fright and fear. The liver and gallbladder stand in interior-exterior relationship, and the unyielding nature is a combined manifestation of both these organs.

3.5. 肾
The Kidney

254. 肾属水〔腎屬水〕 *shèn shǔ shuǐ,* **kidney belongs to water** [ˈkɪdnɪ brˈlɔŋz tə ˈwɔtɚ]: The kidney is associated with water among the five phases.

255. 肾主水〔腎主水〕 *shèn zhǔ shuǐ,* **kidney governs water** [ˈkɪdnɪ ˈɡʌvərnz ˈwɔtər]: The kidney "steams" the fluids, regulates their distribution, and discharges waste water, thereby maintaining normal water metabolism in the body. For this reason, the kidney is said to govern water. Body fluids are derived from fluids taken in by the stomach. Through the spleen's movement and transformation and the lung's regulation of the waterways, they are distributed throughout the body, and waste water is carried down to the bladder before being discharged. The qì transformation of the kidney plays a vital role in this. This is why it is said that the kidney governs water. Impairment of this action due to kidney yáng vacuity can either cause disorders of fluid metabolism, such as scant urine and water swelling, or failure to contain water, characterized by long voidings of clear urine or profuse urination at night. The function of the bladder is to store and discharge urine and is closely related to the kidney. Storage relies on the retentive power of kidney qì, while discharge relies on the power of the kidney to permit flow. This is known as the "opening and closing" function of the kidney that controls the flow of urine down to the bladder, and enables the bladder to store up to a certain amount of urine before permitting its discharge. *Elementary Questions (Sù Wèn, líng lán mì diǎn lùn)* says, "The bladder... stores fluid, and by qì transformation discharges it." In reality, "qì transformation" referred to here is a function of the kidney. According to *Elementary Questions (Sù Wèn, xuān míng wǔ qì piān)*, "Inhibition of the bladder manifests as dribbling urinary block, and its failure to ensure containment, as enuresis." Pathologies associated with the bladder include dribbling urinary block, dribble after voiding, frequent urination, enuresis, or urinary incontinence, which in the absence of disease of the bladder itself are generally attributed to disease of the kidney.

256. 肾与膀胱相表里〔腎與膀胱相表裡〕 *shèn yǔ páng guāng xiāng biǎo lǐ,* **kidney and bladder stand in interior-exterior relationship** [ˈkɪdnɪ ənd ˈblædər stænd ɪn ɪnˈtɪrɪər ɪksˈtɪrɪər rɛˈleʃənʃɪp]: The kidney stands in interior-exterior relationship with the bladder. The kidney channel nets the bladder and the bladder channel nets the kidney. The kidney governs water within the body, and the bladder (essentially by the action of kidney qì) governs the "opening and closing," i.e., the release and temporary storage of urine.

257. 肾藏精〔腎藏精〕 *shèn cáng jīng,* **kidney stores essence** [ˈkɪdnɪ stɔrz ˈɛsəns]: Growth, development, and reproduction rely on the essential qì stored by the kidney. Kidney essential qì is derived from the reproductive essence of the parents (congenital essence), out of which the embryo develops. After birth, it is gradually nurtured by the essence

of food (acquired essence) and reaches fullness in puberty, when men are able to produce semen and women begin menstruating—important signs of the reproductive function coming to maturity. In old age, the kidney essential qì weakens, so that the reproductive function gradually fades away, and the body degenerates. *Elementary Questions* (*Sù Wèn, shàng gǔ tiān zhēn lùn*) states, "[In the male] at the age of two eights [i.e., sixteen], kidney qì is exuberant, the "heavenly tenth" (天癸 *tiān guǐ*) arrives, essential qì flows forth, yīn and yáng are in harmony, and [he] can beget offspring... At the age of seven eights [i.e., fifty-six] heavenly tenth is exhausted, essence diminishes, the kidney grows weak, and the body gradually reaches the extreme [of decline]; at eight eights, the teeth and hair fall out. [In the female] at the age of two sevens, heavenly tenth arrives, the controlling (*rèn*) vessel flows, and the thoroughfare vessel fills, the menses come according to their times, and [she] can bear offspring... At seven sevens, the controlling (*rèn*) vessel empties, the thoroughfare vessel weakens, heavenly tenth is exhausted, the passages of the Earth are cut, the body deteriorates, and she can no longer bear children." In this quotation, heavenly tenth is explained as meaning viability of the reproductive function.

258. 肾主开阖〔腎主開闔〕*shèn zhǔ kāi hé,* **kidney governs opening and closing** [ˈkɪdnɪ ˈɡʌvɚnz ˈopənɪŋ ənd ˈklozɪŋ]: Kidney qì governs the storage of urine in the bladder and its release from the bladder. See **kidney governs water**.

259. 肾开窍于耳〔腎開竅於耳〕*shèn kāi qiào yú ěr,* **kidney opens at the ears** [ˈkɪdnɪ ˈopənz ət ði irz]: The kidney determines hearing ability. The kidney is said to open at the ears since only when kidney qì is abundant is hearing acute. *The Magic Pivot* (*Líng Shū*) states, "The kidney qì reaches the ears, and if the kidney is in harmony, the ears perceive the five sounds."

260. 肾开窍于二阴〔腎開竅於二陰〕*shèn kāi qiào yú èr yīn,* **kidney opens at the two yīn** [ˈkɪdnɪ ˈopənz ət ðə tu jɪn]: The kidney opens at the "two yīn," i.e., the "posterior yīn," which refers to the anus, and the "anterior yīn," which refers to the genitals. The genitals are located in the lower burner, and their function is associated with kidney qì, so that they are referred to as the outer orifices of the kidney. This relationship is also reflected in various diseases. For example, kidney vacuity may lead to changes in urination and defecation such as scant urine, long voidings of clear urine, incontinence, enduring diarrhea (久泄 *jiǔ xiè*), and fecal incontinence. The reproductive system may also be affected, causing impotence, premature ejaculation, or seminal emission.

261. 肾，其华在发〔腎，其華在髮〕*shèn, qí huá zài fà,* **kidney... its bloom is in the hair (of the head)** ['kɪdnɪ, ɪts blum ɪz ɪn ðə hɛr (əv ðə hɛd)]: The general condition of the hair, hair growth, and hair loss are all associated with the strength of the kidney essential qì. Loss of hair in old age is one sign of debilitation of essential qì. However, the hair also relies on the nourishing action of the blood, so it is also said, "The hair [of the head] is the surplus of the blood."

262. 肾生骨髓〔腎生骨髓〕*shèn shēng gǔ suí,* **kidney engenders the bone and marrow** ['kɪdnɪ ɪn'dʒendəz ðə bon ənd 'mæro]: The growth, development, and healing of the bones depends on the nourishment and activation provided by kidney essential qì. Insufficiency of kidney essential qì may result in retarded closure of the fontanel gate and soft bones in infants. It may also lead to marrow vacuity characterized by wilting legs that prevent the patient from walking, or pain or stiffness of the lower lumbar spine preventing the patient from lying either prone or supine. Furthermore, the teeth are the surplus of the bones. In clinical practice, slow growth of teeth in children and the premature loosening and loss of teeth in adults are found to be due to insufficiency of kidney essential qì. Hence, some tooth diseases are vacuity patterns that can be treated through the kidney. Because the kidney governs the bones and engenders marrow, and the brain is known as the "sea of marrow," a close link can be seen between the kidney and the brain.

263. 肾主骨〔腎主骨〕*shèn zhǔ gǔ,* **kidney governs the bones** ['kɪdnɪ 'gʌvənz ðə bonz]: See kidney engenders bone and marrow.

264. 肾，其充在骨〔腎，其充在骨〕*shèn, qí chōng zài gǔ,* **kidney... its fullness is in the bone** ['kɪdnɪ, ɪts 'fʊlnɪs ɪz ɪn ðə bon]: See kidney engenders bone and marrow.

3.6. 脑、子宫、三焦
The Brain, Uterus, and Triple Burner

265. 脑〔腦〕*nǎo,* **brain** [bren]: An extraordinary organ located in the skull. According to traditional doctrine of visceral manifestation, "the brain is the sea of marrow; all marrow belongs to the brain, flowing up to the brain and down to the coccyx." The brain is most closely related to the kidney, which engenders the marrow.

266. **子宫**〔子宫〕*zǐ gōng,* **uterus** [ˈjutərəs]: One of the extraordinary organs; its main function is menstruation and childbearing, which are related to kidney essential qì, the thoroughfare (*chōng*) and controlling (*rèn*) vessels, and the heart, liver, and spleen.

267. **女子胞**〔女子胞〕*nǚ zǐ bāo,* **uterus** [ˈjutərəs]: See preceding item.

268. **三焦主决渎**〔三焦主决渎〕*sān jiāo zhǔ jué dú,* **triple burner governs the sluices** [ˈtrɪpl̩ bɝnɚ ˈɡʌvɚnz ðə ˈslusɪz]: The triple burner represents the waterways: *Elementary Questions (Sù Wèn)* explains, "The triple burner holds the office of the sluices; the waterways emanate from it." This is interpreted to mean that the main functions of the triple burner are the processing of fluids by qì transformation and ensuring free flow through the waterways. As such, qì transformation in the triple burner is a generic expression for the roles played by the lung, spleen, kidney, stomach, small intestine, large intestine, and bladder in regulating the body's water metabolism. *The Magic Pivot (Líng Shū)* states, "When the upper burner is open and permits effusion, it causes the five flavors of food to diffuse, nourishes the skin, makes the body firm, and keeps the [body] hair moistened, like the sprinkling of mist and dew. Such is the action of qì." (上焦开发，宣五谷味，熏肤、充身、泽毛，若雾露之溉，是谓气。) This fits the imagery of the phrase "the upper burner is like mist" (上焦如雾), which in practice refers to the diffusion of defense qì and distribution of fluids by the lung. *The Magic Pivot (Líng Shū)* states, "The center burner... strains off the waste, and steams the fluids, and forms essence [from these]. This then flows upward into the lung channel, where it is transformed into blood." (中焦...泌糟粕，蒸津液，化其精微，上注肺脉，乃化为血。) This statement supports the phrase, "The center burner is like foam" (中焦如沤), which refers to the movement and formation of the essence of grain and water by the stomach and spleen, the source of blood formation. "In the lower burner, the small intestine connects through to the bladder... It transforms waste that is then sent down to the large intestine... and separates out the juices, sending them down to the bladder." (下焦者，别回肠，注于膀胱...成糟粕而俱下于大肠，...济泌别汁，循下焦而渗入膀胱焉。) The intestines, kidney, and bladder are located in the lower burner. The small intestine governs humor, the large intestine governs liquid, and the kidney governs the opening and closing. Their combined functions explain the phrase "the lower burner is like sluices" (下焦如渎).

习题
Questions

Answer the following questions in English:

171. Which viscus governs water? ....

172. With which viscus are the spirit, tongue, blood, and vessels all closely associated? ....

173. Which viscus is said to govern qi? ....

174. Which bowel is said to govern intake? ....

175. Which viscus stores the blood? ....

176. Which is the heart's corresponding bowel in the exterior?
....

177. Which bowel governs the separation of the clear and turbid?
....

178. Which viscus engenders the bone and marrow? ....

179. Which viscus is said to have its bloom in the nails? ....

180. With which viscus does the gallbladder stand in interior-exterior relationship? ....

181. Which viscus opens at the eyes? ....

182. Of which viscus is the hair (of the head) the bloom? ....

183. Which bowel governs the conveyance and transformation of waste?

184. Opening and closing are governed by which viscus? ....

185. Which viscus stores essence? ....

186. Which is the unyielding viscus? ....

187. Which extraordinary organ is the sea of marrow? ....

188. Which bowel is said to hold the office of the sluices? ....

189. What phase does the liver belong to? ....

190. Which viscus has its fullness in the bone? ....

191. Which bowel governs intake? ....

192. Which viscus opens at the ears? ....

193. To which extraordinary vessel is the uterus most closely related?
....

194. Which bowel governs humor? ....

195. With which viscus are the skin and [body] hair associated?
....

196. What are the two yīn? ....

197. Which viscus governs the upbearing of the clear? ....

198. With which viscus are the sinews associated? ....

199. What phase does the lung belong to? ....

200. What is the relationship between the lung and the large intestine?
....

Give the Pīnyīn and English for the following Chinese terms:

201. 子宫 ....
202. 胃主受纳 ....
203. 三焦 ....
204. 肾藏精 ....
205. 肾开窍于耳 ....
206. 脑 ....
207. 肾与膀胱相表里 ....
208. 肺主皮毛 ....
209. 肺主气 ....
210. 肝开窍于目 ....
211. 肺主通调水道 ....
212. 心开窍于舌 ....
213. 肝主筋 ....
214. 脾属土 ....
215. 肝藏血 ....
216. 肾主开阖 ....
217. 脾主运化 ....
218. 肝属木 ....

219. 三焦主决渎 ....

220. 心主血脉 ....

Supply the Chinese and English for the following:

221. *Shèn kāi qiào yú èr yīn.* ....

222. *Gān zhǔ shū xiè.* ....

223. *Dà cháng zhǔ chuán huà zāo pò.* ....

224. *Nǚ zǐ bāo.* ....

225. *Dà cháng zhǔ jīn.* ....

226. *Wèi zhǔ jiàng zhuó.* ....

227. *Shèn zhǔ gǔ.* ....

228. *Xiǎo cháng zhǔ yè.* ....

229. *Shèn, qí chōng zài gǔ.* ....

230. *Wèi zhǔ fǔ shú.* ....

231. *Pí shǔ tǔ.* ....

232. *Gān shǔ mù.* ....

233. *Xiǎo cháng zhǔ fēn bié qīng zhuó.* ....

234. *Pí, qí huá zài chún sì bái.* ....

235. *Pí kāi qiào yú kǒu.* ....

Give the Chinese and Pīnyīn for the following:

236. The liver governs the sinews. ....

237. Movement and transformation. ....

238. The heart opens at the tongue. ....

239. The lung governs depurative downbearing. ....

240. The spleen governs the flesh and limbs. ....

241. The lung opens at the nose. ....

242. The spleen governs the upbearing of the clear. ....

243. The large intestine governs the conveyance and transformation of waste. ....

244. The heart governs the blood and vessel. ....

245. The liver belongs to wood. ....

246. The triple burner governs the sluices. ....

247. The heart stores the spirit. ....

248. The small intestine governs humor. ....

249. The lung governs qì. ....

250. The kidney... its fullness is in the bone. ....

251. Uterus. ....

252. The spleen opens at the mouth. ....

253. The kidney opens at the two yīn. ....

254. The lung belongs to metal. ....

255. The liver governs free coursing. ....

256. The kidney belongs to water. ....

257. The heart and small intestine stand in interior-exterior relationship.
....

258. The four limbs. ....

259. The kidney stores essence. ....

260. The stomach governs downbearing of the turbid. ....

第四章 四诊
Four Examinations

269. 证（候）〔證（候）〕 *zhèng hòu,* **sign** [saɪn]: Any indication of disease, e.g., pain or other localized discomfort, heat effusion, poor appetite, abnormalities of stool, urine, menses, etc. In most cases, a sign is insufficient to determine the nature of the disease. Also called "symptom" (症状 *zhèng zhuàng*), the term used in Western medicine. Note that the Chinese terms 证 *zhèng* and 证候 *zhèng hòu* are used in another sense where they are translated as "pattern" (see Chapter 6).

4.1. 望诊
Inspection

4.1.1. 望神 Inspecting the Spirit

270. 得神〔得神〕 *dé shén,* **spiritedness** ['spɪrɪtɪdnɪs]: General vitality. If the patient has bright eyes, normal bearing, clear speech, and responds coherently to inquiry, he or she is said to be spirited. Spiritedness indicates that right qì is undamaged and the condition is relatively minor. Although certain aspects of the patient's health may be seriously affected, swift improvement may be expected.

271. 失神〔失神〕 *shī shén,* **spiritlessness** ['spɪrɪtləsnɪs]: Poor vitality, i.e., the presence of signs of lack of general vitality such as mental debilitation, apathy, abnormal bearing, torpid expression, dark complexion and dull eyes, low voice, slow halting speech, and incoherent response to inquiry. Spiritlessness indicates a relatively serious condition in which right qì has suffered damage. Although no critical signs may be present, extreme care is necessary in deciding treatment.

272. 假神〔假神〕 *jiǎ shén,* **false spiritedness** [fɔls 'spɪrɪtɪdnɪs]: False signs of vitality that suddenly appear in patients suffering from enduring and severe illness. Such signs, which include sudden garrulousness

and improvement in appetite and facial complexion, are the "last radiance of the setting sun" (回光反照 *huí guāng fǎn zhào*) or the "last flicker of the lamp" (残灯复明 *cán dēng fù míng*) and bode imminent death.

273. 神昏〔神昏〕 *shén hūn*, **clouded spirit** ['klɑʊdɪd 'spɪrɪt]: Stupor or complete loss of consciousness; a sign of a critical condition. It may occur in externally contracted heat (febrile) disease (e.g., bowel heat patterns) or internal damage by the seven affects. It is always treated by opening the orifices before any other aspects of the condition are treated.

4.1.2. 望形态 Inspecting Form and Bearing

274. 形体肥胖〔形體肥胖〕 *xíng tǐ féi pàng*, **obesity** [ə'bisətɪ]: Fatness, corpulence. Traditional literature contains little reference to weight control. With the influence of modern medicine, greater attention is being paid to the problem. Obesity is attributed to phlegm-damp or qì vacuity, or as is often the case, a combination of the two.

275. 肌肉瘦削〔肌肉瘦削〕 *jī ròu shòu xuè*, **emaciation** [ɪm͵esɪ'eʃən]: Marked thinning of the body, usually accompanied by other signs of disease. Emaciation appears in a variety of illnesses that present as vacuity or repletion patterns (emaciation is not only a vacuity sign).

276. 脱肉破䐃〔脱肉破䐃〕 *tuō ròu pò jiǒng (jùn)*, **shedding of flesh and loss of bulk** ['ʃɛdɪŋ əv flɛʃ ənd lɔs əv bʌlk]: Severe emaciation, a sign of debilitation of spleen qì. It is seen in enduring illness.

277. 向里蜷卧〔向裡踡臥〕 *xiàng lǐ quán wò*, **lying in curled-up posture** ['laɪɪŋ ɪn 'kɝ˞ldʌp 'pastʃɚ]: Seen in yīn patterns and cold patterns.

278. 身重〔身重〕 *shēn zhòng*, **heavy body; generalized heaviness** ['hɛvɪ 'badɪ, 'dʒɛnərə͵laɪzd 'hɛvɪnɪs]: A sensation of heaviness with inhibited physical movement. Heavy body is due to dampness in the fleshy exterior caused by exposure to external dampness, wind contending with water (风水相搏 *fēng shuǐ xiāng bó*), or yáng vacuity water flood.

279. 四肢困倦〔四肢困倦〕 *sì zhī kùn juàn*, **fatigued cumbersome limbs** [fə'tigd 'kʌmbɚsʌm lɪmz]: Limbs that lack strength and feel unwieldy. A sign of dampness and spleen vacuity.

280. 头身困重〔頭身困重〕 *tóu shēn kùn zhòng*, **heavy cumbersome head and body** ['hɛvɪ 'kʌmbɚsʌm hɛd ənd 'badɪ]: See heavy body; heavy-headedness.

281. 身重不易转侧〔身重不易轉側〕 *shēn zhòng bù yì zhuǎn cè*, **heavy body with difficulty in turning sides** ['hɛvɪ 'badɪ wɪð 'dɪfɪ͵kʌltɪ ɪn 'tɝ˞nɪŋ saɪdz]: See heavy body.

282. 扬手掷足〔揚手擲足〕*yáng shǒu zhí zú,* **flailing of the arms and legs** ['fleɪɪŋ əv ði ɑrmz ənd lɛgz]: Wild uncontrollable movement of the limbs. A sign of severe agitation.

283. 躁〔躁〕*zào,* **agitation** [ˌædʒɪ'teʃən]: A subjective feeling of vexation outwardly expressed by pronounced abnormal movement. Compare heart vexation.

284. 易怒〔易怒〕*yì nù,* **irascibility** [ɪˌræsɪ'bɪlətɪ]: A sign of binding depression of liver qì.

285. 狂躁〔狂躁〕*kuáng zào,* **mania and agitation** ['menɪə ənd ˌædʒɪ'teʃ-ən]: Agitation with signs of mania.

286. 循衣摸床〔循衣摸床〕*xún yī mō chuáng,* **picking at bedclothes** ['pɪkɪŋ ət 'bɛdkloðz]: An aimless plucking at bedclothes observed in an extreme stage of disease.

287. 撮空理线〔撮空理線〕*cuō kōng lǐ xiàn,* **groping in the air and pulling [invisible] strings** ['gropɪŋ ɪn ði ɛr ənd 'pʊlɪŋ ɪn'vɪzɪbl̩ strɪŋz]: See picking at bedclothes.

288. 口眼喎斜〔口眼喎斜〕*kǒu yǎn wāi xié,* **deviated eyes and mouth** ['divɪetɪd ɑɪz ənd maʊθ]: Tension in the sinews of one side of the face and relaxation in those of the other side manifesting in skewing of the mouth and inability to close the eyes. Deviated eyes and mouth are attributed to wind or wind-phlegm obstructing the channels.

289. 瘛瘲〔瘛瘲〕*qì zòng,* **tugging and slackening** ['tʌgɪŋ ənd 'slækənɪŋ]: Also called *convulsion of the limbs; tugging wind.* Alternating tensing and relaxation of the sinews, often observed in externally contracted heat (febrile) disease, epilepsy, and lockjaw.

290. 四肢抽搐〔四肢抽搐〕*sì zhī chōu chù,* **convulsion of the limbs** [kən'vʌlʃən əv ðə lɪmz]: tugging and slackening.

291. 抽风〔抽風〕*chōu fēng,* **tugging wind** ['tʌgɪŋ]: tugging and slackening.

292. 痉厥〔痙厥〕*jìng jué,* **tetanic reversal** [tɛ'tænɪk rɪ'vɜsl̩]: See tetany.

293. 抽动〔抽動〕*chōu dòng,* **jerking** ['dʒɝkɪŋ]: Spontaneous movement of the sinews and flesh.

294. 筋惕肉瞤〔筋惕肉瞤〕*jīn tì ròu shùn,* **jerking sinews and twitching flesh** ['dʒɝkɪŋ 'sɪnjuz ənd 'twɪtʃɪŋ flɛʃ]: Spasmodic jerking of the sinew and flesh, mostly occurring when copious sweating damages yáng, causing blood vacuity and wear on liquid that deprives the sinews of nourishment.

295. 筋脉拘急〔筋脈拘急〕*jīn mài jū jí,* **tension of the sinews** ['tɛnʃən əv ðə 'sɪnjuz]: Tension of the sinews that prevents normal bending and

stretching. Sinew hypertonicity is mostly attributable to contraction of wind-cold in general vacuity or to blood or liquid vacuity depriving the sinew vessels of nourishment. It is observed in lockjaw, tetany, impediment, fright wind, and wind stroke.

296. 筋脉拘挛〔筋脈拘攣〕 *jīn mài jū luán,* **hypertonicity of the sinews** [ˌhaɪpəˈtə'nɪsɪtɪ əv ðə 'sɪnjuz]: tension of the sinews.

297. 颈项强直〔頸項強直〕 *jǐng xiàng jiàng zhí,* **rigidity of the neck** [rɛ'dʒɪdətɪ əv ðə nɛk]: Tension in the muscles of the neck. It is attributed to a) contraction of wind, cold, or damp evil in the greater yáng (*tài yáng*) channel, b) invasion of disease evil through wounds of the skin and flesh, or c) damage to yīn through loss of blood, great sweating, or great heat [effusion] with insufficiency of liquid and blood depriving the sinews of nourishment. Rigidity of the neck is observed in cold damage, wind stroke, tetany, and crick in the neck.

298. 角弓反张〔角弓反張〕 *jiǎo gōng fǎn zhāng,* **arched-back rigidity** [artʃt bæk rɪ'dʒɪdətɪ]: Rigidity of the neck and back that causes them to arch or bow backward. It occurs in child fright wind, lockjaw, and other forms of tetany.

299. 口噤〔口噤〕 *kǒu jìn,* **clenched jaw** [klɛntʃd dʒɔ]: Inability to open the mouth. A sign of tetanic disease, wind stroke, and fright wind.

300. 昏倒〔昏倒〕 *hūn dǎo,* **clouding collapse** ['klaʊdɪŋ kə'læps]: Fainting or falling unconscious. It is observed in epilepsy, wind-stroke, ascendant hyperactivity of liver yáng, and liver fire flaming upward.

301. 半身不遂〔半身不遂〕 *bàn shēn bù suì,* **hemiplegia** [ˌhɛmɪ'plidʒ(ɪ)ə]: Paralysis of one half of the body. Hemiplegia is the result of wind stroke and is observed in all wind stroke visceral patterns, bowel patterns, and channel patterns, usually in conjunction with deviated eyes and mouth.

302. 头摇〔頭搖〕 *tóu yáo,* **shaking of the head** ['ʃekɪŋ əv ðə hɛd]: Tremor or wobbling of the head that the patient cannot control. There are repletion and vacuity patterns.

4.1.3. 望色泽 Inspecting the Complexion

303. 面色白〔面色白〕 *miàn sè bái,* **white facial complexion** [waɪt 'feʃl̩ kəm'plɛkʃən]: Any pale complexion, generally indicating cold or vacuity. Distinction is made between pale white, somber white, and bright white.

304. 面色淡白〔面色淡白〕 *miàn sè dàn bái,* **pale white facial complexion** [pel waɪt 'feʃl̩ kəm'plɛkʃən]: A colorless complexion. "Pale" de-

notes the absence of color, whereas "white" is the color associated with metal among the five phases. It normally indicates blood vacuity.

305. 面色苍白〔面色蒼白〕 *miàn sè cāng bái,* **somber white facial complexion** ['sɑmbɚ waɪt 'feʃl̩ kəm'plɛkʃən]: A complexion that is white with a tinge of blue or gray. A white complexion with a hint of dull blue or gray, often seen, for example, in desertion patterns.

306. 面色㿠白〔面色㿠白〕 *miàn sè huǎng bái,* **bright white facial complexion** [braɪt waɪt 'feʃl̩ kəm'plɛkʃən]: A very white complexion. With facial vacuity edema it generally indicates yáng qì vacuity and occurs after massive bleeding, in chronic nephritis, or in wheezing and panting patterns.

307. 面色黄〔面色黃〕 *miàn sè huáng,* **yellow facial complexion** ['jɛlo 'feʃl̩ kəm'plɛkʃən]: A sign of dampness or vacuity. Yellowing of the whites of the eyes (sclerae) and generalized yellowing of the skin indicate jaundice.

308. 面色萎黄〔面色萎黃〕 *miàn sè wěi huáng,* **withered-yellow facial complexion** ['wɪðɚd 'jəlo 'feʃl̩ kəm'plɛkʃən]: A lusterless brownish yellow facial complexion. It indicates vacuity or dampness.

309. 面色无华〔面色無華〕 *miàn sè wú huá,* **lusterless facial complexion** ['lʌstɚlɪs 'feʃl̩ kəm'plɛkʃən]: A complexion that lacks color and vitality.

310. 面色青紫〔面色青紫〕 *miàn sè qīng zǐ,* **green-blue or purple facial complexion** [grin blu ɔr 'pɝpl̩ 'feʃl̩ kəm'plɛkʃən]: A sign of wind-cold, blood stasis, pain, and qì block patterns. It is observed in child fright wind and epilepsy.

311. 面色红〔面色紅〕 *miàn sè hóng,* **red facial complexion** [rɛd 'feʃl̩ kəm'plɛkʃən]: A complexion redder than normal; a sign of heat.

312. 面赤〔面赤〕 *miàn chì,* **red face** [rɛd fes]: See red facial complexion.

313. 面色黑〔面色黑〕 *miàn sè hēi,* **black facial complexion** [blæk 'feʃl̩ kəm'plɛkʃən]: A sign of severe or intractable disease, associated with kidney vacuity and blood stasis. A complexion that is soot-black (black with a tinge of yellow), dark gray, or purple-black may occur in enduring illness, in insufficiency of kidney essence, or in static blood accumulation patterns.

314. 斑疹〔斑疹〕 *bān zhěn,* **maculopapular eruption** [ˌmækjəlo'pæpjəlɚ ɪ'rʌpʃən]: Eruption of macules or papules. Macules are colored (usually red) patches that are unraised above the surface of the skin and vary in size. Papules are like grains of millet in shape and size (or may be larger) that are raised above the surface of the skin. The appearance of maculopapular eruptions in externally contracted heat (febrile) diseases

indicates heat entering construction-blood. In miscellaneous internal damage diseases, they usually indicate blood heat.

4.1.4. 舌诊 Tongue Inspection

315. 舌质〔舌質〕*shé zhì,* **tongue body** ['tʌŋ–bɑdɪ]: The tongue itself as opposed to the tongue fur.

316. 舌体〔舌體〕*shé tǐ,* **tongue body** ['tʌŋ–bɑdɪ]: See preceding item.

317. 舌胖大〔舌胖大〕*shé pàng dà,* **enlarged tongue** [ɪn'lɑrdʒd tʌŋ]: A tongue that is swollen to a size slightly larger than normal, most clearly indicated by dental impressions on the margins. An enlarged tongue indicates qì vacuity or the presence of water-damp (dampness, phlegm-rheum).

318. 舌淡胖嫩〔舌淡胖嫩〕*shé dàn pàng nèn,* **pale tender-soft enlarged tongue** [pel 'tɛndɚ-sɔft ɪn'lɑrdʒd tʌŋ]: A tongue that is larger than normal and is usually pale and tender looking. Note that "tender" here does not mean painful when touched, but soft to the touch like a child's flesh. For clinical significance, see previous item.

319. 舌边齿痕〔舌邊齒痕〕*shé biān chǐ hén,* **dental impressions on the margins of the tongue** ['dəntl ɪm'prɛʃənz ɔn ðə 'mɑrdʒɪnz əv ðə tʌŋ]: See enlarged tongue.

320. 舌瘦瘪〔舌瘦癟〕*shé shòu biě,* **shrunken tongue** ['ʃrʌŋkən tʌŋ]: A thin, shrunken tongue indicates insufficiency of yīn liquid or a dual vacuity of yīn and qì. A shrunken tongue resulting from damage to yīn humor by exuberant heat is crimson in color and dry. In dual vacuity of yīn and qì, the tongue is pale in color.

321. 舌起芒刺〔舌起芒刺〕*shé qǐ máng cì,* **prickly tongue** ['prɪklɪ tʌŋ]: Abnormal projections on the tongue surface. Prickles often occur with red speckles and are invariably accompanied by a scorched yellow or black tongue fur. They indicate exuberant heat.

322. 舌裂〔舌裂〕*shé liè,* **fissured tongue** ['fɪʃɚd tʌŋ]: A tongue bearing deep longitudinal furrows or creases. The fissures vary in depth and position. With a dry tongue, they indicate insufficiency of the fluids. They may also occur in exuberant heat patterns with a crimson tongue.

323. 舌卷〔舌卷〕*shé juǎn,* **curled tongue** [kɜ˞ld tʌŋ]: A flexed tongue that impedes speech. It is attributed to heart fire flaming upward, warm evil falling inward into the pericardium, or pronounced liver channel heat. In the latter case, it occurs with retracted testicles.

324. 吐弄舌〔吐弄舌〕*tù nòng shé,* **protrusion and worrying of the tongue** [prə'truʒən ənd 'wɜ˞ɪɪŋ əv ðə tʌŋ]: Protrusion of the tongue

is a state in which the tongue is loosely stretched and hangs out of the mouth. Worrying is when the tongue moves in a circular motion whereby the tip is extended from and retracted back into the mouth, or licks the upper and lower lips or the corners of the mouth.

325. 吐舌〔吐舌〕*tù shé,* **protrusion of the tongue** [prə'truʒən əv ðə tʌŋ]: See protrusion and worrying of the tongue.

326. 弄舌〔弄舌〕*nòng shé,* **worrying of the tongue** ['wɝɪŋ əv ðə tʌŋ]: See protrusion and worrying of the tongue.

327. 舌强〔舌強〕*shé jiàng,* **stiff tongue** [stɪf tʌŋ]: A tongue that is stiff, moves sluggishly, and inhibits speech. A stiff tongue occurs in a number of severe conditions such as heat entering the pericardium, phlegm confounding the orifices of the heart, and liver wind stirring internally. Other signs are therefore decisive in determining the nature of the disease. In Western medicine, a stiff tongue generally indicates diseases of the central nervous system.

328. 舌强语謇〔舌強語謇〕*shé jiàng yǔ jiǎn,* **stiff tongue and impeded speech** [stɪf tʌŋ ənd ɪm'pɪdɪd spitʃ]: See preceding item.

329. 舌淡〔舌淡〕*shé dàn,* **pale tongue** [pel tʌŋ]: A pale tongue indicates vacuity of qì and blood. A well-moistened pale enlarged tongue with accompanying cold signs indicates yáng qì vacuity.

330. 舌红〔舌紅〕*shé hóng,* **red tongue** [rɛd tʌŋ]: A tongue redder than normal. A red tongue indicates either vacuity heat or repletion heat.

331. 舌绛〔舌絳〕*shé jiàng,* **crimson tongue** ['krɪmzən tʌŋ]: A deep red or maroon tongue. Like a red tongue, it is associated with heat, but the added depth of color indicates that the heat is located in the construction or blood aspect.

332. 镜面舌〔鏡面舌〕*jìng miàn shé,* **mirror tongue** ['mɪrɚ tʌŋ]: A completely smooth tongue, free of liquid and fur. It indicates severe yīn humor depletion. A smooth red or deep red tongue indicates damage to yīn by intense heat. If pale in color, a smooth tongue indicates damage to both qì and yīn.

333. 舌光红〔舌光紅〕*shé guāng hóng,* **smooth bare red tongue** [smuð bɛr rɛd tʌŋ]: A mirror tongue.

334. 舌紫〔舌紫〕*shé zǐ,* **purple tongue** ['pɝpl̩ tʌŋ]: A purple coloration of the tongue indicates an impaired flow of blood and qì and resultant congealing blood stasis. A purple tongue is observed in either heat or cold patterns.

335. 瘀点〔瘀點〕*yū diǎn,* **stasis speckles** ['stesɪs 'spɛklz]: Green-blue or purple speckles on the tongue that indicate the presence of static blood. Also called stasis macules.

336. 瘀斑〔瘀斑〕*yū bān,* **stasis macules** ['stesɪs 'mækjulz]: See stasis speckles.

337. 苔厚〔苔厚〕*tāi hòu,* **thick fur** [θɪk fɜ·]: A tongue fur that does not allows the underlying tongue surface to show through; it indicates a strong evil.

338. 苔薄〔苔薄〕*tāi bó,* **thin fur** [θɪn fɜ·]: A tongue fur that allows the underlying tongue surface to show through faintly. A thin white tongue fur may be normal or may be a sign of initial-stage external contraction. The pathological significance of other thin furs is judged by their color and texture.

339. 舌苔干燥〔舌苔乾燥〕*shé tāi gān zào,* **dry tongue fur** [drɑɪ 'tʌŋ–fɜ·]: A dry fur generally indicates heat.

340. 舌净〔舌淨〕*shé jìng,* **clean tongue** [klin tʌŋ]: A tongue bearing a tongue fur that is neither turbid nor gray-brown in appearance. Indicates the absence of turbid evils.

341. 苔垢〔苔垢〕*tāi gòu,* **grimy fur** ['grɑɪmɪ fɜ·]: A tongue fur that is turbid and gray-brown in appearance. A grimy slimy fur indicates, on the one hand, the presence of turbid evils such as damp turbidity and phlegm turbidity, and on the other, stomach qì vacuity.

342. 苔腻〔苔膩〕*tāi nì,* **slimy fur** ['slɑɪmɪ fɜ·]: A sign of dampness, phlegm, and food accumulations.

343. 苔剥〔苔剝〕*tāi bō,* **peeling fur** ['pilɪŋ fɜ·]: A patchy fur interspersed with mirror-like, furless areas is known as peeling fur. This generally indicates insufficiency of yīn humor and stomach qì vacuity.

344. 白苔〔白苔〕*bái tāi,* **white fur** [wɑɪt fɜ·]: A clean moist thin white fur is normal and healthy, but may also appear at the onset of illness, indicating that the evil has not yet entered the interior and right qì remains undamaged. A glossy white fur indicates cold; thin glossy white fur indicates external wind-cold or internal cold. A thick glossy white fur indicates cold-damp or cold-phlegm. A dry white fur indicates transformation of cold evil into heat. A very dry thin white fur indicates insufficiency of fluids; thick dry fur indicates transformation of dampness into dryness. A white mealy fur with a red tongue body (see next term) indicates "dampness trapping hidden (deep-lying) heat" (湿遏热伏 *shī è rè fú*). A thick slimy white fur indicates phlegm-damp and is usually accompanied by sliminess in the mouth (口腻 *kǒu nì*), oppression in the chest, and torpid stomach intake.

345. 舌苔白如积粉〔舌苔白如積粉〕*shé tāi bái rú jī fěn,* **mealy white tongue fur** [ˈmilɪ wɑɪˈt tʌŋ–fɝ]: On a red tongue body, a white mealy tongue fur indicates dampness trapping hidden heat, which is treated by first transforming the dampness to allow the heat to escape rather than with the excessive use of cool medicinals.

346. 黄苔〔黃苔〕*huáng tāi,* **yellow fur** [ˈjɛlo fɝ]: A yellow fur usually signifies heat. Because heat patterns vary in severity and may involve different evils, different forms of yellow fur are distinguished. A thin dry yellow fur indicates damage to liquid by heat evil, posing the need to safeguard liquid. A slimy yellow fur usually indicates damp-heat. An "old yellow" (老黄 *lǎo huáng,* i.e., dark yellow) fur and a "burnt yellow" (焦黄 *jiāo huáng,* i.e., blackish yellow) fur indicate binding of repletion heat. A mixed white and yellow fur indicates the initial stages of the transformation of cold into heat that is associated with evils entering the interior.

347. 黑苔〔黑苔〕*hēi tāi,* **black fur** [blæk fɝ]: A black fur may occur in cold, heat, repletion, and vacuity patterns, but most commonly indicates an exuberant disease evil (病邪盛 *bìng xié shèng*). A rough, dry, black fur, somewhat parched in appearance, together with a red or crimson tongue body, indicates damp-heat transforming into dryness or damage to yīn by intense heat. Usually, a thick slimy black fur indicates a phlegm-damp complication. A glossy black fur signifies either stomach or kidney vacuity. A slimy yellow fur with a grayish black fur generally indicates an exuberant damp-heat evil. A mixed gray and white fur or a gray thin slimy glossy fur generally indicates cold-damp.

348. 苔化〔苔化〕*tāi huà,* **transforming fur** [trænsˈfɔrmɪŋ fɝ]: A tongue fur that is disappearing; a sign that the disease is regressing.

4.1.5. 望头面部 Inspecting the Head and Face

349. 囟门高突〔囟門高突〕*xìn mén gāo tú,* **bulging fontanel gate** [ˈbʌldʒɪŋ ˈfɑntəˌnɛl get]: A condition characterized by bulging at the anterior fontanel (traditionally called the "fontanel gate"). It may indicate cold or heat.

350. 囟门下陷〔囟門下陷〕*xìn mén xià xiàn,* **depressed fontanel gate** [dɪˈprɛst ˈfɑntəˌnɛl get]: A condition in infants in which the fontanel gate forms an indentation. It is attributed to qì-blood vacuity and vacuous visceral qì failing to rise to nourish the head, which stems from congenital insufficiency, enduring diarrhea, or chronic fright wind.

351. **囟门迟闭**〔囟門遲閉〕*xìn mén chí bì,* **retarded closure of the fontanel gate** [rɪˈtɑrdɪd ˈkloʒɚ əv ðə ˈfɑntəˌnɛl get]: The failure of the bones of the head to join together in infants.

352. **头摇**〔頭搖〕*tóu yáo,* **shaking of the head** [ˈʃekɪŋ əv ðə hɛd]: Tremor or wobbling of the head that the patient cannot control; observed in repletion and vacuity patterns.

353. **头发早白**〔頭髮早白〕*tóu fà zǎo bái,* **premature graying of the hair** [ˈprɛmətʃɚ ˈgreɪŋ əv ðə hɛr]: Partial or complete whitening of the hair in youth or middle age. It is attributable to liver-kidney depletion and insufficiency of yīn-blood depriving the hair of nourishment.

354. **发枯**〔髮枯〕*fà kū,* **dry hair** [drɑɪ hɛr]: A condition in which the hair lacks moisture and sheen. It is attributed to kidney vacuity and blood heat with yīn-blood failing to nourish the hair.

355. **发落**〔髮落〕*fà luò,* **hair loss** [ˈhɛr–lɔs]: Falling out of the hair. The hair [of the head] is the external bloom of the kidney and is the surplus of the blood. Hair loss is attributed to kidney vacuity or blood vacuity depriving the hair of nourishment.

356. **眼无光彩**〔眼無光彩〕*yǎn wú guāng cǎi,* **dull eyes** [dʌl ɑɪz]: See spiritlessness.

357. **直视**〔直視〕*zhí shì,* **forward-staring eyes** [ˈfɔrwɚd ˈstɛrɪŋ ɑɪz]: A condition in which the eyes look forward fixedly and are spiritless. It is mostly attributed to liver wind stirring internally and is observed in wind stroke, fright wind, and epilepsy.

358. **两目上视**〔兩目上視〕*liǎng mù shàng shì,* **upward staring eyes** [ˈʌpwɚd ˈstɛrɪŋ ɑɪz]: Attributed to liver wind stirring internally. In greater yáng (*tài yáng*) expiration patterns, eyes fixed in an upturned direction are called 戴眼 *dài yǎn,* "upcast eyes."

359. **目上视**〔目上視〕*mù shàng shì,* **upward staring eyes** [ˈʌpwɚd ˈstɛrɪŋ ɑɪz]: See preceding item.

360. **斜视**〔斜視〕*xié shì,* **squint** [skwɪnt]: Deviation from the normal direction of one or both eyeballs that prevents the eyes from being directed at one object at the same time. It is attributed to wind evil striking the network vessels, wind-phlegm obstructing the network vessels, wind-heat attacking the upper body, liver yáng transforming into wind, or blood stasis.

361. **目赤**〔目赤〕*mù chì,* **red eyes** [rɛd ɑɪz]: Red whites of the eye of either or both eyes. It is attributable to wind-heat, liver fire flaming upward, and liver-kidney yīn depletion.

362. 目黄〔目黃〕*mù huáng*, **yellow eyes** [ˈjɛlo ɑɪz]: Yellowing of the whites of the eye (sclera), indicating jaundice.

363. 目窠上微肿〔目窠上微腫〕*mù kē shàng wēi zhŏng*, **slight swelling of the eye nest** [slɑɪt ˈswɛlɪŋ əv ði ɑɪ nɛst]: Mild swelling of the upper and lower eyelids. It is attributable to the spleen failing to control water and the kidney failing to perform qì transformation, or to externally contracted wind evil contending with water.

364. 目窠内陷〔目窠內陷〕*mù kē nèi xiàn*, **sunken eyes** [ˈsʌŋkən ɑɪz]: Often a sign of severe damage to liquid and humor desertion.

365. 眼球外突〔眼球外突〕*yăn qiú wài tú*, **bulging eyes** [ˈbʌldʒɪŋ ɑɪz]: Occurs in goiter due to exuberant liver fire, and can occur in severe cases of wheezing patterns.

366. 鼻翼煽动〔鼻翼煽動〕*bí yì shān dòng*, **flaring nostrils** [ˈflɛrɪŋ ˈnɑstrɪlz]: Dilatation of the nostrils on inhalation; a sign associated with rapid breathing due to lung heat.

367. 口唇淡白〔口唇淡白〕*kŏu chún dàn bái*, **pale lips** [pel lɪps]: A sign of dual vacuity of qì and blood.

368. 口唇青紫〔口唇青紫〕*kŏu chún qīng zǐ*, **green-blue or purple lips** [grin blu or ˈpɝpl lɪps]: Green-blue or purple lips are seen in both blood stasis and cold patterns and indicate impaired flow of blood and qì.

369. 口唇干焦〔口唇乾焦〕*kŏu chún gān jiāo*, **parched lips** [pɑrtʃt lɪps]: Parched lips indicate damage to liquid.

370. 口角不闭〔口角不閉〕*kŏu jiăo bù bì*, **gaping corners of the mouth** [ˈgepɪŋ ˈkɔrnəz əv ðə mɑʊθ]: Gaping corners of the mouth with shrinking of the philtrum signify imminent desertion of right qì.

371. 口角流涎〔口角流涎〕*kŏu jiăo liú xián*, **drooling from the corners of the mouth** [ˈdrulɪŋ frəm ðə ˈkɔrnəz əv ðə mɑʊθ]: Drooling from the corners of the mouth during sleep generally indicates spleen vacuity or stomach heat. Drooling from one side of the mouth is associated with deviation of the mouth in facial paralysis.

372. 喉中有痰声〔喉中有痰聲〕*hóu zhōng yŏu tán shēng*, **sound of phlegm in the throat** [sɑʊnd əv flɛm ɪn ðə θrot]: Observed with deviation of the eyes and mouth and in severe cases with clenched jaw in wind stroke.

373. 咽喉肿痛〔咽喉腫痛〕*yān hóu zhŏng tòng*, **sore swollen throat** [sɔr ˈswolən θrot]: Usually a sign of lung-stomach heat flaming upward.

374. 牙齿干燥如枯骨〔牙齒乾燥如枯骨〕*yá chǐ gān zào rú kū gŭ*, **teeth dry as desiccated bones** [tiθ drɑɪ əs ˈdɛsɪˌketɪd bonz]: A sign of desiccation of kidney yīn.

375. **齿龈结瓣**〔齒齦結瓣〕*chǐ yín jié bàn*, **petaled gums** ['pɛtl̩d gʌmz]: Gums that are patterned by the presence of coagulated blood, observed in warm disease when evil causes frenetic movement of hot blood and consequent spilling of blood in the upper body.

376. **齿龈虚浮**〔齒齦虛浮〕*chǐ yín xū fú*, **vacuous puffy gums** ['vækjuəs 'pʌfɪ gʌmz]: A sign of kidney vacuity.

377. **齿牙松动**〔齒牙鬆動〕*chǐ yá sōng dòng*, **loosening of the teeth** ['lusənɪŋ əv ðə tiθ]: A sign of kidney vacuity.

378. **耳轮枯焦**〔耳輪枯焦〕*ěr lún kū jiāo*, **withered helices** ['wɪðəᵊd 'hɛləsiz]: A sign of exhaustion of qì and blood and of impending expiration of kidney qì.

4.1.6. 望痰 Inspecting Phlegm

379. **痰多清稀**〔痰多清稀〕*tán duō qīng xī*, **copious clear thin phlegm** ['kopɪəs klɪr θɪn flɛm]: A sign of cold. "All disease with water humors that are clear, pure, and cold are ascribed to cold" (诸病水液澄澈清冷，皆属于寒 *zhū bìng shuǐ yè shéng chè qīng lěng, jiē shǔ yú hán*).

380. **咳痰黄稠**〔咳痰黃稠〕*ké tán huáng chóu*, **cough with thick yellow phlegm** [kɔf wɪð θɪk 'jɛlo flɛm]: A sign of heat.

381. **痰少不易咯**〔痰少不易咯〕*tán shǎo bú yì kǎ*, **scant phlegm expectorated with difficulty** [skænt flɛm ɪks'pɛktə,retɪd wɪð 'dɪfɪ,kʌltɪ]: A sign of heat or dryness.

382. **痰中带血**〔痰中帶血〕*tán zhōng dài xuè*, **phlegm containing blood** [flɛm kən'tenɪŋ blʌd]: A sign of effulgent yīn vacuity fire or lung heat damaging the network vessels.

383. **咯血**〔咯血〕*kǎ xuè*, **expectoration of blood** [ɪks,pɛktə'reʃən əv blʌd]: The bringing up of blood from the chest. The term has two meanings: (1) *Confucian Filiality* (*Rú Mén Shì Qīn*) describes this sign as the expectoration of a blood clot or fresh blood preceded by a sensation of fishy-smelling blood in the throat. Such expectoration of blood is mostly attributable to effulgent yīn vacuity fire or lung dryness-heat. (2) In some books, such as *On Blood Patterns* (*Xuè Zhèng Lùn*), this term refers to expectoration of phlegm streaked with threads of blood, which arises when effulgent heart channel fire disquiets the blood vessels.

384. **鼻流清涕**〔鼻流清涕〕*bí liú qīng tì*, **runny nose with clear snivel (nasal mucus)** ['rʌnɪ noz wɪθ klɪr 'snɪvl̩ ('nezl̩ 'mjukəs)]: Seen in common cold due to wind damage.

385. **鼻塞**〔鼻塞〕*bí sè*, **nasal congestion** ['nezl̩ kən'dʒɛstʃən]: Seen in common cold.

386. 多嚏〔多嚏〕*duō tì*, **sneezing** [sniziŋ]: A sudden, involuntary expulsion of air through the nose and mouth due to irritation in the nostrils.

387. 呕吐痰饮〔嘔吐痰飲〕*ǒu tù tán yǐn*, **vomiting of phlegm-rheum** ['vamɪtɪŋ əv flɛm rum]: A sign of phlegm-rheum in the stomach; usually occurs in cold patterns.

4.1.7. 望二便 Inspecting Stool and Urine

388. 大便稀溏〔大便稀溏〕*dà biàn xī táng*, **thin sloppy stool** [θɪn 'slɑpɪ stul]: A sign of cold-damp.

389. 便血〔便血〕*biàn xuè*, **bloody stool** ['blʌdɪ stul]: Stool containing red blood.

390. 大便下血〔大便下血〕*dà biàn xià xuè*, **precipitation of blood with the stool** [prə,sɪpɪ'teʃən əv blʌd wɪð ðə stul]: Bloody stool, especially when severe.

391. 大便黑色〔大便黑色〕*dà biàn hēi sè*, **black stool** [blæk stul]: Black stool that is thin, sloppy, and glossy; attributable to bleeding in the digestive tract.

392. 下利清谷〔下利清穀〕*xià lì qīng gǔ*, **clear-grain diarrhea; clear-food diarrhea** ['klɪr–gren ,dɑɪə'rɪə; 'klɪr–fud ,dɑɪə'rɪə]: Diarrhea characterized by watery, light brown stool containing partially digested food and having no malodor. Clear-grain diarrhea is accompanied by aversion to cold and cold limbs; it is a sign of spleen-kidney yáng vacuity.

393. 大便水样〔大便水樣〕*dà biàn shuǐ yàng*, **watery stool** ['wɔtərɪ stul]: See preceding item.

394. 大便如羊屎〔大便如羊屎〕*dà biàn rú yáng shǐ*, **stool like sheep's droppings** [stul lɑɪk ʃips 'drɑpɪŋz]: Stool formed into small, dry balls. It results from heat bind (热结 *rè jié*) desiccating the intestines and is observed in stomach reflux and dysphagia-occlusion.

4.2. 闻诊
Listening and Smelling

4.2.1. 听声音 Listening to Sounds

395. **喉中有水鸡声**〔喉中有水雞聲〕*hóu zhōng yǒu shuǐ jī shēng,* **frog rale in the throat** [frɑg rɑl ɪn ðə θrot]: A continuous rale produced by phlegm blocking the respiratory tract, so named because of its similarity to the croaking of frogs in chorus. Frog rale in the throat is characteristic of wheezing patterns.

396. **咳声重浊**〔咳聲重濁〕*ké shēng zhòng zhuó,* **heavy turbid cough sound** [ˈhɛvɪ ˈtɝbɪd kɔf saʊnd]: When a cough sounds heavy and turbid with the gurgling sound of phlegm, it is usually attributed to phlegm turbidity congesting the lung.

397. **懒言**〔懶言〕*lǎn yán,* **laziness to speak** [ˈlezɪnɪs tə spik]: No energy to speak; reduced frequency of speech and lack of vigor in enunciation. It reflects general weakness due to qì vacuity.

398. **气粗**〔氣粗〕*qì cū,* **rough breathing** [rʌf ˈbriðɪŋ]: Breathing characterized by a rough sound in the nose. It usually occurs when contraction of external evils or exuberant internal phlegm turbidity inhibits qì dynamic. In such cases, it forms part of a repletion pattern, but it can also arise in vacuity patterns characterized by faint weak breathing and attributed to lung-kidney qì vacuity.

399. **气促**〔氣促〕*qì cù,* **hasty breathing** [ˈhestɪ ˈbriðɪŋ]: Rapid breathing with short breaths.

400. **短气**〔短氣〕*duǎn qì,* **shortness of breath** [ˈʃɔrtnɪs əv brɛθ]: Breathing characterized by short, rapid, shallow breaths. Shortness of breath is observed in many different diseases and in both vacuity and repletion patterns. In repletion patterns, it is characterized by a rough sound usually associated with distention and fullness in the chest and abdomen, and it is attributable to phlegm or stagnant food affecting the normal bearing of qì. In vacuity patterns, it is generally a sign of major vacuity of original qì in enduring disease and is characterized by weak, faint breathing and associated with physical fatigue and lassitude of spirit.

401. **气急**〔氣急〕*qì jí,* **rapid breathing** [ˈræpɪd ˈbriðɪŋ]: Breathing much more quickly than normal. See panting.

402. **肩息**〔肩息〕*jiān xī,* **raised-shoulder breathing** [rezd ˈʃoldɚ ˈbrið-ɪŋ]: Raising of the shoulders to assist breathing in severe panting. See panting.

403. 少气〔少氣〕*shǎo qì*, **shortage of qì** [ˈʃɔrtɪdʒ əv tʃi]: Weak, short, hasty breathing, a weak voice, and a tendency to take deep breaths in order to continue speaking; mainly attributable to visceral qì vacuity, especially of center and lung-kidney qì, but also observed in phlegm turbidity, water-rheum, food stagnation, and qì stagnation.

404. 叹息〔嘆息〕*tàn xī*, **sighing** [ˈsɑɪɪŋ]: A long, deep, audible exhalation that is commonly observed in binding depression of liver qì, but that may also be observed in qì vacuity patterns.

405. 声音嘶嗄〔聲音嘶嗄〕*shēng yīn sī shà*, **hoarse voice** [hɔrs vɔɪs]: A harsh, husky, muffled, faltering, or forced voice. It is attributable to wind-cold, wind-heat, heat evil congesting the lung (热邪壅肺 *xié rè yōng fèi*), lung-kidney yīn vacuity, or blood stasis and phlegm.

406. 谵言〔譫言〕*zhān yán*, **delirious speech** [dɪˈlɪrɪəs spitʃ]: Talking nonsense in a forceful strident voice. It is a repletion sign and usually occurs in externally contracted heat (febrile) disease.

407. 骂詈无常〔罵詈無常〕*mà lì wú cháng*, **abnormal chiding and cursing** [əbˈnɔrml̩ ˈtʃɑɪdɪŋ ənd ˈkɜ˞sɪŋ]: Shouting and swearing at people in a manner contrary to the patient's normal habits, irrespective of who is present. It a sign of mental disease and is observed in yáng patterns such as phlegm-fire harassing the heart.

408. 呻吟〔呻吟〕*shēn yín*, **groaning** [ˈgronɪŋ]: A sign of distention, oppression, or pain.

409. 独语〔獨語〕*dú yǔ*, **soliloquy; talking alone** [səˈlɪləkwɪ, ˈtɔkɪŋ əˈlon]: Talking to oneself, but ceasing when another approaches. Soliloquy is a sign of a deranged heart-spirit (insanity).

410. 郑语〔鄭語〕*zhèng yǔ*, **muttering; mussitation** [ˈmʌtərɪŋ, ˌmʌsɪˈteʃən]: The act of mumbling to oneself haltingly and with frequent repetitions; observed in yīn collapse or yáng collapse patterns.

411. 肠鸣〔腸鳴〕*cháng míng*, **rumbling intestines** [ˈrʌmblɪŋ ɪnˈtɛstɪnz]: Any sound made by the contents of the intestines.

412. 呃逆〔呃逆〕*è nì*, **hiccup** [ˈhɪkʌp]: Stomach qì ascending counterflow and causing the stomach to continually jerk and produce short sounds in the throat. Hiccup may be caused by excessive consumption of raw or cold or hot spicy foods, or by cold bitter or warm dry medicines. It may also be caused by emotional stimulus, or by stomach vacuity cold in enduring or severe disease. Hiccup can occur in cold, heat, vacuity, and repletion patterns.

4.2.2. 嗅气味 Smelling Odors

413. **嗳气酸腐**〔 噯氣酸腐〕 *ài qì suān fǔ,* **belching of sour putrid qì (gas)** [ˈbɛltʃɪŋ əv saʊr ˈpjutrɪd tʃi (gæs)]: A sign of food damage. Belching, like hiccup, nausea, and vomiting, is a manifestation of stomach qì ascending counterflow.

414. **腹泻秽臭**〔 腹瀉穢臭〕 *fù xiè huì chòu,* **foul-smelling diarrhea** [ˈfaʊl–smɛlɪŋ ˌdaɪəˈɪə]: Usually a sign of large intestinal damp-heat.

4.3. 问诊
Inquiry

4.3.1. 问寒热 Inquiring About Cold and Heat

415. **发热**〔 發熱〕 *fā rè,* **heat effusion; fever** [ˈhit-ɪˌfjuʒən; ˈfivɚ]: Excessive body heat that can be palpated, or a sensation of heat. The Chinese 发热 *fā rè* is wider in meaning than the English "fever," notably including subjective sensations of heat. For this reason, we have introduced the literal translation "heat effusion." Heat effusion (fever) occurring with aversion to cold or aversion to wind at the onset of illness indicates external evils invading the fleshy exterior. If the aversion to cold is more pronounced than the heat effusion, the pattern is one of wind-cold. Pronounced heat effusion with only aversion to wind suggests wind-heat. Heat effusion without aversion to cold occurs in various patterns. Distinction is made between vigorous heat [effusion], tidal heat [effusion], vexing heat in the five hearts, steaming bone tidal heat [effusion], and unsurfaced heat. Note that the term 高热 *gāo rè,* high fever, is a Western medical term.

416. **壮热**〔 壯熱〕 *zhuàng rè,* **vigorous heat [effusion]; vigorous fever** [ˈvɪgərəs ˈhit(-ɪˌfjuʒən) (ˈfivɚ)]: A persistent high fever without aversion to cold that occurs as external evil passes from the exterior into the interior of the body.

417. **身热**〔 身熱〕 *shēn rè,* **generalized heat [effusion]; generalized fever** [ˈdʒɛnərəlaɪzd ˈhit(-ɪˌfjuʒən) (ˈfivɚ)]: Heat felt all over the body.

418. **身热不扬**〔 身熱不揚〕 *shēn rè bù yáng,* **unsurfaced heat; unsurfaced fever** [ʌnˈsɜˈfɪst hit (ˈfivɚ)]: Heat [effusion] (fever) caused by dampness trapping hidden heat; the heat can only be felt after prolonged palpation.

419. 潮热〔潮熱〕*cháo rè,* **tidal heat [effusion]; tidal fever** [ˈtɑɪdl̩ ˈhit[-ɪˌfjuʒən] (ˈfivɚ)]: Heat effusion (fever), sometimes only felt subjectively, occurring at regular intervals, usually in the afternoon or evening (postmeridian tidal heat [effusion]). It may form part of both vacuity (e.g., yīn vacuity) and repletion (e.g., yáng brightness) patterns.

420. 午后潮热〔午後潮熱〕*wǔ hòu cháo rè,* **postmeridian tidal heat [effusion]; postmeridian tidal fever** [ˌpostməˈrɪdɪən tɑɪdl̩ ˈhit(-ɪˌfjuʒən) (ˈfivɚ)]: See tidal heat [effusion].

421. 骨蒸潮热〔骨蒸潮熱〕*gǔ zhēng cháo rè,* **steaming bone tidal heat [effusion]; steaming bone tidal fever** [ˈstimɪŋ bon ˈtɑɪdl̩ ˈhit(-ɪˌfjuʒən) (ˈfivɚ)]: Tidal heat effusion (tidal fever) occurring in the early evening or afternoon. Steaming bone tidal heat [effusion] is so called because the heat is subjectively felt to emanate from the bone or marrow. It is attributable to yīn vacuity.

422. 五心烦热〔五心煩熱〕*wǔ xīn fán rè,* **vexing heat in the five hearts** [ˈvɛksɪŋ hit ɪn ðə fɑɪv hɑrts]: Heat in the center of the soles and palms and in the center of the chest. Vexing heat in the five hearts is observed in vacuity detriment and consumption, and arises from effulgent yīn vacuity fire, vacuity heat failing to clear after illness, or internally depressed fire-heat.

423. 手足心热〔手足心熱〕*shǒu zú xīn rè,* **heat in the (hearts of the) palms and soles** [hit ɪn ðə (hɑrts əv ðə) pɑms ənd solz]: Feeling of heat in the palms and soles. See preceding item.

424. 恶寒〔惡寒〕*wù hán,* **aversion to cold** [əˈvɝʒən tə kold]: A pronounced sensation of cold, not easily eliminated by extra clothing or bedclothes. With heat effusion (fever), it is a sign of wind-cold; without heat effusion, it is associated with cold arising from within due to yáng qì vacuity. External cold striking the bowels and viscera directly can also manifest in aversion to cold without heat effusion, in which case it is accompanied by cold signs in the affected area such as cold stomach duct pain and clear-grain diarrhea.

425. 寒热往来〔寒熱往來〕*hán rè wǎng lái,* **alternating [aversion to] cold and heat [effusion]; alternating fever and chills** [ˈɔltɚˌnetɪŋ (əˈvɝʒən tə) kold ənd ˈhit(-ɪˌfjuʒən); ˈɔltɚˌnetɪŋ ˈfivɚ ənd tʃɪlz]: Bouts of fever interspersed with chills. It is attributed to lesser yáng (*shào yáng*) midstage patterns, malaria, or damp-heat obstructing the triple burner.

426. 恶风〔惡風〕*wù fēng,* **aversion to wind** [əˈvɝʒən tə wɪnd]: A sensation of cold experienced in wind or drafts. Aversion to wind is usually

a sign of external evils assailing the fleshy exterior. Compare aversion to cold.

427. **憎寒**〔憎寒〕*zēng hán,* **abhorrence of cold** [əbˈhɔrəns əv kold]: External shivering with internal heat vexation that occurs when a deeply-lying internal heat evil blocks yáng qì and prevents it from reaching the exterior. Compare aversion to wind; aversion to cold.

4.3.2. 问汗 Inquiring About Sweating

428. **自汗**〔自汗〕*zì hàn,* **spontaneous sweating** [spɑnˈtenɪəs ˈswɛtɪŋ]: Excessive sweating during the daytime, or sweating at the slightest physical exertion. It occurs in patients suffering from qì or yáng vacuity.

429. **盗汗**〔盜汗〕*dào hàn,* **night sweating; thief sweating** [ˈnɑɪt–swɛt-ɪŋ, ˈθif–swɛtɪŋ]: Sweating during sleep that ceases when the patient awakes. It is usually attributed to yīn vacuity.

430. **战汗**〔戰汗〕*zhàn hàn,* **shiver sweating** [ˈʃɪvɚ–ˌswɛtɪŋ]: Sweating accompanied by pronounced shivering is a sign of the struggle between the evil and right in externally contracted heat (febrile) diseases. Shiver sweating is a favorable sign when the disease resolves after it. If the disease does not resolve, then right qì, severely debilitated by the struggle, may desert outward leaving the patient in a critical state. Shivering without sweating is a sign of insufficiency of right qì and heralds the inward fall of the evil.

4.3.3. 问头身 Inquiring About Head and Body

431. **头痛**〔頭痛〕*tóu tòng,* **headache** [ˈhɛdek]: Any pain in the head. Distinction is made between headaches in different parts of the head. A broad distinction is made between medial headache and hemilateral headache. More precise distinctions are made on the basis of channel pathways. Headache is attributable to a variety of causes including wind-cold, wind-heat, wind-damp, qì vacuity, yáng vacuity, blood vacuity, yīn vacuity, ascendant liver yáng, food damage, and liquor damage.

432. **正头痛**〔正頭痛〕*zhèng tóu tòng,* **medial headache** [ˈmidɪəl ˈhɛdek]: A pain felt on the right and left side of the head.

433. **偏头痛**〔偏頭痛〕*piān tóu tòng,* **hemilateral headache** [ˌhɛmɪˈlætə-rəl ˈhɛdek]: A pain felt on one side of the head.

434. **头重**〔頭重〕*tóu zhòng,* **heavy-headedness** [ˌhɛvɪˈhɛdɪdnɪs]: Feeling of heaviness in the head, sometimes combined with dizziness. Heavy-headedness can be caused by wind-damp, damp-heat, phlegm-damp, or insufficiency of center qì.

435. 头重如裹〔頭重如裹〕*tóu zhòng rú guǒ,* **head heavy as if swathed** [hɛd ˈhɛvɪ əz ɪf sweðd]: Heavy-headedness characterized by a feeling of encumbrance, as though the head were swathed in cloth or bandages. It is attributed to wind-damp.

436. 头胀〔頭脹〕*tóu zhàng,* **distention in the head** [dɪsˈtɛnʃən ɪn ðə hɛd]: A feeling of pressure and discomfort in the head. Distention in the head is usually caused by external contraction of dampness evil or by failure to eliminate summerheat-warmth evil. It is variously treated by resolving the exterior, clearing heat, repelling foulness, and transforming dampness.

437. 头痛如掣〔頭痛如掣〕*tóu tòng rú chè,* **headache with pulling sensation** [ˈhɛdek wɪð ˈpulɪŋ sɛnˈseʃən]: Headache characterized by pressure or tension as though the head were squeezed by a tight iron band. Headache with pulling sensation is observed in liver wind stirring internally.

438. 眩晕〔眩暈〕*xuàn yūn,* **dizziness** [ˈdɪzɪnəs]: Visual distortion with a whirling sensation in the head that, in severe cases, can upset the sense of balance. In some literature, flowery vision causing dizziness is known as "dizzy vision," whereas dizziness causing flowery vision is called "dizzy head." It can be caused by the six excesses or by internal damage to qì, blood, or bowels and viscera, the most common causes being wind-fire, phlegm-damp, and vacuity of right (正虚 *zhèng xū*).

439. 头晕〔頭暈〕*tóu yūn,* **dizzy head** [ˈdɪzɪ hɛd]: See dizziness.

440. 目眩〔目眩〕*mù xuàn,* **dizzy vision** [ˈdɪzɪ ˈvɪʒən]: See dizziness.

441. 健忘〔健忘〕*jiàn wàng,* **forgetfulness** [fəˈgɛtfulnɪs]: Tendency to forget matters. Forgetfulness occurs most commonly in vacuity patterns such as depletion of kidney essence and insufficiency of the heart and spleen, but also in repletion patterns such as affect damage and phlegm turbidity harassing the upper body.

442. 心烦〔心煩〕*xīn fán,* **heart vexation** [hɑrt vɛkˈseʃən]: A feeling of unrest or irritability that focuses in the heart region. Vexation is commonly observed in either vacuity or repletion heat. In severe cases, it is associated with agitation, i.e., increased physical movement. Compare agitation.

443. 易惊〔易驚〕*yì jīng,* **susceptibility to fright** [səˈsɛptəˈbɪlɪtɪ tə fraɪt]: Tendency to be easily frightened or get nervous. Susceptibility to fright is associated with liver and gallbladder disease and heart disease. See in particular gallbladder vacuity and disquieted heart spirit.

444. 关节疼痛〔關節疼痛〕*guān jié téng tòng,* **joint pain** [ˈdʒɔɪnt–pen]: Pain in any joint. Enduring joint pain is observed in impediment pat-

terns. Joint pain of limited duration is observed in some externally contracted febrile disease patterns such as wind-cold exterior patterns and
qì-aspect heat.

445. 腰痛〔腰痛〕*yāo tòng*, **lumbar pain** [ˈlʌmbɚ-pen]: Pain in the lumbus, on one or both sides, or affecting the spine. It is attributable to
kidney qì vacuity, external injury, or other causes.

446. 腰酸〔腰痠〕*yāo suān*, **aching lumbus** [ˈekɪŋ ˈlʌmbəs]: Continual
dull pain and discomfort in the lumbus as distinct from lumbar pain,
which generally denotes more acute pain.

447. 腰膝软弱〔腰膝軟弱〕*yāo xī ruǎn ruò*, **limp lumbus and knees**
[lɪmp ˈlʌmbəs ənd niz]: Insufficient strength in the lumbus and knees to
perform normal movements, in severe cases, called limp wilting lumbus and knees (腰膝痿软 *yāo xī wěi ruǎn*), in which movement is
seriously restricted. Limpness of the lumbus and knees, especially limpness of the lumbus, often accompanies aching of the lumbus, hence the
combined terms limp aching lumbus and knees and aching lumbus
and limp knees. Such conditions are attributed to liver-kidney vacuity, cold-damp, or damp-heat (or combinations of liver-kidney vacuity
with cold-damp or damp-heat); they differ from simple aching lumbus,
which is mostly due to kidney vacuity.

448. 腰酸腿软〔腰痠腿軟〕*yāo suān tuǐ ruǎn*, **aching lumbus and limp
legs** [ˈekɪŋ ˈlʌmbəs ənd lɪmp lɛgz]: A combined condition of limp lumbus and knees and aching lumbus.

449. 腰酸膝软〔腰痠膝軟〕*yāo suān xī ruǎn*, **aching lumbus and limp
knees** [ˈekɪŋ ˈlʌmbəs ənd lɪmp niz]: See limp lumbus and knees.

450. 四肢麻木〔四肢麻木〕*sì zhī má mù*, **numbness (and tingling) of
the limbs** [nʌmnɪs (ənd ˈtɪŋlɪŋ) əv ðə lɪmz]: Numbness (or tingling
sensations) in the limbs, usually attributable to wind-damp pestilential
qì, phlegm-damp obstruction, dual vacuity of qì and blood, or blood
stasis.

451. 倦怠乏力〔倦怠乏力〕*juàn dài fá lì*, **fatigue and lack of strength**
[fəˈtig ənd læk əv strɛŋθ]: Tiredness and lack of strength. Fatigue is
observed in dual vacuity of qì and blood, spleen vacuity with damp
encumbrance, and damage to qì by summerheat-heat.

452. 形倦神怠〔形倦神怠〕*xíng juàn shén dài*, **physical fatigue and lassitude of spirit** [ˈfɪzɪkl̩ fəˈtig ənd ˈlæsɪt(j)ud əv ˈspɪrɪt]: See fatigue and
lack of strength.

453. 肢倦〔肢倦〕*zhī juàn*, **fatigued limbs** [fəˈtigd lɪmz]: See fatigue and
lack of strength.

4.3.4. 问二便 Inquiring About Stool and Urine

454. 小便短赤〔小便短赤〕*xiǎo biàn duǎn chì,* **short voidings of reddish urine** [ʃɔrt ˈvɔɪdɪŋz əv ˈrɛdɪʃ ˈjurɪn]: Scant urine that is darker in color than normal; usually indicates repletion heat.

455. 小便短少〔小便短少〕*xiǎo biàn duǎn shǎo,* **short voidings of scant urine** [ʃɔrt ˈvɔɪdɪŋz əv skænt ˈjurɪn]: See short voidings of reddish urine.

456. 小便清长〔小便清長〕*xiǎo biàn qīng cháng,* **long voidings of clear urine** [lɔŋ ˈvɔɪdɪŋz əv klɪr ˈjurɪn]: Copious colorless urine that comes in long voidings. Long voidings of clear urine are a sign of vacuous kidney yáng failing to perform its containing function (insecurity of kidney qì), which is a vacuity cold pattern, or exuberant internal yīn cold, which is a repletion cold pattern.

457. 夜间多尿〔夜間多尿〕*yè jiān duō niào,* **profuse urination at night; nocturia** [prəˈfjus ˌjurɪˈneʃən ət nɑɪt, nɑkˈtʃurɪə]: Waking two, three, or more times a night to urinate, and passing in the night a quarter or more of the whole day's urine; a sign of debilitation of kidney yáng or spleen-kidney yáng vacuity.

458. 小便频数〔小便頻數〕*xiǎo biàn pín shuò,* **frequent urination** [ˌfrikwənt ˌjurɪˈneʃən]: Increased frequency of urination, most commonly due to bladder damp-heat or kidney vacuity (kidney yīn or yáng vacuity).

459. 小便不利〔小便不利〕*xiǎo biàn bù lì,* **inhibited urination** [ɪnˈhɪbɪtɪd ˌjurɪˈneʃən]: Difficult voiding of scant urine; ascribed to nondiffusion of lung qì, devitalized spleen yáng, debilitation of kidney yáng, internal damp-heat obstruction, or qì stagnation with damp obstruction.

460. 尿有余沥〔尿有餘瀝〕*niào yǒu yú lì,* **dribble after voiding** [ˈdrɪbl̩ ˈæftɚ ˈvɔɪdɪŋ]: A dribbling discharge of urine after urination. It is attributed to kidney vacuity, insufficiency of center qì, and bladder damp-heat.

461. 遗尿〔遺尿〕*yí niào,* **enuresis** [ɪnˈjurəsɪs]: Involuntary loss of urine, especially during sleep. It is mostly observed in children, in which case it is attributable to bad eating habits (excessive eating and drinking) or fatigue due to excessive play, reducing the ability to waken from sleep to urinate. It may also be due to kidney yáng vacuity with insecurity of kidney qì, or to spleen-lung qì vacuity affecting regulation of the waterways.

462. 小便失禁〔小便失禁〕*xiǎo biàn shī jìn,* **urinary incontinence** [ˈjurɪˌnɛrɪ ɪŋˈkɑntɪnənz]: Involuntary loss of urine, especially in the day-

time (compare enuresis); most commonly occurs in vacuity patterns, but is sometimes observed in repletion heat patterns.

463. 便秘〔便秘〕*biàn bì*, **constipation** [ˌkɑnstɪˈpeʃən]: Stagnation in the intestines lengthening the interval between bowel movements to three or four days or more. It is attributable to many causes.

464. 大便干结〔大便乾結〕*dà biàn gān jié*, **dry bound stool** [dɹɑɪ bɑʊnd stul]: See constipation.

465. 便难〔便難〕*biàn nán*, **difficult defecation** [ˈdɪfɪˌkʌlt ˌdɛfɪˈkeʃən]: Difficulty in evacuating the bowels with relatively long intervals between motions. It differs from constipation in being characterized by stool that is not necessarily hard, the intervals between defecation may not be so long as in constipation, and abdominal discomfort is not usually present. It is attributable to heat binding in the large intestine, brewing damp-heat, spleen-lung qì vacuity, liver-spleen qì stagnation, spleen-kidney yáng vacuity, or yīn vacuity with blood depletion.

466. 泄泻〔泄瀉〕*xiè xiè*, **diarrhea** [ˌdɑɪəˈrɪə]: Increased frequency of the stool and fluidity of the stool. Diarrhea occurs in vacuity, repletion, cold, and heat patterns.

467. 大便失禁〔大便失禁〕*dà biàn shī jìn*, **fecal incontinence** [ˈfikḷ ɪŋˈkɑntɪnəns]: Involuntary loss of stool. It is attributable to spleen-kidney yáng vacuity, center qì fall, or exuberant heat toxin.

468. 五更泄〔五更泄〕*wǔ gēng xiè*, **fifth-watch diarrhea** [fɪfθ wɑtʃ ˌdɑɪəˈrɪə]: Diarrhea before daybreak. It is attributable to kidney vacuity.

469. 里急后重〔裡急後重〕*lǐ jí hòu zhòng*, **tenesmus; abdominal urgency and rectal heaviness** [təˈnɛzməs, əbˈdɑmɪnḷ ˈɝdʒənsɪ ənd rɛktḷ ˈhɛvɪnɪs]: The urgent desire to evacuate, with difficulty in defecation characterized by heaviness or pressure in the rectum. With stool containing pus and blood, it is a principal sign of dysentery.

470. 大便不爽〔大便不爽〕*dà biàn bù shuǎng*, **ungratifying defecation** [ʌnˈgrætɪˌfaɪɪŋ ˌdɛfɪˈkeʃən]: Defecation that leaves the patient with a feeling that the bowels have not been satisfactorily emptied. It occurs in dysentery and other damp-heat patterns, in food stagnation, and in gastrointestinal accumulation.

471. 久泄〔久泄〕*jiǔ xiè*, **enduring diarrhea** [ɪnˈdjurɪŋ ˌdɑɪəˈrɪə]: Chronic or persistent diarrhea.

472. 脱肛〔脫肛〕*tuō gāng*, **prolapse of the rectum** [ˈprolæps əv ðə ˈrɛktʌm]: The downward fall of the rectum through the anus. Prolapse of the rectum is most prevalent among the young and the aged; it is the

result of center qì fall (a qì vacuity pattern) or of damp-heat in the large intestine.

4.3.5. 问饮食口味 Inquiring About Diet and Taste in the Mouth

473. 口渴〔口渴〕*kǒu kě,* **thirst** [θɝst]: A sense of dryness in the mouth with a greater or lesser desire to drink. Thirst most commonly reflects insufficiency of yīn fluids and/or the presence of heat that causes fluid loss through sweating, as observed in lung-stomach heat, yīn vacuity, and blood vacuity. It may occur when water-damp, phlegm, or static blood causes obstruction. It can also reflect impaired movement of the essence of food and water due to spleen vacuity or impaired transformation of fluids due to kidney vacuity. *Thirst with a desire to drink* is a sign of heat. *Thirst with no desire to drink* (or without large fluid intake) is a sign of water-damp. Thirst with a *desire only to wash the mouth with water without desire to swallow it* is a sign of blood stasis. *Thirst with a liking for hot drinks* is seen in spleen vacuity.

474. 口干〔口乾〕*kǒu gān,* **dry mouth** [drɑɪ mɑʊθ]: A lack of fluid in the mouth, usually, but not necessarily, with a desire to drink. See thirst.

475. 渴不欲饮〔渴不欲飲〕*kě bù yù yǐn,* **thirst with no desire to drink** [θɝst wɪð no dɪˈzaɪr tə drɪŋk]: See thirst.

476. 渴不多饮〔渴不多飲〕*kě bù duō yǐn,* **thirst without large fluid intake** [θɝst wɪˈðaʊt lɑrdʒ ˈfluɪd ˈɪntek]: See thirst.

477. 渴喜凉饮〔渴喜涼飲〕*kě xǐ liáng yǐn,* **thirst with a liking for cool drinks** [θɝst wɪð ə ˈlaɪkɪŋ fɚ kul drɪŋks]: See thirst.

478. 渴喜热饮〔渴喜熱飲〕*kě xǐ rè yǐn,* **thirst with a liking for hot drinks** [θɝst wɪð ə ˈlaɪkɪŋ fɚ hɑt drɪŋks]: See thirst.

479. 大渴引饮〔大渴引飲〕*dà kě yǐn yǐn,* **great thirst with fluid intake** [gret θɝst wɪð ˈfluɪd ˈɪntek]: See thirst.

480. 漱口不欲饮〔漱口不欲飲〕*shù kǒu bù yù yǐn,* **washing the mouth with water without desire to swallow it** [ˈwɔʃɪŋ ðə mɑʊθ wɪð ˈwɔtɚ wɪˈðaʊt dɪˈzaɪr tə ˈswɔlo ɪt]: See thirst.

481. 食欲不振〔食欲不振〕*shí yù bù zhèn,* **poor appetite** [pʊr ˈæpətaɪt]: Reduced desire to eat. Traditionally called *no (little) though of food and drink, no pleasure in eating, inability to get food down,* or *inability to eat.* Poor appetite occurs in a number of situations. (1) With distention after eating, diarrhea, emaciation, and lack of strength, poor appetite is ascribed to spleen-stomach qì vacuity that develops when the stomach's function of decomposing food and the spleen's function of movement

and transformation is impaired. (2) Accompanied by oppression in the stomach duct, heavy cumbersome head and body, rumbling intestines, diarrhea, and slimy tongue fur, it is a sign of dampness encumbering the spleen that prevents the normal upbearing of clear yáng and that causes disharmony of stomach qì. (3) With aversion to oily food and accompanied by yellowing of the body, abdominal distention and glomus in the stomach duct, nausea, fatigue, and scant yellow urine, it is a sign of spleen-stomach damp-heat causing disharmony of stomach qì. (4) With belching, abdominal distention, rib-side pain, frequent passing of flatus, and sloppy stool, it is a sign of liver-spleen disharmony. (5) With alternating [aversion to] cold and heat [effusion], chest and rib-side fullness, bitter taste in the mouth, dry throat, and dizzy vision, it is a sign of cold damage lesser yáng (shào yáng) disease.

482. 不思饮食〔不思飲食〕 bù sī yǐn shí, **no thought of food and drink** [no θɔt əv fud ənd drɪŋk]: See poor appetite.

483. 饮食少思〔飲食少思〕 yǐn shí shǎo sī, **little thought of food and drink** [ˈlɪtl̩ θɔt əv fud ənd drɪŋk]: See poor appetite.

484. 纳谷不香〔納穀不香〕 nà gǔ bù xiāng, **no pleasure in eating** [no ˈplɛʒɚ ɪn ˈitɪŋ]: See poor appetite.

485. 纳谷不馨〔納穀不馨〕 nà gǔ bù xīn, **no pleasure in eating** [no ˈplɛʒɚ ɪn ˈitɪŋ]: See poor appetite.

486. 食不下〔食不下〕 shí bù xià, **inability to get food down** [ˌɪnəˈbɪlətɪ tə gɛt fud dɑun]: See poor appetite.

487. 不食〔不食〕 bù shí, **inability to eat** [ˌɪnəˈbɪlətɪ tu it]: See poor appetite.

488. 厌食〔厭食〕 yàn shí, **aversion to food** [əˈvɝʒən tə fud]: A feeling of sickness at the sight or thought of food. It occurs in two situations. (1) Aversion to food is most commonly observed when voracious eating and drinking impairs decomposition, causing food to stagnate in the stomach. Hence, it is said, "Food damage is invariably characterized by aversion to food." It can also occur in mania and withdrawal. (2) When accompanied by vomiting, with absence of menstruation, and with a rapid slippery harmonious pulse in sexually active women, aversion to food is a sign of malign obstruction (vomiting in pregnancy), which is caused by upsurge of thoroughfare (chōng) vessel qì causing disharmony of stomach qì. Poor appetite differs from aversion to food in that it is associated with a reduced feeling of hunger.

489. 贪食〔貪食〕 tān shí, **rapacious eating** [rəˈpeʃəs ˈitɪŋ]: Eating far larger amounts of food than normal.

490. 纳呆〔納呆〕*nà dāi,* **torpid intake** [ˈtɔrpɪd ˈɪntek]: Poor appetite associated with indigestion. Also called torpid stomach intake (胃纳呆滞 *wèi nà dāi zhì*).

491. 嘈杂〔嘈雜〕*cáo zá,* **clamoring stomach** [ˈklæmərɪŋ ˈstʌmək]: A sensation of emptiness and burning in the stomach duct or heart [region] described as being like hunger but not hunger, and like pain but not pain, and accompanied by belching, nausea, swallowing of upflowing acid, and fullness. It is due to a variety of causes.

492. 口中和〔口中和〕*kǒu zhōng hé,* **harmony of mouth** [ˈhɑrməˌnɪ əv maʊθ]: A normal taste in the mouth and absence of dryness and thirst or sliminess. Harmony of mouth is observed in healthy individuals and in patients suffering from mild disease.

493. 口甜〔口甜〕*kǒu tián,* **sweet taste in the mouth** [swit test ɪn ðə maʊθ]: A sensation of sweetness in the mouth not due to foodstuffs. It is attributable either to spleen-stomach heat or to dual vacuity of spleen-stomach qì and yīn.

494. 口酸〔口酸〕*kǒu suān,* **sour taste in the mouth** [saʊr test ɪn ðə maʊθ]: A sensation of sourness in the mouth that is not due to foodstuffs and that in severe cases may be accompanied by a sour smell on the breath.

495. 口苦〔口苦〕*kǒu kǔ,* **bitter taste in the mouth** [ˈbɪtɚ test ɪn ðə maʊθ]: A sensation of a bitter flavor in the mouth not attributable to foodstuffs. Bitter taste is the most commonly reported deviation from harmony of mouth. It is explained by the presence of bile in the mouth. It is a sign of liver or gallbladder disease and usually reflects steaming of gallbladder qì when there is heat in the liver and gallbladder.

496. 呕吐〔嘔吐〕*ǒu tù,* **(retching and) vomiting** [(ˈretʃɪŋ ənd) ˈvamɪtɪŋ]: Ejection of food through the mouth. The Chinese term is composed of two characters, 呕 *ǒu,* meaning retching (sound without matter), and 吐 *tù,* meaning ejection (matter without sound). However, the combined term simply denotes vomiting. While retching denotes a relative absence of expelled matter, "dry retching" (干呕 *gān ǒu*) denotes its complete absence. Retching and vomiting are the manifestations of stomach qì ascending counterflow, and like nausea they may occur in almost any stomach pattern, such as stomach heat or cold, insufficiency of stomach yīn, liver-stomach disharmony, or food damage.

497. 恶心〔惡心〕*ě xīn,* **nausea** [ˈnɔʒə/ˈnɔzɪə]: The desire to vomit. Nausea normally portends vomiting; sometimes continual nausea is associated with constant retching and vomiting. Like vomiting, it is a sign of stomach qì ascending counterflow, which can occur in a variety of stomach

disorders including stomach vacuity and cold, heat, dampness, phlegm, or food stagnation in the stomach.

498. 泛酸〔泛酸〕*fàn suān*, **acid upflow** [ˈæsɪd ˈʌpflo]: An upflow of acid from the stomach into the mouth, which may be ejected or swallowed. If it is expelled from the body, it is called acid vomiting; if it is swallowed, it is called swallowing of upflowing acid.

499. 吞酸〔吞酸〕*tūn suān*, **swallowing of upflowing acid** [ˈswɔloɪŋ əv ˈʌpfloɪŋ ˈæsɪd]: A tendency for acid welling up from the stomach to be swallowed before it can be spat out.

500. 吐酸〔吐酸〕*tù suān*, **vomiting of acid** [ˈvɑmɪtɪŋ əv ˈæsɪd]: Expulsion through the mouth of sour fluid that flows up from the stomach.

501. 吐血〔吐血〕*tù xuè*, **blood ejection** [blʌd ɪdʒˈɛkʃən]: Ejection of blood through the mouth; vomiting or expectoration of blood (i.e., respiratory tract or digestive tract bleeding); sometimes defined as being associated with neither the sound of retching or of coughing. Blood ejection is attributed to liquor damage or food damage, to taxation fatigue that causes exuberant heat in the bowels and viscera, to effulgent yīn vacuity fire, to qì vacuity, or to spleen cold.

502. 泛恶〔泛惡〕*fàn ě*, **upflow nausea** [ˈʌpflo ˈnɔʒə/ˈnɔzɪə]: Desire to vomit either without vomiting or with upflow of clear drool into the mouth.

4.3.6. 问胸腹 Inquiring About the Chest and Abdomen

503. 胸痛〔胸痛〕*xiōng tòng*, **chest pain** [tʃɛst pen]: Any pain in the chest. It is attributed to heart qì vacuity, congealing cold and stagnant qì, heart blood stasis obstruction, dual vacuity of qì and yīn, obstruction by phlegm turbidity, or pulmonary welling-abscess.

504. 胸满〔胸滿〕*xiōng mǎn*, **fullness in the chest** [ˈfʊlnɪs ɪn ðə tʃɛst]: A bloated feeling in the chest. It is due to interior repletion, qì stagnation, or blood stasis.

505. 胸闷〔胸悶〕*xiōng mèn*, **oppression in the chest** [əˈprɛʃən ɪn ðə tʃɛst]: Discomfort and vexation in the chest caused by damp-heat or phlegm-damp obstructing the center burner and inhibiting qì.

506. 胸痞〔胸痞〕*xiōng pǐ*, **glomus in the chest** [ˈglomэs ɪn ðə tʃɛst]: A localized feeling of fullness in the chest, often associated with oppression. Glomus in the chest is observed in pulmonary welling-abscess external contraction, heart impediment, and liver qì depression.

507. 胁痛〔脅痛〕*xié tòng*, **rib-side pain** [ˈrɪbsɑɪd pen]: Pain in the area between the armpits and the lowest rib. The rib-side is traversed by

the foot reverting yīn (*jué yīn*) liver and foot lesser yáng (*shào yáng*) gallbladder channels; hence pain in this area is associated with disease of the liver and gallbladder.

508. 胸胁苦满〔胸脅苦滿〕*xiōng xié kǔ mǎn,* **chest and rib-side fullness** [tʃɛst ənd ˈrɪbsaɪd ˈfʌlnɪs]: Fullness and oppression in the chest and rib-side associated with disturbance of qì dynamic in the foot lesser yáng (*shào yáng*) gallbladder channel and with gallbladder fire.

509. 心悸〔心悸〕*xīn jì,* **heart palpitations** [hɑrt ˌpælpɪˈteʃəns]: Rapid throbbing of the heart. Distinction is made between fright palpitations (*heart palpitations* in the narrow sense) and fearful throbbing. Fright palpitations are brought on by fright or emotional stimulus and are therefore clearly paroxysmal in nature. They occur in both vacuity and repletion patterns. In Western medicine, they are often found to be a nervous disorder. Fearful throbbing occurs continually, and although it is associated with a feeling of fear, it is not brought on by emotional stimulus. It is more severe than fright palpitations and is experienced as a violent throbbing felt not only in the chest, but even as low as the umbilical region. It is observed in patients in a poor state of health and always occurs in vacuity rather than repletion patterns. From the Western medical perspective, it is usually the manifestation of organic rather than nervous disease. In some older books, the terms fright palpitations and fearful throbbing were used interchangeably. Heart palpitations occur in a wide variety of patterns and combinations of patterns. The basic patterns include heart-gallbladder vacuity timidity; dual vacuity of the heart and spleen; effulgent yīn vacuity fire; heart qì vacuity; heart yáng vacuity; dual vacuity of qì and yīn; water qì intimidating the heart; heart blood stasis obstruction; and phlegm-fire harassing the heart.

510. 惊悸〔驚悸〕*jīng jì,* **fright palpitations** [fraɪt ˌpælpɪˈteʃəns]: See heart palpitations.

511. 怔忡〔怔忡〕*zhēng chōng,* **fearful throbbing** [ˈfɪrful ˈθrɑbɪŋ]: Severe heart palpitations that are not brought on by emotional stimulus. Fearful throbbing is so called because its severity itself causes alarm. See heart palpitations.

512. 心下痞〔心下痞〕*xīn xià pǐ,* **glomus below the heart** [ˈgloməs bɪˈlo ðə hɑrt]: A feeling below the heart of fullness and oppression with a sensation of blockage.

513. 脘腹痛喜按〔脘腹痛喜按〕*wǎn fù tòng xǐ àn,* **pain in the stomach duct and abdomen that likes pressure** [pen ɪn ðə ˈstʌmək-dʌkt ənd

ˈæbdəmən ðət laɪks ˈprɛʃɚ]: Any pain in the greater or smaller abdomen that is relieved by applying pressure. It is a sign of vacuity.

514. **脘腹痛拒按**〔脘腹痛拒按〕*wǎn fù tòng jù àn,* **pain in the stomach duct and abdomen that refuses pressure** [pen ɪn ðə ˈstʌmək-dʌkt ənd ˈæbdəmən ðət rɪˈfjuzɪz ˈprɛʃɚ]: Any pain in the greater or lower abdomen that is exacerbated by applying pressure. It is a sign of repletion.

515. **腹满**〔腹滿〕*fù mǎn,* **abdominal fullness** [əbˈdamɪnl̩ ˈfulnɪs]: A subjective feeling of fullness in the abdomen without pronounced visible or palpable expansion.

516. **腹痛**〔腹痛〕*fù tòng,* **abdominal pain** [əbˈdamɪnl̩ pen]: Pain in the stomach duct, in the umbilical region, in the smaller abdomen, or in the lesser abdomen. It is attributable to external contraction of one of the six excesses, dietary irregularities, affect damage, stagnation of qì dynamic, blood stasis obstructing the vessels, worm accumulations, etc.

517. **腹痛喜温**〔腹痛喜溫〕*fù tòng xǐ wēn,* **abdominal pain that likes warmth** [əbˈdamɪnl̩ pen ðət laɪks wɔrmθ]: Abdominal pain that is relieved by warmth; a sign of cold.

518. **腹痛拒按**〔腹痛拒按〕*fù tòng jù àn,* **abdominal pain that refuses pressure** [əbˈdamɪnl̩ pen ðət rɪfˈjuzɪz ˈprɛʃɚ]: Abdominal pain that is exacerbated by pressure; a sign of repletion.

519. **脐周窜痛**〔臍周竄痛〕*qí zhōu cuàn tòng,* **scurrying pain around the umbilicus** [ˈskɝ-ɪɪŋ pen əˈraʊnd ði ˌʌmbɪˈlaɪkəs]: When intermittent, it may indicate worms.

520. **少腹痛**〔少腹痛〕*shào fù tòng,* **lesser-abdominal pain** [ˈlɛsɚ-əbˌdamɪnl̩ pen]: Pain in the lesser abdomen (i.e., part of the abdomen below the umbilicus on either or both sides). It is due to cold stagnating in the liver channel, binding depression of liver qì, large intestinal damp-heat, or lower burner vacuity cold.

521. **小腹痛**〔小腹痛〕*xiǎo fù tòng,* **smaller-abdominal pain** [ˈsmɔlɚ-əbˌdamɪnl̩ pen]: Pain in the smaller abdomen (i.e., the part of the abdomen below the umbilicus) due to various factors including damp-heat, static blood, and kidney vacuity.

4.3.7. 问耳目 Inquiring About the Ears and Eyes

522. **耳聋**〔耳聾〕*ěr lóng,* **deafness** [ˈdɛfnɪs]: Loss of hearing. Deafness can be congenital; otherwise it is the result of external contractions or internal damage. Sudden deafness usually forms a repletion pattern, whereas deafness of gradual onset is usually due to vacuity.

523. 重听〔重聽〕*zhòng tīng,* **hardness of hearing; hearing impairment** [hɑrdnɪs əv hɪrɪŋ; 'hɪrɪŋ ɪm'pɛrmənt]: Poor hearing with incorrect perception of sounds.

524. 耳鸣〔耳鳴〕*ěr míng,* **tinnitus; ringing in the ears** [tɪ'nɑɪtɪs, 'rɪŋɪŋ ɪn ðə ɪrz]: Subjective ringing, buzzing, or rushing sounds heard in the ears. Distinction is made between repletion and vacuity. Repletion patterns are attributed to ascendant counterflow of liver fire or phlegm fire. Vacuity patterns are attributed to depletion of kidney yīn or center qì fall. In repletion patterns, tinnitus is of rapid onset and is characterized by the sound of frogs or of the tide. In vacuity patterns, it is like the sound of cicadas or a flute or pipe.

525. 耳鸣如蝉声〔耳鳴如蟬聲〕*ěr míng rú chán shēng,* **ringing in the ears like the sound of cicadas** ['rɪŋɪŋ ɪn ðɪ irz lɑɪk ðə sɑʊnd əv sɪ'kedəz]: See tinnitus.

526. 目痛〔目痛〕*mù tòng,* **eye pain** [ɑɪ pen]: Any pain of the eye. Pain in the eye during the day is a yáng pattern; pain during the night is a yīn pattern. Pain accompanied by vexation and oppression indicates qì repletion; pain accompanied by aversion to cold indicates qì vacuity. Intermittent dull pain indicates stirring of yīn vacuity fire; pain like the pricking of a needle that continues unabated indicates fire evil. Pain accompanied by dryness signifies wearing of the fluids or water depletion and blood vacuity. Red sore eyes with copious sticky discharge indicate wind-heat congestion. Mild redness and soreness with inhibited stool and urine indicates repletion fire blazing internally. Pain that refuses pressure and likes cold compresses indicates repletion, whereas pain that likes pressure and hot compresses indicates vacuity.

527. 目花〔目花〕*mù huā,* **flowery vision** ['flɑʊrɪ 'vɪʒən]: A general term embracing various kinds of visual disturbances such as blurring, distortion, floaters, nearsightedness, etc.

528. 目糊〔目糊〕*mù hú,* **blurred vision** [blɝd 'vɪʒən]: See flowery vision.

529. 目干涩〔目乾澀〕*mù gān sè,* **dry eyes** [drɑɪ ɑɪz]: Lack of fluid to ensure the smooth movement of the eyelids, usually attributable to insufficiency of lung yīn with vacuity fire flaming upward, to liver-kidney yīn depletion, or to insufficiency of liver blood.

530. 恶光羞明〔惡光羞明〕*wù guāng xiū míng,* **aversion to light** [ə'vɝʒən tə lɑɪt]: Abnormal insensitivity to or intolerance of light—and sometimes also of warmth (aversion to lights and fire)—that causes a desire to close the eyes.

4.3.8. 问睡眠 Inquiring About Sleep

531. **失眠**〔失眠〕*shī mián*, **insomnia** [ɪn'sɑmnɪə]: Also called sleepless-ness. Total or partial reduction in sleeping time. Insomnia may take the form of difficulty getting to sleep (initial insomnia), tendency to awake and difficulty getting back to sleep, or tendency to sleep on and off through the night (failure to sleep soundly). In severe cases, there may be nightlong sleeplessness. Insomnia arises through a variety of path-omechanisms, most of which involve heart blood vacuity, dual vacu-ity of the heart and spleen, dual vacuity of qì and blood, water qì intimidating the heart, noninteraction of the heart and kidney, heart-gallbladder qì vacuity, effulgent yīn vacuity fire, hyperac-tive heart fire, liver depression transforming into fire, gallbladder fire, and phlegm-heat harassing the inner body.

532. **不得卧**〔不得臥〕*bù dé wò*, **sleeplessness** ['slipləsnɪs]: See insomnia.

533. **不寐**〔不寐〕*bù mèi*, **sleeplessness** ['slipləsnɪs]: See insomnia.

534. **多梦**〔多夢〕*duō mèng*, **profuse dreaming** [prə'fjus 'drimɪŋ]: Dream-ing more often than normal. Profuse dreaming occurs with insomnia in dual vacuity of the heart and spleen and noninteraction of the heart and kidney. When patients suffering from susceptibility to fright, emotional instability, heart palpitations, or fearful throbbing wake from dreaming with a start, it is a sign of heart and gallbladder qì vacuity. When patients suffering from dizziness, heart palpitations, irascibility, copious phlegm, and oppression in the chest have confused dreams, this is a sign of phlegm-fire.

535. **昏睡**〔昏睡〕*hūn shuì*, **clouding sleep** ['klɑʊdɪŋ slip]: A pronounced somnolence that occurs in heat entering the pericardium, whose other signs include generalized heat [effusion] that is most pronounced at night, a crimson tongue, rapid pulse, and sometimes maculopapular eruptions.

536. **嗜眠**〔嗜眠〕*shì mián*, **somnolence** ['sɑmnələns]: Pronounced drowsi-ness and tendency to sleep for long periods; due to phlegm-damp or wind-phlegm.

537. **食后困顿**〔食後困頓〕*shí hòu kùn dùn*, **drowsiness after eating** ['drɑʊzɪnɪs 'æftɚ 'itɪŋ]: Desire to sleep occurring after eating, or, in severe cases, before the end of a meal. It is caused by spleen qì vacuity or phlegm-damp.

4.3.9. 男子、妇女 Men and Women

538. **失精**〔失精〕*shī jīng*, **seminal loss** ['sɛmɪnl̩ lɔs]: Any involuntary loss of semen. The main causes are effulgent sovereign and ministerial fire,

heart vacuity and liver depression, insecurity of kidney qì, noninteraction of the heart and kidney, and spleen vacuity qì fall.

539. 遗精〔遺精〕*yí jīng*, **seminal emission** [ˈsɛmɪnl̩ ɪˈmɪʃən]: Seminal loss, especially during sleep.

540. 滑精〔滑精〕*huá jīng*, **seminal efflux** [ˈsɛmɪnl̩ ˈɛflʌks]: Seminal loss occurring night and day.

541. 梦遗〔夢遺〕*mèng yí*, **dream emission** [ˈdrim-ɪˌmɪʃən]: Seminal emission while dreaming; the mildest form of seminal emission, mostly attributed to disease of the heart.

542. 不梦而遗〔不夢而遺〕*bù mèng ér yí*, **seminal emission without dreaming** [ˈsɛmɪnl̩ ɪˈmɪʃən wɪðaut ˈdrimɪŋ]: Seminal emission without dreaming. It is mostly attributed to disease of the kidney.

543. 阳痿〔陽痿〕*yáng wěi*, **impotence; yáng wilt** [ˈɪmpətəns; jæŋ/jɑŋ wɪlt]: Inability to perform intercourse owing to inability to achieve or maintain erection. Impotence is caused by debilitation of the life gate fire, liver-kidney vacuity fire, dual vacuity of the heart and spleen, binding depression of liver qì, liver channel damp-heat pouring downward, spleen-stomach damp-heat, or fright damaging the kidney.

544. 早泄〔早洩〕*zǎo xiè*, **premature ejaculation** [ˈprɛmətʃɚ ɪˌdʒækjəˈleʃən]: Ejaculation shortly after insertion, followed by a subsidence of the erection that prevents further intercourse. Premature ejaculation is attributed to hyperactivity of the ministerial fire, to insecurity of kidney qì, to dual vacuity of the heart and spleen, to liver channel damp-heat, or to binding depression of liver qì.

545. 卵缩〔卵縮〕*luǎn suō*, **retracted testicles** [rɪˈtræktɪd ˈtɛstɪkl̩z]: Testicles drawn upward and into the body. Retracted testicles are usually attributed to disease of the foot reverting yīn (*jué yīn*) liver channel. *The Magic Pivot* (*Líng Shū, Jīng Mài*) states, "When reverting yīn (*jué yīn*) qì expires, the sinews expire. The reverting yīn (*jué yīn*) is the liver vessel. The liver is the union of the sinews. The sinews gather at the yīn organs (genitals) and net the root of the tongue. When the vessel loses its luxuriance, the sinews become tense. When the sinews become tense, they pull the tongue and testicles. Hence, green-blue lips, curled tongue, and retracted testicles mean the death of the sinews."

546. 月经失调〔月經失調〕*yuè jīng shī tiáo*, **menstrual irregularities** [ˈmɛnstruəl ɪˌrɛgjəˈlærətɪz]: Abnormalities of the length of the menstrual cycle or of volume, color, or consistency of menstrual flow. See the following eight items.

547. 月经过多〔月經過多〕*yuè jīng guò duō*, **profuse menstruation** [prəˈfjus ˌmɛnstruˈeʃən]: Greater menstrual flow or longer menstrual

period than normal. Profuse menstruation is attributed to qì vacuity, blood heat, or taxation fatigue causing insecurity of the thoroughfare (*chōng*) and controlling (*rèn*) vessels.

548. 月经过少〔月經過少〕*yuè jīng guò shǎo*, **scant menstruation** [skænt mɛnstru'eʃən]: A smaller menstrual flow or shorter menstrual period than normal (in some cases reduced to spotting). Because the flow is not smooth and continuous, scant menstruation is often called inhibited menstruation. It is attributed to blood vacuity, blood cold and blood stasis, phlegm-damp, or kidney vacuity.

549. 月经不利〔月經不利〕*yuè jīng bù lì*, **inhibited menstruation** [ɪn'hɪ-bɪtɪd ˌmɛnstru'eʃən]: See scant menstruation.

550. 月经先期〔月經先期〕*yuè jīng xiān qī*, **advanced menstruation (early periods)** [əd'vænst ˌmɛnstru'eʃən ('ɝ·lɪ 'pɪrɪədz)]: The arrival of the menstrual period eight days or more before the normal time (i.e., within 20 days of the onset of the previous period in women who normally have a standard 28-day cycle). Attributed to blood heat, liver depression, or qì vacuity.

551. 月经后期〔月經後期〕*yuè jīng hòu qī*, **delayed menstruation (late periods)** [dɪ'led ˌmɛnstru'eʃən (let 'pɪrɪədz)]: Late menstrual periods. The arrival of the menstrual period eight days or more after the normal time (i.e., roughly 36 days after the onset of the previous period in women who normally have a standard 28-day cycle). It is attributed to blood vacuity, blood cold, kidney vacuity, qì stagnation, or blood stasis.

552. 经行先后无定期〔經行先後無定期〕*jīng xíng xiān hòu wú dìng qī*, **menstruation at irregular intervals** [ˌmɛnstru'eʃən ət ɪ'rɛgjələ 'ɪntɚvəlz]: Menstruation that is sometimes advanced and sometimes delayed; attributed to liver qì depression, kidney vacuity, or spleen vacuity. Also called chaotic menstruation.

553. 乱经〔亂經〕*luàn jīng*, **chaotic menstruation** [ke'atɪk ˌmɛnstru-'eʃən]: See menstruation at irregular intervals.

554. 闭经〔閉經〕*bì jīng*, **menstrual block; amenorrhea** ['mɛnstruəl blɑk; əˌmɛnə'rɪə]: Absence of menstruation. Between menarche (start of menses in puberty) and menopause (end of menses in middle age), menstruation normally ceases only in pregnancy. Menstrual block is the continuing absence of menstruation after the age of 18 or the abnormal cessation of menstrual periods for at least three months in women who are neither pregnant nor lactating. In rare cases, lifelong absence of menstruation is unaccompanied by impairment of reproductive function (in other words, women in rare cases bear children without ever having

periods). Menstrual block is usually due to blood vacuity, kidney vacuity, qì stagnation and blood stasis, or to congealing cold-damp.

555. 带下〔帶下〕*dài xià,* **vaginal discharge** ['vædʒənl̩ 'dɪstʃɑrdʒ]: The emission of a viscid fluid via the vagina. Scant white vaginal discharge often occurs in healthy women. Only discharge that is profuse, bears an unnatural color, or gives off a malign odor is pathological. A copious clear white discharge without malodor is called white vaginal discharge and is caused by cold-damp pouring downward with spleen vacuity. A foul-smelling copious thick yellow discharge is called yellow vaginal discharge and is due to damp-heat pouring downward. A thick discharge that is white and red in color and bears a faint fishy smell is called red vaginal discharge, and arises when depressed liver qì transforms into heat, which damages the network vessels of the uterus. Modern research shows that continued red vaginal discharge is in some cases a sign of cancer. Malodorous vaginal discharge is a sign of damp toxin when it resembles rice water (water in which rice has been washed), yellow-green like pus, or is multicolored, and attended by pudendal itch and soreness.

556. 子宫下垂〔子宮下垂〕*zǐ gōng xià chuí,* **prolapse of the uterus** ['prolæps əv ðə 'jutərəs]: Downward displacement of the uterus, in severe cases beyond the mouth of the vagina. Prolapse of the uterus is attributed to qì vacuity fall or to excessive childbirth, difficult childbirth, or excessive straining during childbirth. Also called yīn protrusion and eggplant disease.

557. 胎动不安〔胎動不安〕*tāi dòng bù ān,* **stirring fetus** ['stɝɪŋ 'fitəs]: A disease pattern characterized by movement of the fetus, pain and sagging sensation in the abdomen, and, in severe cases, discharge of blood from the vagina; a sign of possible or impending miscarriage; can be caused by knocks and falls, qì vacuity, blood vacuity, kidney vacuity, or blood heat causing damage to the thoroughfare (*chōng*) and controlling (*rèn*) vessels.

558. 恶露不绝〔惡露不絕〕*è lù bù jué,* **persistent flow of the lochia** [pə'sɪstənt flo əv 'lɑkɪə]: Flow of the lochia in excess of 20 days. Persistent flow of lochia is attributed to qì vacuity, blood heat, or blood stasis.

4.4. 切诊
Palpation

4.4.1. 脉诊 Pulse Examination

559. 寸口〔寸口〕*cùn kǒu,* **wrist pulse; inch opening** [rɪst pʌls; ɪntʃ ˈopənɪŋ]: The wrist pulse.

560. 把脉〔把脈〕*bǎ mài,* **take the pulse** [tek ðə pʌls]: To feel the (wrist) pulse.

561. 切脉〔切脈〕*qiè mài,* **take the pulse** [tek ðə pʌls]: To feel the (wrist) pulse.

562. 寸〔寸〕*cùn,* **inch** [ɪntʃ]: The section of the wrist pulse closest to the hand; when the pulse is taken with three fingers, this section is felt with the index finger.

563. 关〔關〕*guān,* **bar** [bɑr]: The section of the wrist pulse between the inch and cubit; palpated with the middle finger.

564. 尺〔尺〕*chǐ,* **cubit** [ˈkjubɪt]: The section of the wrist pulse closest to the elbow; palpated with the fourth (ring) finger.

565. 浮脉〔浮脈〕*fú mài,* **floating pulse** [ˈflotɪŋ pʌls]: A pulse superabundant at the superficial level, but insufficient at the deep level, described as being "like wood floating on water" (如木漂水 *rú mù piāo shuǐ*). A floating pulse is felt as soon as the fingers touch the skin, but becomes markedly less perceptible when further pressure is applied. Although classically associated with exterior patterns, the floating pulse may be indistinct in patients of heavy build, with weak constitutions, or suffering from severe water swelling, even when an exterior pattern is present. A floating pulse may also occur in enduring illnesses or after a major loss of blood, indicating a severe insufficiency of right qi rather than an exterior pattern.

566. 沉脉〔沉脈〕*chén mài,* **sunken pulse; deep pulse** [ˈsʌŋkən, dip pʌls]: A pulse that is distinct only at the deep level. A sunken pulse is associated essentially with interior patterns, although the exterior patterns of external diseases may temporarily present with a tight sunken pulse when the body's yáng qì is obstructed.

567. 迟脉〔遲脈〕*chí mài,* **slow pulse** [slo pʌls]: A pulse that has three or less beats per respiration (一息 *yī xí*). The slow pulse is principally associated with cold and with yáng vacuity. It may occur in any disease involving insufficiency of yáng qì or obstruction of qì dynamic, such as cold, phlegm turbidity, and static blood. Occurring in pregnancy, this pulse signifies uterine vacuity cold or insecurity of fetal qì.

568. 数脉〔數脈〕*shuò mài,* **rapid pulse** ['ræpɪd pʌls]: A pulse that has six beats per respiration is a rapid pulse; one having between five and six beats is termed a slightly rapid pulse. The rapid pulse is usually quite smooth-flowing, so it is often confused with a slippery pulse. However, the term "rapid" refers exclusively to the pace, whereas "slippery" denotes a quality. The rapid pulse is associated with heat, but may sometimes be an indication of vacuity. A forceful rapid pulse indicates repletion heat and is most commonly seen in externally contracted heat (febrile) disease. A forceless fine rapid pulse indicates effulgent yīn vacuity fire and is generally seen in depletion patterns, such as are described in Western medicine as pulmonary tuberculosis. A forceless large rapid pulse generally indicates qì vacuity. Most healthy infants have rapid pulses, and a slippery rapid pulse is a normal sign in pregnancy.

569. 虚脉〔虛脈〕*xū mài,* **vacuous pulse** ['vækjuəs pʌls]: A forceless soft, usually large pulse that feels empty.

570. 实脉〔實脈〕*shí mài,* **replete pulse** [rɪ'plit pʌls]: A large pulse that is forceful at all levels; its beats are equally forceful when arriving as when departing.

571. 滑脉〔滑脈〕*huá mài,* **slippery pulse** ['slɪpərɪ pʌls]: A smooth-flowing pulse classically described as "pearls rolling in a dish" (如盘走珠 *rú pán zǒu zhū*). A slippery pulse is commonly seen in pregnancy, particularly in the early stages where extra blood is needed to nourish the fetus. It is also sometimes seen in healthy people, indicating an abundance of qì and blood. Phlegm-rheum patterns and food accumulation may also be characterized by a slippery pulse.

572. 涩脉〔澀脈〕*sè mài,* **rough pulse** [rʌf pʌls]: A pulse opposite to the slippery pulse, i.e., one that does not flow smoothly and that is classically described as being like "a light knife scraping bamboo" (如轻刀刮竹 *rú qīng dāo guā zhú*). The rough pulse is sometimes termed a choppy or dry pulse in English. It tends to be somewhat fine, is generally slightly slower than the normal pulse, and has been described as being "fine, slow, short, dry, and beating with difficulty." The rough pulse is often seen in blood stasis patterns and dual vacuity of blood and qì.

573. 弦脉〔弦脈〕*xián mài,* **stringlike pulse** ['strɪŋlɑɪk pʌls]: A pulse that is long and taut and feels like a zither string to the touch. The stringlike pulse is associated with diseases of the liver and gallbladder and in particular with ascendant liver yáng. It is also associated with pain and with phlegm-rheum patterns.

574. 濡脉〔濡脈〕*rú mài,* **soggy pulse** [ˈsɔɡɪ pʌls]: A soft pulse lacking in force. A soggy pulse tends to be floating and is fine, though less distinctly so than a fine pulse. The soggy pulse is associated with dual vacuity of blood and qì and with damp encumbrance.

575. 洪脉〔洪脈〕*hóng mài,* **surging pulse** [ˈsɜˈdʒɪŋ pʌls]: A pulse that is broad and large and that is forceful at all levels, especially the superficial. The arrival is longer and more forceful than the departure, which accounts for the descriptions, "Arriving forcefully, departing feebly" (来盛去衰 *lái shèng qù shuāi*), "like tempestuous billowing waves dashing against the shore" (如波涛拍岸 *rú bō táo pāi àn*), "surging over the whole of the finger[tip]." It is characterized by a strong initial swell followed by a sharp, but calm, ebbing away. A surging pulse indicates exuberant heat and is usually a sign of repletion. It is observed in enduring diseases (such as tuberculosis) or in vacuity patterns due to massive bleeding; it indicates that right qì is extremely weak and that the condition is deteriorating.

576. 微脉〔微脈〕*wēi mài,* **faint pulse** [fent pʌls]: A pulse so fine and weak that it is barely perceptible. It indicates vacuity desertion or qì and blood vacuity.

577. 细脉〔細脈〕*xì mài,* **fine pulse** [faɪn pʌls]: A pulse that feels like a well-defined fine thread under the fingers. The fine pulse indicates dual vacuity of qì and blood or of yīn and yáng, and in particular points to blood and yīn vacuity.

578. 弱脉〔弱脈〕*ruò mài,* **weak pulse** [wik pʌls]: A pulse that is sunken and without force. A weak pulse is associated with vacuity of qì and blood.

579. 大脉〔大脈〕*dà mài,* **large pulse** [lɑrdʒ pʌls]: A broad pulse, i.e., the opposite of a fine pulse. Compare surging pulse.

580. 散脉〔散脈〕*sàn mài,* **dissipated pulse** [ˈdɪsɪˌpetɪd pʌls]: A large floating pulse without root. A dissipated pulse is large at the superficial level, but ceases to be felt as soon as the slightest pressure is applied. It indicates the dissipation of qì and blood and the impending expiration of the essential qì of the bowels and viscera.

581. 紧脉〔緊脈〕*jǐn mài,* **tight pulse** [taɪt pʌls]: A stringlike pulse that has marked forcefulness. "Stringlike" denotes a quality, whereas "tight" denotes a quality and a strength. A tight pulse is always stringlike, whereas a stringlike pulse is not necessarily tight. A tight pulse is associated with cold and pain.

582. 芤脉〔芤脈〕*kōu mài,* **scallion-stalk pulse** [ˈskælɪən–stɔk pʌls]: A large floating pulse that is empty in the middle when pressure is applied,

like pressing a scallion (or green onion) stalk (如按葱管 *rú àn cōng guǎn*). Lǐ Zhōng-Zǐ (李中梓) states, "It is as if the finger is feeling a scallion. At the superficial level, the skin of the scallion is felt. At the mid-level, the empty middle of the scallion is felt. At the deep level, the finger touches the under side of the scallion." This is why this pulse is likened to a scallion stalk. The scallion-stalk pulse is a sign of heavy blood loss and usually occurs in major bleeding.

583. 革脉 〔革脈〕 *gé mài,* **drumskin pulse** ['drʌmskɪn pʌls]: A pulse that is floating and beats against the palpating fingers. A drumskin pulse is hard on the outside and empty in the middle like the skin of a drum. It signifies blood collapse and loss of essence.

584. 牢脉 〔牢脈〕 *láo mài,* **firm pulse; confined pulse** [fɜˑm pʌls, kənˈ-faɪnd pʌls]: A forceful sunken pulse. It is associated with cold pain. In clinical practice, the name "firm pulse" is rarely used. Instead it is called a stringlike sunken pulse or a sunken full pulse.

585. 疾脉 〔疾脈〕 *jí mài,* **racing pulse** ['resɪŋ pʌls]: A pulse having seven or more beats per respiration, i.e., at least one beat or more per respiration than the rapid pulse. It is a sign of exhaustion of yīn and yáng and original qì about to desert, and is observed in acute febrile disease and vacuity taxation. It is usually a critical sign. A racing pulse in a healthy pregnant woman is a sign of imminent birth.

586. 动脉 〔動脈〕 *dòng mài,* **stirred pulse** ['stɜˑd pʌls]: A pulse that is forceful, rapid, and slippery, wobbling like a bean (如豆，厥厥动摇 *rú dòu, jué jué dòng yáo*). According to some sources, the stirred pulse is only felt at the bar (not generally recognized nowadays). The stirred pulse is a sign of pain or fright and may be seen in sweating, heat effusion (fever), diarrhea, and flooding and spotting. A stirred pulse is also observed in pregnancy.

587. 伏脉 〔伏脈〕 *fú mài,* **hidden pulse** ['hɪdn̩ pʌls]: A pulse even deeper than the sunken pulse, considerable pressure being needed to feel it. It is associated with fulminant desertion of yáng qì and deep-lying cold, and it generally appears in conjunction with severe vomiting, diarrhea, and pain.

588. 缓脉 〔緩脈〕 *huǎn mài,* **moderate pulse** ['mɑdərət pʌls]: A pulse with four beats per respiration (slightly faster than a slow pulse) and that is soft and harmonious in its form. If it is gentle and even, it is a normal pulse signifying the presence of stomach qì; if it is forceless, it mostly indicates dampness or spleen-stomach vacuity.

589. 促脉 〔促脈〕 *cù mài,* **skipping pulse** ['skɪpɪŋ pʌls]: A pulse that is urgent and forceful and that pauses at irregular intervals. It indicates:

a) exuberant heat repletion; b) blood, qì, phlegm, or food stagnation; or c) painful swelling.

590. 结脉〔結脈〕*jié mài,* **bound pulse** [bɑʊnd pʌls]: A pulse that is moderate or slow and pauses at irregular intervals. *The Pulse Canon (Mài Jīng)* states that it "indicates exuberant yīn and bound qì, congested qì and stagnant phlegm, or concretions, conglomerations, accumulations, and gatherings."

591. 代脉〔代脈〕*dài mài,* **intermittent pulse** [ˌɪntərˈmɪtənt pʌls]: A moderate weak pulse that pauses at regular intervals. It indicates debilitation of the visceral qì and is seen in heart disease, fear and fright, and severe knocks and falls.

592. 长脉〔長脈〕*cháng mài,* **long pulse** [lɔŋ pʌls]: A long pulse is one that can be felt beyond the inch and cubit positions. It runs straight from head to tail and feels like a long stick. A long pulse that is harmonious and moderate is a sign of effulgent center qì. *Elementary Questions (Sù Wèn, Mài Yào Jīng Wēi Lùn)* states, "If the pulse is long, qì is in order." If the pulse is long, stringlike, and hard, and feels like a rope pulled taut, this is a repletion pattern in which evil and right are both exuberant and that is seen in repletion heat binding internally or exuberant heat stirring wind. *The Bin-Hu Sphygmology (Bīn Hú Mài Xué)* states, "[The] long [pulse] governs superabundance; it is seen in qì counterflow and exuberant fire."

593. 短脉〔短脈〕*duǎn mài,* **short pulse** [ʃɔrt pʌls]: A short pulse is one that is felt only at the bar position. The short pulse signifies dual vacuity of blood and qì or impaired flow of blood and qì.

594. 有力〔有力〕*yǒu lì,* **forceful** [ˈfɔrsfʊl]: Possessing strength. Compare forceless.

595. 无力〔無力〕*wú lì,* **forceless** [ˈfɔrsləs]: Lacking in strength. The term "forceless" is most commonly used in the pulse examination to describe any pulse that beats without force. "Forceless" is a descriptive word, not the name of a pulse type. A pulse described as forceless should not be confused with a weak pulse.

4.4.2. 触诊 Body Examination

596. 肢冷〔肢冷〕*zhī lěng,* **cold limbs** [kold lɪmz]: Any condition of palpable cold in the limbs. Mild cases are referred to as lack of warmth in the limbs and severe cases, with cold up to the elbows and knees, as reversal cold of the limbs or counterflow cold of the limbs.

597. 四肢欠温〔四肢欠溫〕*sì zhī qiàn wēn,* **lack of warmth in the limbs** [læk əv wɔrmθ ɪn ðə lɪmz]: See cold limbs.

598. 四肢不温〔四肢不溫〕*sì zhī bù wēn,* **lack of warmth in the limbs** [læk əv wɔrmθ ɪn ðə lɪmz]: See cold limbs.

599. 四肢厥冷〔四肢厥冷〕*sì zhī jué lěng,* **reversal cold of the limbs** [rɪ'vɝsl̩ kold əv ðə lɪmz]: See cold limbs.

600. 四肢逆冷〔四肢逆冷〕*sì zhī nì lěng,* **counterflow cold of the limbs** ['kɑʊntɚˌflo kold əv ðə lɪmz]: See cold limbs.

601. 厥逆〔厥逆〕*jué nì,* **reverse-flow** [rɪ'vɝs flo]: reversal cold of the limbs.

602. 形寒〔形寒〕*xíng hán,* **physical cold** ['fɪzɪkl̩ kold]: Outwardly manifest signs of cold, e.g., aversion to cold, desire for warm beverages, curled-up lying posture, cold limbs, etc. *Elementary Questions (Sù Wèn, tiáo jīng lùn)* states, "When yáng is vacuous, there is external cold." "Physical cold" is what is meant by "external cold."

See Inquiring about Cold and Heat, page 74.

603. 五心烦热〔五心煩熱〕*wǔ xīn fán rè,* **vexing heat in the five hearts** ['vɛksɪŋ hit ɪn ðə faɪv hɑrts]: Heat in the palms of the hands, soles of the feet, and center of the chest (all yīn aspects of the body). It is a sign of yīn vacuity.

604. 痞块〔痞塊〕*pǐ kuài,* **glomus lump** ['glomns lʌmp]: Any palpable abdominal mass. These are classified in ancient literature as concretions, conglomerations, accumulations, and gatherings. The presence of a glomus lump invariably heralds pronounced abdominal distention.

605. 腹胀〔腹脹〕*fù zhàng,* **abdominal distention** [əb'dɑmɪnl̩ dɪs'tɛnʃən]: Enlargement of the abdomen (objectively detectable). See drum distention. Distention also refers to a subjective feeling of fullness. See abdominal fullness.

606. 浮肿〔浮腫〕*fú zhǒng,* **puffy swelling** ['pʌfɪ 'swɛlɪŋ]: Water swelling or vacuity puffiness. A distinction is sometimes made between swelling and puffiness, swelling being repletion and puffiness being vacuity. Puffy swelling is caused by debilitation of the visceral qì of the lung, spleen, and kidney. When the lung is vacuous, water is not transformed; when the spleen is vacuous, water is not dammed; when the kidney is vacuous, water is not governed. When the spleen is affected, there is puffy swelling of the flesh; when the lung is affected, there is rapid panting. See water swelling.

607. 灼热〔灼熱〕*zhuó rè,* **scorching heat** ['skɔrtʃɪŋ hit]: Intense heat that is palpable (such as in sores), or intense heat subjectively felt by the patient (as a burning pain on urination).

习题
Questions

Answer the following questions in English:

261. Yellow eyes are a sign of what disease? ....

262. In what disease patterns are bulging eyes observed? ....

263. With what condition is drooling from the corners of the mouth associated? ....

264. What is the significance of teeth dry as desiccated bones? ....

265. Is a cough with thick yellow phlegm observed in heat or cold patterns? ....

266. What is vigorous heat [effusion] a sign of? ....

267. What does steaming bone tidal heat indicate? ....

268. When a patient experiences a sensation of cold in wind or drafts, he is said to have what sign? ....

269. Shiver sweating is considered unfavorable if what fails to happen after it? ....

270. Are conditions popularly described in Chinese as the "last flicker of the lamp" ones of spiritedness or false spiritedness? ....

271. What disease does nasal congestion occur in? ....

272. What does clear-grain diarrhea indicate? ....

273. Does laziness to speak indicate qì vacuity or blood vacuity? ....

274. What is hasty breathing? ....

275. Raised-shoulder breathing is a sign of what? ....

276. In what patterns does sighing occur? ....

277. Hiccup, belching, and vomiting are all associated with which of the six bowels? ....

278. What is the name we give to a gurgling sound in the intestines?

279. What do we call the sign observed when a patient talks to himself haltingly and with frequent repetitions? ....

280. What pulse is described as wobbling like a bean? ....

281. What do we call a pulse that is urgent and forceful and that pauses at irregular intervals? ....

282. What is the other term for "fever" used in this book? ....

283. In what disease pattern is anger usually observed? ....

284. What is the term referring to uncontrollable movement of the limbs? ....

285. In what kind of pattern is lying in curled-up posture observed? ....

286. What is generalized heaviness a sign of? ....

287. Of what disease is hemiplegia a sign? ....

288. What is tugging and slackening? ....

289. What does an enlarged tongue with dental impressions on the margins indicate? ....

290. What is the difference between a moderate pulse and a slow pulse? ....

291. What are the three types of white complexion? ....

292. In what tongue color are both vacuity and repletion heat likely to be reflected? ....

293. In what ways is blood stasis reflected in the tongue? ....

294. What does a mirror tongue indicate? ....

295. What does a prickly tongue indicate? ....

296. What does a mealy white tongue fur indicate? ....

297. Which color of tongue fur is observed in healthy patients? ....

298. Is a bulging fontanel gate observed in infants or adults? ....

299. What are the causes of dry hair? ....

300. What is the name given to the sign in which the patient feels as though his head were wrapped in cloth or bandages? ....

301. Name one cause of lumbar pain. ....

302. Is blood stasis a possible cause of numbness and tingling of the limbs? ....

303. Are long voidings of clear urine normal? ....

304. Is enuresis mostly observed in children or adults? ....

305. Name one cause of fecal incontinence. ....

306. Is tenesmus observed in cholera or dysentery? ....

307. If a patient washes the mouth with water without desire to swallow it, what does he or she have? ....

308. What does the term "transforming tongue fur" refer to? ....

309. What do we call defecation that leaves the patient with a feeling that the bowels have not been satisfactorily emptied? ....

310. Is "little desire for food and drink" the same as "poor appetite"?

311. Eating far larger amounts of food than normal is called what? ....

312. What sign is said to be like hunger but not hunger, and like pain but not pain? ....

313. What do we call it when acid wells up and is swallowed before the patient can spit it out? ....

314. Seminal emission without dreaming is usually attributable to disease of which viscus? ....

315. Name one cause of premature ejaculation. ....

316. What is the difference between clouding sleep and somnolence? ....

317. What is another name for "chaotic menstruation"? ....

318. Name one cause of chest pain. ....

319. What do we call severe heart palpitations that are not brought on by emotional stimulus? ....

320. Does pain in the stomach duct and abdomen that refuses pressure indicate vacuity or repletion? ....

321. What does hardness of hearing mean? ....

322. Name one cause of dry eyes. ....

323. What is the difference between abdominal fullness and abdominal distention? ....

324. Do the terms "sleeplessness" and "insomnia" mean the same thing? ....

325. What is another English term for "ringing in the ears"? ....

326. Seminal emission and seminal efflux are both kinds of what? ....

327. In pregnancy, what do signs such as pain and sagging in the abdomen and discharge of blood via the vagina mean? ....

328. What do we call a slow pulse that pauses at irregular intervals? ....

329. What do we call a pulse that feels superabundant at the superficial level but that is insufficient at the deep level? ....

330. A pulse that has three or less beats per respiration is called what?

331. Is a vacuous pulse usually large or fine? ....

332. A rapid pulse indicates what? ....

333. Which pulse is described as being like a "a light knife scraping bamboo"? ....

334. What pulse is described as "arriving forcefully, departing feebly"? ....

335. What pulse is described as being like "tempestuous billowing waves dashing against the shore"? ....

336. What pulse indicates dissipation of qì and blood and the impending expiration of the essential qì of the bowels and viscera? ....

337. What is the difference between a stringlike pulse and a tight pulse? ....

338. Is a weak pulse the same as a forceless pulse? ....

339. Which is more serious, lack of warmth in the limbs or reversal cold of the limbs? ....

340. What does "scorching heat" mean? ....

341. Name the three positions of the wrist pulse. ....

342. What do we call it when a patient has her periods over a week after they are due? ....

343. Does the lochia occur before or after childbirth? ....

344. What is the traditional term for downward displacement of the uterus? ....

345. What is the term we use to denote the inability of males to perform intercourse owing to inability to achieve or maintain erection? ....

346. What does abdominal pain that likes warmth indicate? ....

347. With which viscus and what bowel is rib-side pain associated? ....

348. Heart palpitations, insomnia, and profuse dreaming occurring to-gether would indicate disease of which viscus? ....

349. Would spontaneous loss of semen in the daytime be called seminal emission or seminal efflux? ....

350. What are the causes of menstrual block (amenorrhea)? ....

351. Name one cause of drowsiness after eating. ....

352. What is the cause of intermittent dull eye pain? ....

353. What may intermittent scurrying pain around the umbilicus indicate? ....

354. Nausea and vomiting indicate counterflow of the qì of which of the six bowels? ....

355. Prolapse of the rectum is most prevalent in what age groups? ....

356. What do we call diarrhea occurring before daybreak? ....

357. Name one cause of dribble after voiding of urine. ....

358. What is the clinical significance of night sweating? ....

359. What is aversion to cold without heat effusion due to?
....

360. What do we call heat in the center of the soles and palms and in the center of the chest? ....

Give the Pīnyīn and English for the following Chinese terms:

361. 四肢欠温 ....

362. 五心烦热 ....

363. 四肢逆冷 ....

364. 代脉 ....

365. 动脉 ....

366. 弦脉 ....

367. 月经过少 ....

368. 失精 ....

369. 不梦而遗 ....

370. 昏睡 ....

371. 目痛 ....

372. 少腹痛 ....

373. 脘腹痛拒按 ....

374. 重听 ....

375. 惊悸 ....

376. 牢脉 ....

377. 恶心 ....

378. 胸满 ....

379. 纳谷不香 ....

380. 大便不爽 ....

381. 脱肛 ....

382. 五更泄 ....

383. 夜间多尿 ....

384. 小便短赤 ....

385. 腰痛 ....

386. 健忘 ....

387. 腰膝软弱 ....

388. 心烦 ....

389. 憎寒 ....

390. 盗汗 ....

391. 气促 ....

392. 大便希溏 ....

393. 咯血 ....

394. 鼻塞 ....

395. 齿龈结瓣 ....

396. 口唇干焦 ....

397. 发枯 ....

398. 苔垢 ....

399. 吐舌 ....

400. 舌胖大 ....

401. 筋惕肉瞤 ....

402. 筋脉拘急 ....

403. 口眼㖞斜 ....

404. 头身困重 ....

405. 肌肉瘦削 ....

406. 有神 ....

407. 四肢困倦 ....

408. 狂躁 ....

409. 易怒 ....

410. 撮空理线 ....

Supply the Chinese and English for the following:

411. *Chén mài*. ....

412. *Jí mài*. ....

413. *Sì zhī jué lěng*. ....

414. *Duăn mài.* ....
415. *Cù mài.* ....
416. *Xiăo biàn qīng cháng.* ....
417. *Zhàn hàn.* ....
418. *Cháo rè.* ....
419. *Miàn sè bái.* ....
420. *Tāi hòu.* ....
421. *Yāo suān xī ruăn.* ....
422. *Kŏu jìn.* ....
423. *Cán dēng fù míng.* ....
424. *Shé juăn.* ....
425. *Zì hàn.* ....
426. *Yáng shŏu zhí zú.* ....
427. *Miàn sè qīng zĭ.* ....
428. *Jĭng xiàng jiàng zhí.* ....
429. *Jiăo gōng făn zhāng.* ....
430. *Shé biān chĭ hén.* ....
431. *Huáng tāi.* ....
432. *Tóu yáo.* ....
433. *Fà luò.* ....
434. *Liăng mù shàng shì.* ....
435. *Mù chì.* ....
436. *Kŏu jiăo liú xián.* ....
437. *Eĭ lún kū jiāo.* ....
438. *Ké tán huáng chóu.* ....
439. *Dà biàn rú yáng shĭ.* ....
440. *Tán zhōng dài xuè.* ....
441. *Shēng yīn zhòng zhuó.* ....
442. *Hóu zhōng yŏu shuĭ jī shēng.* ....
443. *Lăn yán.* ....

444. *Jiān xī.* ....

445. *Zhān yán.* ....

446. *Cháng míng.* ....

447. *Zhèng yǔ.* ....

448. *Fā rè.* ....

449. *Tóu zhòng rú guǒ.* ....

450. *Xuàn yūn.* ....

451. *Qí zhōu cuàn tòng.* ....

452. *Bù dé wò.* ....

453. *Yuè jīng shī tiáo.* ....

454. *Zǎo xiè.* ....

455. *Guān jié téng tòng.* ....

456. *Yāo suān.* ....

457. *Xiǎo biàn duǎn chì.* ....

458. *Xiè xiè.* ....

459. *Kǒu kě.* ....

460. *Dà kě yǐn yǐn.* ....

461. *Shí yù bù zhèn.* ....

462. *Kǒu gān.* ....

463. *Xīn jì.* ....

464. *Tù xuè.* ....

465. *Qiè mài.* ....

466. *Shí hòu kùn dùn.* ....

467. *Yuè jīng xiān qí.* ....

468. *È lù bù jué.* ....

469. *Bǎ mài.* ....

470. *Shēn rè bù wài yáng.* ....

471. *Wǔ hòu cháo rè.* ....

472. *Tóu tòng rú chè.* ....

473. *Cùn kǒu.* ....

474. *Shuò mài.* ....

475. *Chí mài.* ....

476. *Hóng mài.* ....

477. *Jié mài.* ....

478. *Fú zhǒng.* ....

479. *Xíng hán.* ....

480. *Pǐ kuài.* ....

Give the Chinese and Pīnyīn for the following:

481. Lying in curled-up posture. ....

482. Clenched jaw. ....

483. Shortness of breath. ....

484. Steaming bone tidal heat [effusion]. ....

485. Black facial complexion. ....

486. Aversion to wind. ....

487. Shrunken tongue. ....

488. Heavy-headedness. ....

489. Harmony of mouth. ....

490. Bitter taste in the mouth. ....

491. Mirror tongue. ....

492. Inhibited urination. ....

493. Hiccup. ....

494. Dribble after voiding. ....

495. Transforming tongue fur. ....

496. Enuresis. ....

497. Fecal incontinence. ....

498. Drumskin pulse. ....

499. Aversion to food. ....

500. Clear-grain diarrhea. ....

501. Faint pulse. ....

502. Difficult defecation. ....

503. No thought of food and drink. ....

504. Inability to eat. ....

505. Rough pulse. ....

506. Acid upflow. ....

507. Oppression in the chest. ....

508. Moderate pulse. ....

509. Deafness. ....

510. Abdominal fullness. ....

511. Chaotic menstruation. ....

512. Replete pulse. ....

513. Abdominal pain that likes warmth. ....

514. Tinnitus. ....

515. Insomnia. ....

516. Aversion to light. ....

517. Dry eyes. ....

518. Profuse menstruation. ....

519. Dream emission. ....

520. Skipping pulse. ....

521. Somnolence. ....

522. Stirring fetus. ....

523. Wrist pulse. ....

524. Scallion-stalk pulse. ....

525. Long pulse. ....

526. Upflow nausea. ....

527. Forceful. ....

528. Puffy swelling. ....

529. Sleeplessness. ....

530. Picking at bedclothes. ....

第五章　疾病
Diseases

Note that some of the terms included in Chapter 4, Four Examinations, such as "headache" and "cough," which are traditionally understood to be disease names, are not repeated in this section.

608. **外感** 〔 外感 〕 *wài gǎn,* **external contraction** [ɪksˈtɜˑnl̩ kənˈtrækʃən]: Disease resulting from contraction of external evils such as wind, cold, or summerheat.

609. **杂病** 〔 雜病 〕 *zá bìng,* **miscellaneous disease** [ˌmɪsəˈlenɪəs dɪˈziz]: Any disease not resulting from contraction of external evils or from knocks and falls, cuts, or bites.

610. **内伤杂病** 〔 內傷雜病 〕 *nèi shāng zá bìng,* **miscellaneous internal damage disease** [ˌmɪsəˈlenɪəs ɪnˈtɜˑnl̩ˈdæmɪdʒ dɪˈziz]: Miscellaneous diseases that result from internal damage by the seven affects.

5.1. 内科疾病
Internal Medicine Diseases

611. **鼻渊** 〔 鼻淵 〕 *bí yuān,* **deep-source nasal congestion** [dip sɔrs ˈnezəl kənˈdʒɛstʃən]: Persistent nasal congestion with turbid snivel (nasal mucus) attributable to wind-cold, wind-heat, or gallbladder heat.

612. **头风** 〔 頭風 〕 *tóu fēng,* **head wind** [ˈhəd-wɪnd]: Persistently remittent, usually intense headache attributed to wind-cold or wind-heat invasion and obstruction of the channels by phlegm or static blood. Head wind may be accompanied by various other signs such as eye pain and loss of vision, runny nose, nausea, dizziness, numbness of the head, or stiffness of the neck.

613. **痨瘵** 〔 癆瘵 〕 *láo zhài,* **consumption** [kənˈsʌmpʃən]: A contagious disease characterized by cough with expectoration of blood, tidal heat effusion, night sweating, and emaciation. In Western medicine, this disease is now referred to as pulmonary tuberculosis.

614. 喘〔喘〕*chuǎn*, **panting** [ˈpæntɪŋ]: Hasty, rapid, labored breathing with discontinuity between inhalation and exhalation, in severe cases with gaping mouth, raised shoulders, flaring nostrils, and inability to lie down. When associated with counterflow movement of qì, it is sometimes called "panting counterflow" (喘逆 *chuǎn nì*). When breathing is unusually rapid, it is sometimes called "hasty panting" (喘促 *chuǎn cù*). When in severe cases it is associated with raising of the shoulders and flaring nostrils, it is "raised-shoulder breathing" (肩息 *jiān xī*). Panting is a manifestation of impaired diffusion and downbearing of lung qì. Since the "lung is the governor of qì" (肺为气之主 *fèi wéi qì zhī zhǔ*) and the "kidney is the root of qì" (肾为气之根 *shèn wéi qì zhī gēn*), panting is associated primarily with disease of the lung and/or kidney. Panting occurs in repletion and vacuity. Repletion panting may occur when externally contracted wind-heat or wind-cold invade the lung, when depressed liver qì invades the lung, or when phlegm resulting from spleen-lung vacuity obstructs the lung. Vacuity panting occurs in dual vacuity of lung yīn and lung qì and also in kidney failing to absorb qì (肾不纳气 *shèn bù nà qì*). Kidney vacuity with phlegm obstruction and yáng vacuity water flood are vacuity-repletion complexes that may also cause panting.

615. 哮〔哮〕*xiāo,* **wheezing** [ˈwizɪŋ]: Hasty rapid breathing with phlegm rale in the throat.

616. 哮喘〔哮喘〕*xiāo chuǎn,* **wheezing and panting** [ˈwizɪŋ ənd ˈpæntɪŋ]: See wheezing and panting.

617. 百日咳〔百日咳〕*bǎi rì ké,* **whooping cough** [ˈhupɪŋ kɔf]: A children's disease readily identifiable by the characteristic whoop of the cough. The whooping sound is similar to the sound made by a hen after laying an egg, hence the alternate name "hen cough" (鸡咳 *jī ké*). Whooping cough is attributed to contraction of a seasonal evil that causes phlegm turbidity to obstruct the airways and inhibit lung qì. If the cough continues, it can damage the network vessels of the lung and cause expectoration of blood.

618. 白喉〔白喉〕*bái hóu,* **diphtheria** [dɪfˈθɪrɪə]: A disease characterized by whitening of the throat. Diphtheria occurs mostly in the autumn or winter after a long period of dryness; it is attributed to seasonal epidemic scourge toxin exploiting vacuity of the lung and stomach. It starts with a sore throat that makes swallowing painful and with the appearance of white speckles on one or both throat nodes (喉核 *hóu hé*, i.e., the tonsils), which spread quickly to create a white membrane that covers the uvula and stretches into the regions inside and outside the throat

pass (侯关 *hóu guān*, i.e., isthmus faucium). The membrane does not easily slough off, cannot be forcefully removed without causing bleeding, and if removed always grows back. Other signs include headache, generalized pain, slight heat effusion (fever) or alternating [aversion to] cold and heat [effusion], lack of spirit, oppression in the chest, vexation and agitation, bad breath, and nasal congestion. If the white membrane spreads into the region inside the throat pass and down to the epiglottis and beyond, signs such as labored breathing, flaring nostrils, green-blue lips, heart palpitations or fearful throbbing, and a bound or intermittent pulse may be observed. Distinction is made between yáng heat and yīn vacuity patterns. Yáng heat patterns are attributed to wind-heat or heat toxin and are characterized by a red sore swollen throat, heat effusion (fever), constipation, and reddish urine; yīn vacuity patterns are attributed to dryness-heat damaging the lung and stomach and are characterized by white putrid throat, low fever, heat in the hearts of the palms and soles, fatigue, shortness of breath, and a fine rapid pulse.

619. 喉痹 〔喉痹〕 *hóu bì,* **throat impediment** [θrot ɪm'pɛdɪmənt]: Critical swelling and soreness of the throat in which the throat becomes severely occluded.

620. 乳蛾 〔乳蛾〕 *rǔ é,* **nipple moth; baby moth** ['nɪpl̩ mɑθ, 'bebɪ mɑθ]: Redness, swelling, and soreness of either or both of the throat nodes (tonsils) with a yellowish white discharge visible on their surface. Baby moth is attributable to a) congesting lung-stomach heat with fire toxin steaming upward; b) qì stagnation and congealing blood together with old phlegm and liver fire binding to form malign blood; or c) liver-kidney yīn-liquid depletion with vacuity fire flaming upward. Accompanying signs include constipation, a thick slimy tongue fur, difficulty in swallowing fluids, and alternating [aversion to] cold and heat [effusion]. This condition corresponds to tonsillitis.

621. 单蛾 〔單蛾〕 *dān é,* **single moth** ['sɪŋgl̩ mɑθ]: Baby moth on one side of the throat.

622. 双蛾 〔雙蛾〕 *shuāng é,* **double moth** ['dʌbl̩ mɑθ]: Baby moth on both sides of the throat.

623. 解颅 〔解顱〕 *jiě lú,* **ununited skull** [ˌʌnjuˈnaɪtɪd skʌl]: Retarded closure of the fontanel gate.

624. 麻疹 〔麻疹〕 *má zhěn,* **measles** ['mizl̩z]: A transmissible disease that mostly affects children and that is characterized by eruption of papules the shape of sesame seeds. The disease is located in the spleen and lung channels and can affect other bowels and viscera. Measles is characterized at onset by heat effusion (fever), cough, copious tearing, and white

speckles inside the mouth. After three days of heat effusion, papules appear behind the ears and on the neck and face, and they spread to the limbs. Eruptions are complete when the papules reach the legs.

625. 痄腮〔痄腮〕*zhà sāi,* **mumps** [mʌmps]: A febrile disease characterized by soft diffuse swelling and tenderness that affects one side of the face or one side after the other. Mumps is attributed to accumulated gastrointestinal heat and to depressed liver with gallbladder fire that arises after contraction of warm toxin and causes blockage of the lesser yáng (*shào yáng*). It occurs in epidemics in the winter and spring, and chiefly affects children.

626. 天花〔天花〕*tiān huā,* **smallpox** [ˈsmɔlpɑks]: A disease characterized by heat effusion (fever), cough, sneezing (喷嚏 *pēn tì*), yawning (呵欠 *hē qiàn*), red face, fright palpitations, cold extremities and ears, and eruption of pox.

627. 痘〔痘〕*dòu,* **pox** [pɑks]: Eruptive diseases such as smallpox and measles.

628. 痹〔痹〕*bì,* **impediment** [ɪmˈpɛdɪmənt]: Any disease pattern that results from blockage of the channels occurring when wind, cold, and dampness invade the fleshy exterior and the joints, and that manifests in signs such as joint pain, sinew and bone pain, and heaviness or numbness of the limbs. *Elementary Questions (Sù Wèn, bì lùn)* states, "When wind, cold, and dampness evils concur and combine, they give rise to impediment." Distinction is made between three pattern types, each of which corresponds to a prevalence of one of those three evils: wind impediment (or moving impediment) characterized by wandering pain and attributed to a prevalence of wind; cold impediment (or painful impediment) characterized by acute pain and attributed to a prevalence of cold; damp impediment (or fixed impediment) characterized by heaviness and attributed to a prevalence of dampness. A fourth type, heat impediment, arises when the three evils transform into heat.

629. 行痹〔行痹〕*xíng bì,* **moving impediment** [ˈmuvɪŋ ɪmˈpɛdɪmənt]: See impediment.

630. 周痹〔周痹〕*zhōu bì,* **generalized impediment** [ˈdʒɛnrəlɑɪzd ɪmˈpɛdɪmənt]: See impediment.

631. 着痹〔著痹〕*zhuó bì,* **fixed impediment** [fɪkst ɪmˈpɛdɪmənt]: See impediment.

632. 热痹〔熱痹〕*rè bì,* **heat impediment** [hit ɪmˈpɛdɪmeənt]: See impediment.

633. 历节风〔歷節風〕*lì jié fēng,* **joint-running wind** [ˈjɔɪnt–ˌrʌnɪŋ wɪnd]: A disease described in *Essential Prescriptions of the Golden Coffer (Jīn*

Guì Yào Lüè), characterized by redness and swelling of the joints, with acute pain and difficulty bending and stretching. Joint-running wind is attributed to transformation of wind-cold-damp into heat in patients suffering from liver-kidney vacuity, and it falls within the scope of impediment.

634. 鹤膝风〔鶴膝風〕*hè xī fēng,* **crane's-knee wind** ['krenz 'ni wind]: A disease marked by a painful suppurative swelling of the knee associated with emaciation of the lower leg. Crane's-knee wind is attributed to depletion of kidney yīn and to depletion of the three yáng channels allowing the invasion of cold-damp, which causes congealing stagnation; in most cases it develops from joint-running wind (*lì jié fēng*). Crane's-knee wind starts with physical cold and heat effusion, slight swelling of the knee, difficulty walking, and local pain. As it progresses, the knee becomes red, swollen, and hot or white with diffuse swelling. The thigh and calf become thin, and the swelling at the knee bursts to produce fluid pus or a thick yellow humor. Crane's-knee wind heals with difficulty.

635. 落枕〔落枕〕*lào zhěn,* **crick in the neck** [krɪk ɪn ðə nɛk]: Stiffness of the neck that results from taxation fatigue (overwork, etc.), twisting, sleeping in the wrong posture, or from exposure to a draft (wind-cold).

636. 痿〔痿〕*wěi,* **wilting** ['wɪltɪŋ]: Any disease pattern characterized by weakness and limpness of the sinews. In severe cases it prevents the lifting of the arms and legs and is accompanied by the sensation that the elbow, wrist, knee, and ankle are dislocated. In advanced cases, atrophy sets in. In clinical practice, the condition is mainly found to affect the legs and prevent the patient from walking, hence it is also called "crippling wilt" (痿躄 *wěi bì*). Wilting patterns include withering and paralysis of the limbs after high fever in neonates and infants, which Western medicine attributes to poliomyelitis.

637. 梅核气〔梅核氣〕*méi hé qì,* **plum-pit qì** ['plʌm–pɪt tʃi]: Dryness and a sensation in the throat of a foreign body that can be neither swallowed or ejected. The intensity of the signs fluctuates. The main cause is binding depression of liver qì. Plum-pit qì corresponds to globus hystericus in Western medicine.

638. 噎膈〔噎膈〕*yē gé,* **dysphagia-occlusion** [dɪs'fædʒɪə ə'kluʒən]: A disease characterized by sensation of blockage on swallowing, difficulty in getting food and drink down, and, in some cases, immediate vomiting of ingested food. The Chinese term is a compound of 噎 *yē,* meaning difficulty in swallowing (dysphagia), and 膈 *gé,* meaning blockage preventing food from going down (occlusion). Dysphagia and

occlusion may occur independently. Dysphagia most commonly but not necessarily develops into occlusion. There are four principal patterns: 1) phlegm and qì obstructing each other, 2) liquid depletion and heat bind, 3) static blood binding internally, and 4) qì vacuity and yáng debilitation.

639. 反胃〔反胃〕 *fǎn wèi*, **stomach reflux** ['stʌmək–ˌriflʌks]: A disease pattern characterized by distention and fullness after eating, either vomiting in the evening of food ingested in the morning or vomiting in the morning of food ingested in the evening (i.e., vomiting a long time after eating) with untransformed food in the vomitus, lassitude of spirit, and lack of bodily strength. Its principal cause is spleen-stomach vacuity cold, but it may also be due to debilitation of the life gate fire or to dual vacuity of qì and yīn.

640. 霍乱〔霍亂〕 *huò luàn*, **cholera; sudden turmoil** ['kɑlərə, 'sʌdn̩ 'tɝˑmɔɪl]: A disease characterized by simultaneous vomiting and diarrhea, usually followed by severe cramps. Dry cholera is characterized by an ungratified urge to vomit and defecate at the same time. Cholera in Chinese medicine comprises what modern Western medicine calls cholera as well as acute gastroenteritis presenting with the same signs. "Sudden turmoil" is a literal translation of the Chinese.

641. 痢疾〔痢疾〕 *lì jí*, **dysentery** [ˌdɪsən'tɛrɪ]: A disease characterized by abdominal pain, tenesmus, and stool containing pus and blood (described as mucoid and bloody stool in Western medicine). Dysentery usually occurs in hot weather and arises when gastrointestinal vacuity and eating raw, cold, or unclean food allow damp-heat or other evils to brew in the intestines. It takes the form of vacuity or repletion. Depending on the cause, distinction is made between summerheat dysentery, damp-heat dysentery, cold dysentery, and heat dysentery. Depending on the nature of the stool, distinction is made between red dysentery (blood in the stool), white dysentery (pus in the stool), and red and white dysentery (赤白痢, stool containing pus and blood).

642. 黄疸〔黃疸〕 *huáng dǎn*, **jaundice** ['dʒɔndɪs]: A condition characterized by the three classic signs of yellow skin, yellow eyes, and yellow urine, i.e., generalized yellowing of the body, yellowing of the whites of the eyes (sclera), and darker-than-normal urine. Jaundice occurs when contraction of seasonal evils or dietary irregularities cause damp-heat or cold-damp to obstruct the center burner, preventing bile from flowing according to its normal course.

643. 痉病〔痙病〕 *jìng bìng*, **tetany** ['tɛtənɪ]: Severe spasm such as rigidity in the neck, clenched jaw, convulsions of the limbs, and arched-back

rigidity. In severe cases, there is clouding reversal (loss of consciousness), which is often referred to as "tetanic reversal" (痙厥 *jìng jué*). Repletion patterns are attributed to wind, cold, dampness, phlegm, or fire congesting the channels, whereas vacuity patterns occur when excessive sweating, loss of blood, or constitutional vacuity causes qì vacuity, shortage of blood, and insufficiency of the fluids, which deprive the sinews of nourishment and allow internal wind to stir. To resolve tetany, repletion patterns are treated primarily by dispelling wind and secondarily by supporting right qì, whereas vacuity patterns are treated primarily by boosting qì and nourishing the blood and secondarily by extinguishing wind. Distinction is made between "soft tetany" (柔痙 *róu jìng*) and "hard tetany" (剛痙 *gāng jìng*), the former being distinguished from the latter by the presence of sweating and absence of aversion to cold. The terms yīn tetany and yáng tetany are synonymous with soft and hard tetany, or may denote tetany with and without counterflow cold of the limbs, respectively. Tetany may occur as a sign of a variety of different diseases, including, but not limited to, tetanus (see lockjaw); occurring in infants and children, it is referred to as fright wind.

644. 小儿惊风〔小兒驚風〕*xiǎo ér jīng fēng*, **child fright wind** [tʃaɪld fraɪt wɪnd]: A disease of infants and children, characterized by convulsions and loss of consciousness. Fright wind is equivalent to tetany in adults. Distinction is made between acute and chronic forms: acute fright wind; chronic fright wind.

645. 惊风〔驚風〕*jīng fēng*, **fright wind** [fraɪt wɪnd]: See child fright wind.

646. 疳〔疳〕*gān*, **gān** [gæn]: **1.** A disease of infancy or childhood characterized by emaciation, dry hair, heat effusion (fever) of varying degree, abdominal distention with visible superficial veins, yellow face and emaciated flesh, and loss of essence-spirit vitality. Pathomechanically, it essentially involves dryness of the fluids due to damage to spleen and stomach that results from dietary intemperance, evils, and in particular, worms. Other viscera besides the spleen may be affected, hence there are the "five gān" (i.e., gān of the heart, gān of the lung, gān of the liver, gān of the spleen, and gān of the kidney). **2.** Various kinds of ulcerations and sores, e.g., "child eye gān" (小儿疳眼 *xiǎo ér gān yán*).

647. 疟疾〔瘧疾〕*nüè jí*, **malaria** [məˈlɛrɪə]: A recurrent disease that is characterized by shivering, vigorous heat [effusion], and sweating and that is classically attributed to contraction of summerheat during the hot season, contact with "mountain forest miasma" (山岚瘴气 *shān*

lán zhàng qì), or contraction of cold-damp. Malaria is explained as evil qì latent at midstage (half-exterior and half-interior). Different forms are distinguished according to signs and causes.

648. 心痹〔心痹〕*xīn bì*, **heart impediment** [hɑrt ɪmˈpɛdɪmənt]: A disease of the heart that is characterized by pain and by suffocating oppression and that is caused by stasis obstruction of the heart vessels. *Elementary Questions (Sù Wèn)* states, "Heart impediment is stoppage in the vessels. ..." The stoppage may actually be due to either a) an inadequate warming and propulsion of the blood as a result of insufficiency of yáng qì or b) an obstruction of the heart vessels by static blood that forms when internal phlegm turbidity impedes blood flow. Signs of heart impediment include dull pain and stifling oppression in the chest, which are attributed to impaired yáng qì perfusion or obstruction of the network vessels by phlegm stasis (blood stasis resulting from the presence of phlegm). Attacks (发作 *fā zuò*) are characterized by gripping pain in the heart (心绞痛 *xīn jiǎo tòng*, angina pectoris), green-blue or purple complexion, cold limbs, and a faint fine pulse verging on expiration, which indicate severe obstruction of heart qì and heart yáng. Heart palpitations, fearful throbbing, fatigued spirit, and shortness of breath are general signs of heart qì vacuity between attacks.

649. 奔豚〔奔豚〕*bēn tún*, **running piglet** [ˈrʌnɪŋ ˈpɪglət]: A sensation of upsurge from the lower abdomen to the chest and throat, accompanied by gripping abdominal pain, oppression in the chest, rapid breathing, dizziness, heart palpitations, and heart vexation. This pattern results from an upsurging of yīn cold qì of the kidney or from liver channel qì fire ascending counterflow (肝经气火上逆).

650. 鼓胀〔鼓脹〕*gǔ zhàng*, **drum distention** [ˈdrʌm–dɪsˌtɛnʃən]: Severe abdominal distention. Drum distention is also called abdominal distention. It is attributed to a variety of causes and usually involves spleen disease affecting the liver or liver and spleen disease affecting the kidney.

651. 消渴〔消渴〕*xiāo kě*, **dispersion-thirst** [dɪsˈpɝʒən θɝst]: **1.** Any disease characterized by thirst, increased fluid intake, and copious urine. Dispersion-thirst is categorized as upper burner, center burner, and lower burner dispersion, depending on the pathomechanism. It includes conditions diagnosed in Western medicine as diabetes mellitus. **2.** Thirst (as in reverting yīn disease).

652. 癥瘕积聚〔癥瘕積聚〕*zhēng jiǎ jī jù*, **concretions, conglomerations, accumulations, and gatherings** [kənˈkriʃənz kənˌglɑməˈreʃənz əˌkjumjəˈleʃənz ənd ˈgæðərɪŋz]: Four kinds of abdominal masses as-

sociated with pain and distention. Concretions and accumulations are masses of definite form and fixed location that are associated with pain of fixed location. They stem from disease in the viscera and blood aspect. Conglomerations and gatherings are masses of indefinite form that gather and dissipate at irregular intervals and are attended by pain of unfixed location. They are attributed to disease in the bowels and qì aspect. Accumulations and gatherings chiefly occur in the center burner. Concretions and conglomerations chiefly occur in the lower burner and in many cases are the result of gynecological diseases. In general, concretions, conglomerations, accumulations, and gatherings arise when emotional depression or dietary intemperance causes damage to the liver and spleen. The resultant organ disharmony leads to obstruction and stagnation of qì, which in turn causes static blood to collect gradually. Most often the root cause is insufficiency of right qì.

653. 疝 〔 疝 〕 *shàn*, **mounting** ['mɑʊntɪŋ]: Any of various diseases characterized by pain or swelling of the abdomen or scrotum. Traditional literature describes many different diseases and patterns labeled as "mounting." Mounting disease can be divided into three categories: (1) Conditions characterized by the protrusion of the abdominal contents through the abdominal wall, the inguen, or the base of the abdominal cavity, and usually associated with qì pain. Also called mounting qì. This corresponds to hernia in Western medicine. (2) Various diseases of the external genitals, including conditions known as hydrocele (水囊肿 *shuǐ náng zhǒng*) and hematoma (血肿 *xuè zhǒng*) of the testis in Western medicine. In traditional literature, scrotal conditions are sometimes referred to as "unilateral sagging (of the testicles)" (偏坠 *piān zhuì*). (3) Certain forms of acute abdominal pain associated with urinary and fecal stoppage.

654. 疝气 〔 疝氣 〕 *shàn qì*, **mounting qì** ['mɑʊntɪŋ tʃi]: See mounting.

655. 中风 〔 中風 〕 *zhòng fēng*, **wind stroke; wind strike** ['wɪnd–strok, 'wɪnd–straɪk]: **1.** A disease characterized by the sudden appearance of hemiplegia, deviated eyes and mouth, and impeded speech that may or may not start with sudden clouding collapse. Wind stroke occurs a) when depletion of yīn essence or sudden anger causes hyperactivity of liver yáng that stirs liver wind; b) when, owing to a predilection for rich, fatty foods, phlegm-heat congests in the inner body and transforms into wind; c) when vacuity of qì and blood causes vacuity wind; or d) when a patient suffering from internal vacuity suddenly contracts external wind. Distinction can be made between: a) channel and network [vessel] stroke, which is marked by deviated eyes and mouth, inhibited

speech, and hemiplegia with no change in spirit-mind; and b) bowel and visceral stroke, marked by sudden collapse and loss of consciousness. Bowel and visceral stroke can be divided into block patterns characterized by clenched jaw and clenched hands and desertion patterns marked by closed eyes and open mouth, limp hand and snoring nose, urinary and fecal incontinence, and in some cases by spontaneous sweating. **2.** An external wind contraction described in *On Cold Damage* (*Shāng Hán Lùn*) as one type of greater yáng (*tài yáng*) disease. *On Cold Damage* (*Shāng Hán Lùn*) states, "Greater yáng disease, with heat effusion, sweating, aversion to wind, and a pulse that is moderate, is called wind stroke."

656. 癫痫〔癲癇〕*diān xián*, **epilepsy** ['ɛpɪˌlɛpsɪ]: A disease characterized by brief episodes (fits) of temporary loss of spirit, white complexion, and fixity of the eyes (双目凝视 *shuāng mù níng shì*), or sudden clouding collapse, foaming at the mouth, upward-staring eyes, clenched jaw, convulsions of the limbs, and in some cases squealing like a goat or pig. After an episode, the patient experiences fatigue and then returns to normal. Epilepsy is attributed to fear and fright or emotional imbalance, dietary irregularities, and taxation damaging the liver, spleen, and kidney channels and causing wind-phlegm to be carried upward by qì.

657. 癫狂〔癲狂〕*diān kuáng*, **mania and withdrawal** ['menɪəə nd 'wɪðdrɔəl]: Mental derangement. Mania denotes states of excitement characterized by noisy, unruly, and even aggressive behavior, offensive speech, constant singing and laughter, irascibility, springing walls and climbing roofs, and inability to remain tidily dressed. This is a yáng pattern of the heart spirit straying outward owing to hyperactivity of yáng qì. Withdrawal refers to emotional depression, indifference, deranged speech, taciturnity, and obliviousness of hunger or satiety. It is a yīn pattern caused by binding of depressed qì and phlegm or heart-spleen vacuity.

658. 破伤风〔破傷風〕*pò shāng fēng*, **lockjaw** ['lɑkdʒɔ]: Tetany that occurs when an external injury or mouth sores permit the invasion of wind evil. Lockjaw begins with lack of strength in the limbs, headache, pain in the cheeks, clenched jaw, difficulty in turning the neck, and heat effusion (fever) and aversion to cold. Subsequently, there is a spasm of the facial muscles that creates the appearance of a strange grimace, tightly clenched jaw, stiff tongue, drooling, intermittent generalized spasm, and arched-back rigidity. The pulse is rapid or tight and stringlike. Finally, speech, swallowing, and breathing all become difficult, and, in the worst cases, the patient dies of asphyxiation.

659. 癃闭〔癃閉〕*lóng bì*, **dribbling urinary block** [ˈdrɪblɪŋ ˈjurɪˌnɛrɪ blɑk]: Dribbling urination or, in severe cases, almost complete blockage of urine flow. Distinction is made between a number of vacuity and repletion patterns. Vacuity patterns include insufficiency of center qì and kidney qì vacuity. The repletion patterns include lower burner damp-heat, lung qì congestion, binding depression of liver qì, and urinary tract stasis blockage.

660. 水肿〔水腫〕*shuǐ zhǒng*, **water swelling** [ˈwɔtɚ–ˌswɛlɪŋ]: Swelling of the flesh that occurs when dysfunction of the spleen, kidney, and lung due to internal or external causes allows water to accumulate. It is attributed to spleen-kidney yáng vacuity or external evils impairing the diffusion of lung qì.

661. 淋证〔淋證〕*lín zhèng*, **strangury pattern** [ˈstræŋgjərɪ–ˌpætɚn]: Any of several disease patterns characterized by urinary urgency, frequent short painful rough voidings, and dribbling incontinence. Strangury is attributed to damp-heat gathering and pouring into the bladder. In persistent conditions or in elderly or weak patients, the cause may be center qì fall or kidney vacuity with impaired qì transformation. Distinction is made between stone strangury, qì strangury, blood strangury, unctuous strangury, and taxation strangury, known collectively as the "five stranguries."

662. 血淋〔血淋〕*xuè lín*, **blood strangury** [ˈblʌd–stræŋgjərɪ]: See strangury.

663. 气淋〔氣淋〕*qì lín*, **qì strangury** [ˈtʃi–stræŋgjərɪ]: See strangury.

664. 膏淋〔膏淋〕*gāo lín*, **unctuous strangury** [ˈʌŋktjuəs ˈstræŋgjərɪ]: Strangury with urine that is like rice water, nasal mucus, or animal fat. See strangury.

665. 石淋〔石淋〕*shí lín*, **stone strangury** [ˈston–stræŋgjərɪ]: See strangury.

666. 劳淋〔勞淋〕*láo lín*, **taxation strangury** [tækˈseʃən ˈstræŋgjərɪ]: See strangury.

667. 淋浊〔淋濁〕*lín zhuó*, **strangury-turbidity** [ˈstræŋgjərɪ tɚˌbɪdɪtɪ]: A generic name for strangury and turbid urine.

668. 转胞〔轉胞〕*zhuǎn bāo*, **shifted bladder** [ˈʃɪftɪd ˈblædɚ]: Urinary stoppage or frequent voiding of small amounts of urine occurring in the seventh or eighth month of pregnancy; attributable to qì vacuity or kidney vacuity.

669. 茄子病〔茄子病〕*qié zi bìng*, **eggplant disease** [ˈɛgplænt-dɪˌzi z]: A traditional term for prolapse of the uterus.

670. 崩漏〔崩漏〕*bēng lòu,* **flooding and spotting** [ˈflʌdɪŋ ənd ˈspatɪŋ]: Any abnormal discharge of blood via the vagina. Flooding (崩 *bēng*) is heavy menstrual flow or abnormal bleeding via the vagina (uterine bleeding); spotting (漏 *lòu*), lit. "leaking" in Chinese, is a slight, often continual discharge of blood via the vagina. If the flow is deep red and clotted, it is usually a sign of heat. Since each may give way to the other, they are commonly referred to together. Flooding and spotting usually occur in puberty or at menopause. They are attributed to insecurity of the thoroughfare (*chōng*) and controlling (*rèn*) vessels, which may stem from a variety of causes.

671. 遏阻〔遏阻〕*è zǔ,* **malign obstruction; morning sickness** [məˈlaɪn əbˈstrʌkʃən, ˈmɔrnɪŋ ˈsɪknɪs]: A condition of aversion to food, nausea, and vomiting during pregnancy, not considered untoward unless it severely affects food intake. Malign obstruction is the manifestation of impaired harmonious downbearing of stomach qì, which may be due to causes such as liver heat, phlegm stagnation, stomach cold, or stomach heat. In Western medicine, it is called *emesis gravidarum* and is commonly referred to as "morning sickness."

672. 恶露不行〔惡露不行〕*è lù bù xíng,* **retention of the lochia** [rɪˈtɛnʃən əv ðə ˈlokɪə]: Absence of normal postpartum discharge. Retention of the lochia is when cold evil exploits the sudden vacuity of qì and blood created by childbirth and invades the uterine vessels, where it congeals and causes blood stasis. It may also arise in patients with constitutional vacuity when damage to qì and blood through childbirth causes sluggish movement of the blood.

673. 恶露不断〔惡露不斷〕*è lù bù duàn,* **persistent flow of the lochia** [pəˈsɪstənt flo əv ðə ˈlokɪə]: Flow of the lochia in excess of 20 days. Persistent flow of lochia is attributed to qì vacuity, blood heat, or blood stasis.

674. 无子〔無子〕*wú zǐ,* **childlessness** [ˈtʃaɪldləsnɪs]: Inability of male or female to produce offspring; sterility.

675. 不孕〔不孕〕*bù yùn,* **infertility** [ɪnfɚˈtɪlɪtɪ]: Inability to become pregnant between menarche and menopause. In clinical practice, a woman who fails to become pregnant within three years of normal conjugal life without the use of contraception is considered infertile. Chinese medicine recognizes congenital factors and acquired factors.

676. 阴挺〔陰挺〕*yīn tǐng,* **yīn protrusion** [jɪn prəˈtruʒən]: A women's disease characterized by heaviness, sagging, and swelling of the anterior yīn or the hanging of the interior outside the body. Yīn protrusion is usually the result of center qì fall or insufficiency of kidney qì, if not

due to holding the breath and straining in childbirth. The center qì fall pattern is one of vacuity and includes signs such as a sagging sensation in the abdomen, heart palpitations, shortness of breath, lassitude of spirit, vaginal discharge, and a floating vacuous pulse. Kidney vacuity is identified by the presence of limp aching lumbus and knees. If there is redness, swelling, and exudation of yellow water, as is often the case when friction causes damage, the pattern is considered to be one of damp-heat pouring downward; this condition may also be identified by a burning sensation on urination, heart vexation, spontaneous sweating, a dry mouth with bitter taste, and a slippery rapid pulse.

677. 肺痈〔肺癰〕*fèi yōng*, **pulmonary welling-abscess** [ˈpʌlməˌnɛrɪ ˈwɛl-ɪŋ–ˌæbsɪs]: A welling-abscess (*yōng*) in the lung. It occurs when externally contracted wind evil and heat toxin brew and obstruct the lung, and when the heat causes congestion and blood stasis, which binds to form a welling-abscess (*yōng*) that in time starts to suppurate. The classic sign is coughing up pus and blood. Pulmonary welling-abscess (*yōng*) is associated with heat effusion (fever) and shivering, and with cough, chest pain, rapid respiration, expectoration of sticky fishy-smelling purulent phlegm, and in severe cases expectoration of phlegm and blood.

678. 肠痈〔腸癰〕*cháng yōng*, **intestinal welling-abscess** [ɪnˈtɛstɪnl̩ ˈwɛl-ɪŋ–ˌæbsɪs]: Welling-abscess of the intestine; attributed to congealing blood that stems from damp-heat or from general qì and blood stagnation. It corresponds to appendicitis or periappendicular abscess in Western medicine.

679. 肺痿〔肺痿〕*fèi wěi*, **lung wilting** [lʌŋ ˈwɪltɪŋ]: A chronic condition characterized by a dull-sounding cough, ejection of thick turbid foamy drool, panting at the slightest exertion, dry mouth and pharynx, emaciation, red dry tongue, and a vacuous rapid pulse. In some cases, there may be tidal heat [effusion], and, in severe cases, the skin and hair may become dry. It is attributed to dryness-heat and enduring cough damaging the lung, or damage to fluid due to other disease depriving the lung of moisturization.

680. 衄〔衄〕*nǜ*, **spontaneous external bleeding** [spɑnˈteniəs ɪksˈtɜ·nl̩ ˈblidɪŋ]: Bleeding not attributable to external injury, especially nosebleed. It includes nosebleed, spontaneous bleeding of the nipple, spontaneous bleeding of the ear, spontaneous bleeding of the flesh, spontaneous bleeding of the gums, and spontaneous bleeding of the tongue.

681. 瘿〔瘿〕*yǐng*, **goiter** [ˈgɔɪtɚ]: Swelling at the front and sides of the neck that moves up and down as the patient swallows. In Western medicine, goiter is usually enlargement of the thyroid gland.

682. 脚气〔腳氣〕*jiǎo qì*, **leg qì** [lɛg tʃi]: A disease characterized by numbness, pain, limpness, and in some cases any of a variety of possible signs such as hypertonicity or swelling, withering, redness and swelling of the calf, heat effusion, and in advanced stages by abstraction of spirit-mind, heart palpitations, panting, oppression in the chest, nausea and vomiting, and deranged speech. Leg qì arises when externally contracted damp evil and wind toxin or accumulating dampness due to damage by excessive consumption of rich food engenders heat and pours down into the legs. Chest and abdominal signs are attributed to leg qì surging into the heart (脚气冲心 *jiǎo qì chōng xīn*). In Western medicine leg qì corressponds to beriberi, which is attributed to vitamin B_1 deficiency.

5.2. 外科疾病
External Medicine Diseases

683. 疮疡〔瘡瘍〕*chuāng yáng*, **sore** [sɔr]: A generic term for diseases of external medicine, such as welling-abscess, flat-abscess, clove sore, boil, streaming sore, and scrofula, generally caused by toxic evils invading the body, evil heat scorching the blood, and congestion of qì and blood. Sores are treated differently according to whether they are yīn or yáng, according to their stage of development, and according to the channel affected.

684. 痈〔癰〕*yōng*, **welling-abscess** [ˈwɛlɪŋ–ˌæbsɪs]: A large suppuration in the flesh characterized by a painful swelling and redness that is clearly circumscribed, and that before rupturing is soft and characterized by a thin shiny skin. Before suppuration begins, it can be easily dispersed; when pus has formed, it easily ruptures (易溃 *yì kuì*); after rupture, it easily closes and heals. It may be associated with generalized heat [effusion], thirst, yellow tongue fur, and a rapid pulse.

685. 疽〔疽〕*jū*, **flat-abscess** [ˈflæt–æbsɪs]: A deep malign suppuration in the flesh, sinew, and even the bone, attributed to toxic evil obstructing qì and blood.

686. 疖〔癤〕*jié*, **boil** [bɑɪl]: A small, round, superficial swelling that is hot and painful, suppurates within a few days, and easily bursts. It is attributable to heat toxin or to summerheat-heat and usually occurs in the summer and autumn.

687. 疔疮〔疔瘡〕*dīng chuāng,* **clove sore** ['klov–sɔr]: A small, hard sore with a deep root like a clove or nail, appearing most commonly on the face and ends of the fingers. A clove sore occurs when fire toxin enters the body through a wound, and then heat brews and binds in the skin and flesh. It may also occur when anger, anxiety, and preoccupation or excessive indulgence in rich food or alcohol lead to accumulated heat in the bowels and viscera, which effuses outward to the skin. A clove sore may sometimes have a single red threadlike line stretching from the sore toward the trunk. This is known as a "red-thread clove sore." Severe forms are known as toxin clove sores, whose toxin can spread to penetrate the blood aspect and attack the bowels and viscera, causing clouded spirit. This is called "running yellow" (走黄 *zǒu huáng*).

688. 瘰疬〔瘰癧〕*luǒ lì,* **scrofula** ['skrɑfjələ]: Lumps beneath the skin on the side of the neck and under the armpits. These are often referred to in older books as "saber and pearl-string lumps" (马刀侠瘿 *mǎ dāo jiā yǐng*) because of the saber-like formation they can make below the armpit and the necklace-like formation they make on the neck. Scrofula occurs when phlegm gathers in the neck, armpits, or groin. The phlegm is produced when vacuity fire occurring in lung-kidney vacuity scorches the fluids. In some cases, wind-fire evil toxin is also a factor.

689. 痰核〔痰核〕*tán hé,* **phlegm node** ['flɛm–nod]: Any lump below the skin that feels soft and slippery under the finger, is associated with no redness, pain, or swelling, and (unlike scrofula) does not suppurate.

690. 流注〔流注〕*liú zhù,* **streaming sore** ['strimɪŋ–sɔr]: A suppuration deep in the body that is so called because of the tendency of its toxin to move from one place to another, as if flowing through the flesh. A streaming sore begins with a lump or diffuse swelling of the flesh. Pus forms, and after rupture and thorough drainage, the sore can heal.

691. 疥〔疥〕*jiè,* **scab** [skæb]: A disease characterized by small papules the size of a pinhead that are associated with insufferable penetrating itching and that, when scratched, may suppurate or crust without producing any exudate. Scab commonly occurs between the fingers and may also be observed on the inside of the elbow, in the armpits, on the lower abdomen, in the groin, and on the buttocks and thighs, and, in severe cases, over the whole body. It is attributed to damp-heat depressed in the skin and is transmitted by contact.

692. 癞〔癩〕*lài,* **lài** [lɑɪ]: **1.** Leprosy. **2.** Scab, lichen, etc., that lead to hair loss on the affected area.

693. 癣〔癬〕*xiǎn,* **lichen** ['lɑɪkən]: A skin disease characterized by elevation of the skin, serous discharge, scaling, and itching. Lichen is asso-

ciated with wind, heat, and dampness. Lichen characterized by dryness and scaling of the skin is called "dry lichen" (干癣 *gān xiǎn*), whereas lichen that exudes a discharge is called damp lichen (湿癣 *shī xiǎn*).

694. **口（中生）疮**〔口（中生）瘡〕*kǒu (zhōng shēng) chuāng,* **mouth sore** [mɑʊθ sor]: A pale yellow or gray-white ulceration appearing singly or multiply on the inside of the mouth (lips, cheeks, or palate). Usuall oval in shape, a mouth sore is surrounded by a red areola and has a cratered surface. It is associated with scorching pain, affects eating and swallowing, and is recurrent. It is attributed to repletion fire, spleen heat engendering phlegm, or dual vacuity of the spleen and kidney. Mouth sores are called aphthous stomatitis in Western medicine.

695. **口舌生疮**〔口舌生瘡〕*kǒu shé shēng chuāng,* **sores of the mouth and tongue** [sorz əv ðə mɑʊθ ənd tʌŋ]: See mouth sore.

696. **冻疮**〔凍瘡〕*dòng chuāng,* **frostbite** ['frɑstbɑɪt]: Severe damage to the skin and flesh that occurs when cold and wind cause qì and blood to congeal and stagnate. Frostbite usually affects the hands, feet, and ears. The affected areas present a somber white complexion that gradually turns purple-red and forms macules. This is associated with a burning sensation, itching, and numbness. In severe cases, the macules rupture, giving way to sores that heal with difficulty. Frostbite can be prevented by adequate clothing and physical movement.

697. **丹毒**〔丹毒〕*dān dú,* **erysipelas; cinnabar toxin [sore]** [ˌɛrɪˈsɪpələs, ˈcɪnəbɑr ˈtɑksɪn (sor)]: A condition characterized by sudden localized reddening of the skin, giving it the appearance of having been smeared with cinnabar. Cinnabar toxin usually affects the face and lower legs, is most common among children and the elderly, and usually occurs in spring and summer. Cinnabar toxin is known by different names according to form and location. When it affects the head, it is called "head fire cinnabar" (抱头火丹 *bào tóu huǒ dān*). When it assumes a wandering pattern, it is called "wandering cinnabar" (赤游丹 *chì yóu dān*), as is observed in newborns. Cinnabar toxin of the lower legs is called "fire flow" (流火 *liú huǒ*) or "fire cinnabar leg" (火丹脚 *huǒ dān jiǎo*). Cinnabar toxin occurs when damaged skin and insecurity of defense qì allow evil toxin to enter the body and cause heat in the blood aspect, which becomes trapped in the skin. If the toxin is accompanied by wind, the face is affected; if accompanied by dampness, the lower legs are affected. Thus, the facial type tends to be wind-heat, whereas the lower leg type is damp-heat. The disease develops swiftly.

698. **扭伤**〔扭傷〕*niǔ shāng,* **sprain** [spren]: Damage to the sinew and flesh and to blood vessels around the joints such as the shoulder, elbow,

wrist, lumbus, hip, knee, and ankle joints, due to twisting, pulling, or knocks and falls. Sprains are characterized by pain, by swelling, and by discoloration of the skin due to stasis and blockage. Red indicates damage to the skin and flesh; blue-green indicates damage to the sinews; purple indicates blood stasis. Slight local swelling and tenderness indicate mild injury. Pronounced swelling and difficulty in flexing the joint are signs of a severe sprain.

习题
Questions

Answer the following questions in English:

531. What disease is characterized by a whitening of the throat?
....

532. What is tonsillitis traditionally called in Chinese medicine?
....

533. What disease is characterized by vomiting and diarrhea, and in some cases by severe cramps? ....

534. What disease is characterized by the sensation of an upsurge from the lower abdomen to the chest and throat that is accompanied by gripping abdominal pain, oppression in the chest, rapid breathing, dizziness, heart palpitations, and heart vexation? ....

535. What are the four kinds of abdominal masses discussed in Chinese medical literature? ....

536. Into what traditional disease category do hydrocele and hematoma of the testis fall? ....

537. What disease is characterized by the sudden appearance of hemiplegia, deviated eyes and mouth, and impeded speech?
....

538. What disease is characterized by sudden clouding collapse, foaming at the mouth, upward-staring eyes, clenched jaw, and convulsion of the limbs, and in some cases, squealing like a goat or pig?
....

539. Explain the terms flooding and spotting. ....

540. What disease is characterized by aversion to food, nausea, and vomiting in pregnancy? ....

541. What disease is characterized by a sudden localized reddening of the skin? ....

542. What is the traditional name for a small, hard sore with a deep root? ....

543. What is the name of the disease characterized by lumps beneath the skin on the side of the neck and under the armpits? ....

544. What is the difference between a flat-abscess and a welling-abscess?
....

545. What skin disease is characterized by elevation of the skin, a serous discharge, scaling, and itching? ....

546. What does the term "streaming sore" refer to?
....

547. Into which disease category does enlargement of the thyroid gland fall? ....

548. What disease is characterized by recurrent episodes of shivering, vigorous heat, and sweating? ....

549. Into what traditional disease category does diabetes mellitus fall?
....

550. Fright wind in children corresponds to what disease in adults?
....

551. What disease is characterized by stiffness of the neck that results from taxation fatigue (overwork, etc.), twisting, sleeping in the wrong posture, or from exposure to a draft (wind-cold)? ....

552. Vomiting in the evening of food ingested in the morning or vomiting in the morning of food ingested in the evening is a sign of what disease? ....

553. What is globus hystericus called in Chinese medicine?
....

554. What disease is characterized by weakness and limpness of the sinews accompanied by the sensation that the elbow, wrist, knee, and ankle are dislocated? ....

555. What contagious disease is characterized by cough with expectoration of blood, tidal heat effusion, night sweating, and emaciation?

556. Wheezing occurs with what? ....

557. What disease is characterized by persistent nasal congestion with turbid snivel and is attributable to wind-cold, wind-heat, or gall-bladder heat? ....

558. Any disease not resulting from external evils is called what? ....

559. What disease in children is characterized by papules that appear behind the ears and on the neck and face and that spread to the limbs? ....

560. What disease is characterized by persistently remittent, usually intense headache, and is attributed to wind-cold or wind-heat invasion and obstruction of the channels by phlegm or static blood? ....

Give the Pīnyīn and English for the following Chinese terms:

561. 噎膈 ....

562. 痹证 ....

563. 痿证 ....

564. 淋证 ....

565. 疳 ....

566. 鼓胀 ....

567. 疝 ....

568. 癃闭 ....

569. 肠痈 ....

570. 膏淋 ....

571. 疖 ....

572. 疽 ....

573. 天花 ....

574. 百日咳 ....

575. 癥瘕积聚 ....

576. 落枕 ....

577. 哮喘 ....

578. 头风 ....

579. 水肿 ....

580. 破伤风 ....

Supply the Chinese and English for the following:

581. *Shí lín.* ....

582. *Bēng lòu.* ....

583. *Fèi wěi.* ....

584. *Fèi yōng.* ....

585. *Luǒ lì.* ....

586. *Chuāng yáng.* ....

587. *Yǐng.* ....

588. *Tán hé.* ....

589. *Xiǎn.* ....

590. *Diān kuáng.* ....

591. *Huǎng dǎn.* ....

592. *Jìng bìng.* ....

593. *Rǔ é.* ....

594. *Gān.* ....

595. *Lì jí.* ....

596. *Jīng fēng.* ....

597. *Huò luàn.* ....

598. *Shàn qì.* ....

599. *Dòu.* ....

600. *Fǎn wèi.* ....

Give the Chinese and Pīnyīn for the following:

601. Strangury pattern. ....

602. Pulmonary welling-abscess. ....

603. Shifted bladder. ....

第六章　证候
Patterns

699. 证（候）〔證（候）〕 *zhèng hòu*, **pattern** ['pætɚn]: A manifestation of human sickness that reflects the nature, location, or cause of sickness. For example, the simultaneous presence of heat effusion, aversion to cold, and floating pulse forms an exterior pattern due to an external contraction; vigorous heat effusion, vexation and thirst, red tongue with yellow fur, and constipation constitutes an "interior repletion pattern." Also called "disease pattern" and "pathocondition."

700. 病证〔病證〕 *bìng zhèng*, **disease pattern** [dɪ'ziz-ˌpætɚn]: See pattern.

701. 症〔症〕 *zhèng*, **pathocondition** ['pæθəkɑnˌdɪʃən]: See pattern.

6.1. 八纲辨证
Eight-Principle Pattern Identification

702. 八纲辨证〔八綱辨證〕 *bā gāng biàn zhèng*, **eight-principle pattern identification** [et 'prɪnsɪpl̩ 'pætɚn–aɪˌdɛntɪfɪˌkeʃən]: Identification of disease patterns by eight fundamental principles, namely interior and exterior, cold and heat, vacuity and repletion, and yīn and yáng. Interior and exterior are the principles of depth of the disease; cold and heat are the nature of disease; vacuity and repletion are the weakness of right qì and strength of evil qì. Yīn and yáng, which embrace the other six principles, are general categories of disease. Interior, cold, and vacuity are yīn, whereas exterior, heat, and repletion are yáng. Each principle is associated with specific signs. By matching the patient's signs to them, it is possible to determine (1) the depth and nature of the disease and (2) the relative strength of the forces that resist disease and those that cause it. Eight-principle pattern identification is a preliminary organization of examination data: treatment should be determined only when other methods of pattern identification have provided a more detailed picture of the patient's condition.

703. **表证**〔表證〕*biǎo zhèng*, **exterior pattern** [ɪks'tɪrɪə–ˌpætən]: The manifestation of disease in the exterior of the body, caused by any of the six excesses entering the body's exterior; characterized by sudden onset and by aversion to cold (or the milder aversion to wind), heat effusion (fever), headache, a thin tongue fur, and a floating pulse. Other possible signs are headache, nasal congestion, and aching pain in the limbs and joints. Distinction is made between exterior cold, exterior heat, exterior vacuity, and exterior repletion.

704. **表寒**〔表寒〕*biǎo hán*, **exterior cold** [ɪks'tɪrɪə kold]: Exterior cold patterns are characterized by pronounced cold signs with a distinct aversion to cold. The pulse is tight and floating; the tongue fur is thin, white, and moist. "When cold prevails there is pain," and in exterior cold patterns, headache and generalized pain and heaviness are also pronounced. Runny nose with clear snivel (nasal mucus) and expectoration of clear thin phlegm are common signs. Exterior cold patterns are caused by contraction of wind-cold evil.

705. **表热**〔表熱〕*biǎo rè*, **exterior heat** [ɪks'tɪrɪə hit]: Exterior heat patterns are characterized by pronounced heat signs, such as a red sore pharynx and a relatively red tongue with dry fur. In addition to the regular external signs, the pulse is floating and rapid. Other signs include cough and the production of thick white or yellow phlegm. Most exterior heat patterns are attributable to contraction of wind-heat evil. Note that identification of exterior heat patterns is based on assessment of heat and cold "signs" rather than the actual body temperature. Heat effusion (fever) as a sign does not necessarily correspond to heat in the sense of the eight principles.

706. **表虚**〔表虛〕*biǎo xū*, **exterior vacuity** [ɪks'tɪrɪə və'kjuətɪ]: Exterior patterns with persistent sweating and heat effusion (fever). Exterior vacuity results from construction-defense disharmony in which the body's resistance to external evils is lowered and, despite sweating, fails to expel the evil. Such conditions are reflected in a moderate (i.e., not tight) floating pulse.

707. **表实**〔表實〕*biǎo shí*, **exterior repletion** [ɪks'tɪrɪə rɪ'pliʃən]: Exterior patterns without sweating are exterior repletion patterns. In most cases, exterior repletion patterns are exterior cold patterns caused by contraction of exuberant cold evil that obstructs defense qi and blocks the interstices; they manifest in a tight floating pulse.

708. **里证**〔裡證〕*lǐ zhèng*, **interior pattern** [ɪn'tɪrɪə–ˌpætən]: Any disease pattern that indicates disease of the interior. (1) Any disease pattern of the bowels or viscera, in contradistinction to externally contracted

heat (febrile) disease, e.g., liver disease characterized by dizziness and rib-side pain; heart disease characterized by heart palpitations or fearful throbbing; spleen disease characterized by abdominal distention and diarrhea; and kidney disease characterized by lumbar pain and seminal emission. (2) In externally contracted heat (febrile) disease, an interior pattern arises when an evil that has caused an exterior pattern passes into the interior. Rarely, external evils may strike the interior directly; in most cases, they pass through the exterior. Hence febrile disease interior patterns are identified when aversion to wind or cold—which may or may not be accompanied by heat effusion (fever) or sweating—gives way to high fever or tidal heat [effusion], vexation and agitation, thirst, clouded spirit, abdominal pain or distention, diarrhea or constipation, short voidings of reddish urine or inhibited urination, dry yellow tongue fur, and a rapid sunken pulse.

709. 半表半里证〔半表半裡證〕*bàn biǎo bàn lǐ zhèng,* **midstage pattern; half-interior half-exterior pattern** [ˈmɪdstedʒ ˈpætɚn, hælf ɪnˈtɪriɚ hæf ɪksˈtɪriɚ-ˌpætɚn]: A disease pattern that occurs when an exterior evil fails to reach the interior and right qì is too weak to fight it. The signs are alternating [aversion to] cold and heat [effusion], chest and rib-side fullness, heart vexation, no desire for food and drink, bitter taste in the mouth, dry pharynx, dizzy vision, and stringlike pulse. The etiology of midstage patterns is considered in detail under lesser yáng (*shào yáng*) disease.

710. 寒证〔寒證〕*hán zhèng,* **cold pattern** [ˈkold-ˌpætɚn]: Any disease pattern characterized by cold signs such as aversion to cold, a somber white or green-blue facial complexion, slow or tight pulse, no thirst or desire for warm fluid, and long voidings of clear urine. It is attributed to exuberant yīn evil or to yáng vacuity. (1) Prevalence of yīn due to an exuberant yīn evil accounts for pronounced cold signs such as abdominal pain, fulminant (i.e., sudden and violent) vomiting or diarrhea, green-blue facial complexion, and a tight pulse. (2) Yáng vacuity accounts for signs more commonly encountered in clinical practice, such as liking for quiet, curled-up lying posture, long voidings of clear urine, clear-grain diarrhea, counterflow cold of the limbs, and a slow pulse.

711. 热证〔熱證〕*rè zhèng,* **heat pattern** [ˈhit-ˌpætɚn]: Any disease pattern characterized by heat signs. Heat patterns arise when a yáng evil invades the body or when yīn humor becomes insufficient. Thus, heat patterns are caused by a surfeit of yáng or a deficit of yīn, which form repletion heat or vacuity heat patterns, respectively. Repletion heat patterns are characterized by red complexion, red eyes, vigorous heat [ef-

fusion], agitation, thirst, desire for cold fluids, hard stool, short voidings of reddish urine, a red or crimson tongue with a yellow fur, and a rapid pulse or a rapid large surging pulse. Vacuity heat patterns are marked by vexing heat in the five hearts (palms, soles, and chest), steaming bone tidal heat [effusion], dry throat and mouth, smooth bare red tongue (mirror tongue), and a fine rapid pulse.

712. 虚证〔虛證〕 *xū zhèng,* **vacuity pattern** [vəˈkjuətɪ–ˌpætən]: Any disease pattern caused by weakness of the body's forces and absence of an evil. Vacuity patterns are attributed to insufficiencies of qì, blood, yīn, and yáng that arise from damage to right qì either through enduring illness, loss of blood, seminal loss, and great sweating, or by invasion of an external evil (yáng evils readily damage yīn humor and yīn evils readily damage yáng qì), constitutional weakness, or the wear and tear that comes with age. Since these insufficiencies frequently affect specific bowels or viscera, further distinction is made between such forms as heart yīn vacuity, liver blood vacuity, kidney yáng vacuity, lung qì vacuity, etc.

713. 虚损〔虛損〕 *xū sǔn,* **vacuity detriment** [vəˈkjuətɪ–ˌdɛtrɪmənt]: Any form of severe chronic insufficiency of yīn-yáng, qì-blood, and bowels and viscera that arises through internal damage by the seven affects, taxation fatigue, diet, excesses of drink and sex, or enduring illness.

714. 虚劳〔虛勞〕 *xū láo,* **vacuity taxation** [vəˈkjuətɪ–tækˈseʃən]: Any pattern of severe vacuity (of qì, blood, bowels, or viscera), including notably steaming bone and consumption. The term comes from *Essential Prescriptions of the Golden Coffer (Jīn Guì Yào Lüè, Xuè Bì Xū Láo Bìng Mài Zhèng Bìng Zhì)* and was explained in *The Origin and Indicators of Disease (Zhū Bìng Yuán Hòu Lùn)* as referring to any of various qì, blood, or organ vacuity patterns on the one hand and contagious diseases such as steaming bone and corpse transmission (传尸 *chuán shī,* i.e., consumption) on the other. Since then, it has become a convention to refer to the former patterns as vacuity detriment, whereas the latter patterns are referred to as consumption.

715. 实证〔實證〕 *shí zhèng,* **repletion pattern** [rɪˈpliʃən–ˌpætən]: Any condition in which the presence of an evil is resisted by the body; the opposite of vacuity pattern. Repletion patterns are attributed to external evils, water-damp, phlegm-rheum, static blood, worm accumulations, or food accumulations. They reflect the nature of the evil (e.g., cold being characterized by pale or green-blue complexion, clear thin cold fluids) and the location (e.g., stomach disease being marked by vomiting, belching, etc., or exterior disease being characterized by heat effu-

sion (fever), aversion to cold, and sweating). Most importantly, however, there are signs of right qì fighting the evil, such as pulses that are forceful at the deep level (e.g., rapid surging pulses, slippery stringlike pulses, and large replete pulses), pain or discomfort that refuses pressure, and sudden onset of disease.

716. 阴证〔陰證〕*yīn zhèng,* **yīn pattern** ['jɪn–ˌpætǝn]: Interior, cold, and vacuity patterns. Commonly observed signs include pale complexion, generalized heaviness, curled up lying psture, physical cold and cold limbs, fatigue and lack of strength, timid low voice, bland taste in the mouth, absence of thirst, fishy-smelling stood, short voidings of clear urine, pale tender-soft enlarged tongue, and sunken slow pulse that may be weak or fine and rough.

717. 阳证〔陽證〕*yáng zhèng,* **yáng pattern** ['jæŋ/jɑŋ–ˌpætǝn]: Exterior, heat, and repletion patterns. Commonly observed signs include red complexion, aversion to cold and heat effusion, scorching hot skin, vexed spirit, rough turbid voice, abnormal chiding and cursing, rough breathing, hasty panting and phlegm rale, dry mouth with thirst and intake of fluid, dry bound stool, rough painful urination, short voidings of red urine, red or crimson tongue with yellow or black fur or with prickles, and a pulse that is floating and rapid, large and surging, or slippery and replete.

718. 阴虚〔陰虚〕*yīn xū,* **yīn vacuity** ['jɪn–vǝˌkuɪtɪ]: The manifestation of insufficiency of the yīn aspect and depletion of liquid and blood. When yīn is vacuous, internal heat arises; hence there is low fever, heat in the hearts of the palms and soles, postmeridian heat effusion, emaciation, night sweating, dry mouth and throat, short voidings of reddish urine, red tongue with little or no fur, and a forceless fine rapid pulse. Yīn vacuity may be focused in any of the five viscera, especially in the kidney. See also liver yīn vacuity; heart yīn vacuity; spleen yīn vacuity; lung yīn vacuity; kidney yīn vacuity.

719. 阳虚〔陽虚〕*yáng xū,* **yáng vacuity** ['jæŋ/jɑŋ–vǝˌkuɪtɪ]: The manifestation of insufficiency of yáng qì; reduction in the warming and activating power of the body. Signs include fatigue and lack of strength, shortage of qì and laziness to speak, fear of cold, cold limbs, spontaneous sweating, pale white complexion, long voidings of clear urine, sloppy stool, pale tender-soft tongue, and a large vacuous or faint fine pulse. Yáng vacuity is treated by warming yáng and boosting qì.

720. 亡阴〔亡陰〕*wáng yīn,* **yīn collapse** [jɪn kǝ'læps]: Also called *yīn desertion* and *fulminant desertion of yīn humor.* A critical pattern of wearing of yin-blood. The chief signs are copious sweat, palpably hot

skin, and warm limbs or reversal cold of the limbs with heat in the hearts of the soles and palms. Other signs include agitation or, in severe cases, clouded spirit on the one hand and desire for cool fluids on the other. Breathing is short and hasty with difficulty catching the breath. The tongue is dry and red, whereas the pulse is weak and rapid.

721. **阴脱**〔陰脫〕*yīn tuō,* **yīn desertion** [jɪn dɪˈzɝʃən]: yīn collapse.

722. **阴液暴脱**〔陰液暴脫〕*yīn yè bào tuō,* **fulminant desertion of yīn humor** [ˈfʌlmɪnənt dɪˈzɝʃən əv jɪn ˈhjumɚ]: yīn collapse.

723. **亡阳**〔亡陽〕*wáng yáng,* **yáng collapse** [jæŋ/jɑŋ n kəˈlæps]: Also called *yáng desertion.* A disease pattern of critical debilitation of yáng qì marked by sweating and cold skin and by reversal cold of the limbs. The patient is apathetic or (rarely) agitated, and in severe cases his spirit is clouded. Either there is no thirst or there is a desire for warm fluids. The pulse is either hidden, sunken, fine, and faint, or agitated and racing. The tongue is pale.

724. **阳脱**〔陽脫〕*yáng tuō,* **yáng desertion** [jæŋ/jɑŋ dɪˈzɝʃən]: yáng collapse.

725. **脱证**〔脫證〕*tuō zhèng,* **desertion pattern** [dɪˈzɝʃən–ˌpætɚn]: Any kind of desertion, such as yīn desertion or yáng desertion.

6.2. 气血辨证
Qì and Blood Pattern Identification

6.2.1. 气的辨证 Qì Pattern Identification

726. **气虚**〔氣虛〕*qì xū,* **qì vacuity** [ˈtʃi–vəˌkjuətɪ]: Weakness of qì; the manifestation of insufficiency of original qì. Qì vacuity is associated with poor organ function, general weakening through illness or overwork, dietary imbalance, or damage to yīn-blood. General signs include fatigue and lack of strength, spontaneous sweating at the slightest movement, bright white facial complexion, dizziness, faint voice, shortness of breath, and a weak fine soft pulse. If qì's securing function breaks down, there may be flooding and spotting or bloody stool, prolapse of the rectum or prolapse of the uterus, or reduced resistance to evils. A focus among the bowels and viscera is usually detectable and is identified by weak organ function. Since qì is yáng in nature, qì vacuity and yáng vacuity present with similar signs. Yáng vacuity is characterized

by qì vacuity signs as well as cold signs such as cold limbs, aversion to cold, cold sweating, and slow pulse.

727. 气滞〔氣滯〕*qì zhì,* **qì stagnation** [ˈtʃi–stægˌneʃən]: Decrease in the normal activity of qì that is attributed to the obstructive effect of mental and emotional problems, external injury, evil qì (cold, dampness), static blood, or qì vacuity and that is capable of causing static blood, water-damp, or phlegm-rheum. Qì stagnation is characterized by distention and fullness or oppression in the affected area. "Where there is stop-page, there is pain" (不通则痛 *bù tōng zé tòng*). The pain associated with qì stagnation is of unfixed location or is "scurrying" (窜痛 *cuàn tòng*) as distinct from pain of fixed location associated with blood stasis. Often, discomfort associated with qì stagnation is temporarily relieved by belching (嗳气 *ài qì*) or the passing of flatus (排气 *pái qì*). When there is insufficiency of spleen yáng qì, in which its uplift is diminished, there are sinking effects such as prolapse of the rectum, enduring diar-rhea, prolapse of the uterus, or, in infants, a depressed fontanel gate. The spleen occupies the center, its qì governs upbearing; damage to the spleen by dietary intemperance, taxation fatigue, or enduring illness can cause spleen qì to fall. See spleen qì vacuity.

728. 气逆〔氣逆〕*qì nì,* **qì counterflow** [tʃi ˈkaʊntəˌflo]: A reversal of the normal bearing of qì. The qì of the lung and of the stomach nor-mally flows downward. When lung qì runs counterflow, there is hasty breathing and cough; when stomach qì runs counterflow, there is vom-iting and hiccup, etc. Liver qì normally bears upward and effuses (生发 *shēng fā*). However, when depressed anger damages the liver, then upbearing and effusion become excessive or liver fire ascends counter-flow, causing headache, dizziness, clouding collapse, or blood ejection.

729. 气闭〔氣閉〕*qì bì,* **qì block** [tʃi blak]: Blockage and derangement of qì dynamic due to congestion of wind, phlegm, fire, or stasis evil that manifests in signs such as coma, clenched jaw, clenched fists, and urinary and fecal stoppage.

6.2.2. 血的辨证 Blood Pattern Identification

730. 血瘀〔血瘀〕*xuè yū,* **blood stasis** [blʌd ˈstesɪs]: Impairment or cessa-tion of the normal free flow of blood. Blood stasis may arise when knocks and falls, bleeding, qì stagnation, qì vacuity, blood cold, or blood heat impair free flow in specific locations of the body. It man-ifests in a variety of ways including pain, abdominal masses, bleeding (especially from the vagina), and abdominal distention. The observable signs of blood stasis are: pain of fixed location; masses and swellings;

bleeding; stasis speckles on the tongue; dry lusterless skin; soot-black complexion, etc.

731. 血虚〔血虛〕*xuè xū,* **blood vacuity** [blʌd vəˈkjuətɪ]: Also called *insufficiency of yīn-blood.* The manifestation of insufficiency of the yīn-blood. Blood vacuity can be the result of excessive blood loss or the spleen failing to move and transform. A further cause is failure to eliminate static blood and engender new blood. Blood vacuity is characterized by a pale white or withered-yellow facial complexion, dizzy head, flowery vision, relatively pale tongue, and a fine pulse. Other commonly observed signs include heart palpitations or fearful throbbing, insomnia, and numbness of the extremities. Blood vacuity signs can reflect the insufficient supply of blood to nourish specific channels and bowels or viscera. See heart blood vacuity; liver blood vacuity.

732. 阴血不足〔陰血不足〕*yīn xuè bù zú,* **insufficiency of yīn-blood** [ˌɪnsʌˈfɪʃənsɪ əv jɪn blʌd]: blood vacuity.

733. 亡血〔亡血〕*wáng xuè,* **blood collapse** [blʌd kəˈlæps]: Acute, critical vacuity of the blood.

734. 血热〔血熱〕*xuè rè,* **blood heat** [blʌd hit]: A condition characterized by heat and blood signs, mostly occurring in externally contracted heat (febrile) diseases, though not uncommon in miscellaneous diseases. When blood heat scorches the vessels and causes extravasation of the blood, there is retching of blood, expectoration of blood, bloody stool or urine, nosebleed, or menstrual irregularities. This pathomechanism is called frenetic movement of hot blood. Bleeding is often profuse and the blood is either bright red or purple-black in color. Blood heat can also cause red papules and macules. General signs of blood heat such as heart vexation, thirst, red or deep red tongue, and rapid pulse all indicate heat. Coma may occur in severe cases.

735. 血热妄行〔血熱妄行〕*xuè rè wàng xíng,* **frenetic movement of hot blood** [frəˈnɛtɪk ˈmuvmənt əv hɑt blʌd]: See blood heat.

736. 血寒〔血寒〕*xuè hán,* **blood cold** [blʌd kold]: Congealing cold and stagnant qì that inhibits movement of blood, causing stasis. Blood cold is observed in the following conditions: mounting qì; concretions, conglomerations, accumulations, and gatherings; delayed menstruation; scant menstruation; frostbite. Blood cold mostly arises through blood congealing in the liver vessel.

6.2.3. 气血同病 Dual Disease of Qì and Blood

737. 气滞血瘀〔氣滯血瘀〕*qì zhì xuè yū,* **qì stagnation and blood stasis** [tʃi stægˈneʃən ənd blʌd ˈstesɪs]: The simultaneous occurrence of

qì stagnation and blood stasis, characterized by signs such as menstrual block, stasis clots in the menstrual discharge, abdominal pain at the onset of menstruation, or painful distention of the breasts. Qì stagnation and blood stasis may also arise together as a result of external injury. When qì fails to move the blood, qì stagnation may cause—and be further exacerbated by—blood stasis. This frequently occurs in conditions described by Western medicine as chronic nephritis and ulcerative diseases.

738. 气血俱虚 〔氣血俱虚〕 *qì xuè jù xū,* **dual vacuity of qì and blood** [ˈd(j)uəl vəˈkjuətɪ əv tʃi ənd blʌd]: The simultaneous occurrence of qì and blood vacuity. Because "blood is the mother of qì," blood vacuity causes qì vacuity. Thus, blood vacuity patients often display qì vacuity signs such as shortness of breath and lack of strength. Dual vacuity is treated by dual supplementation of qì and blood, and since "qì engenders blood" (气能生血 *qì néng shēng xuè*), the accent is placed on supplementing qì. Thus, the condition Western medicine identifies as anemia is characterized by classic blood vacuity signs such as lusterless facial complexion, pale-colored nails, dizzy head, and heart palpitations, as well as qì vacuity signs such as shortness of breath and lack of strength. Dual vacuity of qì and blood may also develop from failure of vacuous qì to contain the blood. In such cases, the resulting persistent bleeding causes signs such as fatigue and lack of strength, pale tongue, and a soft soggy pulse. Qì failing to contain the blood is second only to blood heat as a cause of bleeding.

739. 气随血脱 〔氣隨血脫〕 *qì suí xuè tuō,* **qì deserting with the blood** [tʃi dɪˈzɝtɪŋ wɪð ðə blʌd]: Qì desertion that develops as a result of heavy blood loss. Blood is the mother of qì (血为气之母 *xuè wéi qì zhī mǔ*), i.e., original qì requires the nourishing action of the blood in order to perform its functions. When heavy blood loss (**blood desertion**) in severe cases deprives original qì of its support, qì also deserts. This condition may be characterized by a bright white or somber white complexion and a rapid pulse that is forceless at the deep level or else by a great dripping sweat and a faint pulse on the verge of expiration.

6.3. 脏腑辨证
Bowel and Visceral Pattern Identification

6.3.1. 心的证候 Heart Patterns

740. 心气虚〔心氣虛〕*xīn qì xū*, **heart qì vacuity** [hɑrt tʃi vəˈkjuətɪ]: The manifestation of insufficiency of heart qì; a disease pattern characterized by heart palpitations, shortness of breath, fatigue, and lack of strength, which reflects general qì vacuity and inhibited movement of blood. Heart qì vacuity usually appears in gradually developing, enduring illness.

741. 心阳虚〔心陽虛〕*xīn yáng xū*, **heart yáng vacuity** [hɑrt jæŋ/jɑŋ vəˈkjuətɪ]: Heart qì vacuity with pronounced cold signs and blood stasis signs. The chief signs are heart palpitations, shortness of breath, stifling oppression and possibly pain in the chest exacerbated by exertion, as well as aversion to cold and cold limbs. Other signs include lassitude of spirit and lack of strength, shortage of qì and laziness to speak, spontaneous sweating, and bright white or dark stagnant complexion. In some cases, there may be profuse sleeping. The tongue is pale and soft or pale green-blue. The pulse is slow, possibly faint, or rapid and forceless. It may be skipping, bound, or intermittent. Heart yáng vacuity often occurs in conjunction with kidney yáng vacuity, the combined pattern being referred to as heart-kidney yáng vacuity, in which physical cold and cold limbs are more pronounced and are accompanied by kidney yáng vacuity signs such as scant urine or water swelling.

742. 心血虚〔心血虛〕*xīn xuè xū*, **heart blood vacuity** [hɑrt blʌd vəˈkjuətɪ]: The manifestation of insufficiency of heart blood; a disease pattern characterized by disquieting of the heart spirit and insufficiency of yīn-blood. It may occur when fire that forms as a result of excess among the five minds (五志 *wǔ zhì*, i.e., emotions or mental states) damages yīn or when enduring illness causes damaging wear on yīn-blood. Heart blood vacuity is often accompanied by signs of spleen vacuity, and the combined pattern is known as heart-spleen blood vacuity. The chief signs of heart blood vacuity are heart palpitations or fearful throbbing, insomnia, profuse dreaming, and forgetfulness. Other signs include dizziness, a lusterless withered-yellow or pale white complexion, pale lips, and night sweating. The tongue is pale white. The pulse is fine and weak or fine and rapid.

743. 心阴虚〔心陰虛〕*xīn yīn xū*, **heart yīn vacuity** [hɑrt jɪn vəˈkjuətɪ]: The manifestation of insufficiency of heart yīn, characterized chiefly

by heart palpitations, heart vexation, insomnia, and profuse dreaming. Other signs include vexing heat in the five hearts, postmeridian tidal heat [effusion], reddening of the cheeks, night sweating, dry mouth and throat, and forgetfulness. The tongue is red with little liquid and little or no fur. The pulse is fine and rapid. Heart yīn vacuity regularly occurs in conjunction with kidney yīn, the combined pattern being called heart-kidney yīn vacuity.

744. 心火上炎〔心火上炎〕*xīn huǒ shàng yán,* **heart fire flaming upward** ['hɑrt-fɑɪr 'flemɪŋ 'ʌpwə˞d]: A vacuity or repletion pattern of the heart characterized by upper body signs. Classic signs of heart fire flaming upward include reddening of the tip of the tongue, vexation, and erosion of the oral and glossal mucosa. The pulse is rapid. Heart fire flaming upward is the result of hyperactive heart fire or heart yīn vacuity. It may occur with liver fire in effulgent heart-liver fire, which is a repletion pattern, or with kidney yīn vacuity in noninteraction of the heart and kidney, which is an effulgent yīn vacuity fire pattern. Sometimes, heart fire may spread to the small intestine. Signs associated with effulgent heart-liver fire include headache, red eyes, agitation, and irascibility, in addition to the general signs of heart fire flaming upward. Noninteraction of the heart and kidney is characterized by vexation, insomnia, and occasionally by dryness of the pharynx and mouth, red face due to upbearing fire, a red mirror tongue, and a fine rapid pulse. Heart fire spreading heat to the small intestine is characterized by painful dribbling urination with reddish urine.

745. 心火亢盛〔心火亢盛〕*xīn huǒ kàng shèng,* **hyperactive heart fire** [ˌhɑɪpə'ræktɪv 'hɑrt-fɑɪr]: Also called intense heart fire and exuberant heart fire. A heart disease pattern characterized by signs such as heat vexation, insomnia, and mouth sores; this pattern arises when the six excesses lie depressed in the inner body and transform into fire, when the patient is given to excessive consumption of hot acrid foods or warm supplementing medicinals, or when affect-mind causes internal damage that resultss in transformation into fire. The main signs, heart vexation, insomnia, and mouth sores, are accompanied by red face, thirst, yellow urine, dry stool, blood ejection and spontaneous external bleeding, manic agitation and delirious speech, heat effusion, and skin sores that are red, swollen, and painful. The tongue is red or red at the tip, the tongue fur is yellow, and the pulse is rapid.

746. 心火炽盛〔心火熾盛〕*xīn huǒ chì shèng,* **intense heart fire** [ɪn'tɛns 'hɑrt–fɑɪr]: hyperactive heart fire.

747. 心火盛〔心火盛〕*xīn huǒ shèng,* **exuberant heart fire** [ɪˈgzubərənt ˈhɑrt-faɪr]: hyperactive heart fire.

748. 心血瘀阻〔心血瘀阻〕*xīn xuè yū zǔ,* **heart blood stasis obstruction** [hɑrt blʌd ˈstesɪs əbˈstrʌkʃən]: A disease pattern of the heart that stems from binding depression of liver qì and lung qì congestion, as well as spleen, kidney, and lung vacuity. It is characterized by heart palpitations and periodic heart pain like the stabbing of a needle. Other signs include oppression in the chest, green-blue or purple nails, a tongue that is purple in color or bears stasis speckles, and a rough or interrupted pulse. See also heart impediment.

749. 心神不安〔心神不安〕*xīn shén bù ān,* **disquieted heart spirit** [dɪsˈkwaɪətɪd hɑrt ˈspɪrɪt]: Spirit disturbed as a result of the heart's failure to store it. The spirit is stored by the heart and is often referred to as the heart spirit. Disquieted heart spirit arises in heart disease when the heart fails to store the spirit; it manifests heart palpitations, fearful throbbing, susceptibility to fright, heart vexation, and insomnia. It is observed in many heart patterns.

750. 心火移热于小肠〔心火移熱於小腸〕*xīn huǒ yí rè yú xiǎo cháng,* **heart fire spreading heat to the small intestine** [hɑrt faɪr ˈsprɛdɪŋ hit tə ðə smɔl ɪnˈtɛstɪn]: A disease pattern characterized by painful dribbling urination with reddish urine. See heart fire flaming upward.

751. 水气凌心〔水氣凌心〕*shuǐ qì líng xīn,* **water qì intimidating the heart** [wɔtɚ tʃi ɪnˈtɪmɪdetɪŋ ðəhɑrt]: Upsurge of water qì causing disturbances of the heart. Spleen-yáng vacuity and impairment of qì transformation causing water to be retained in the body and thereby giving rise to water qì, which can manifest as phlegm-rheum or water swelling. When the water surges upward and lodges in the chest and diaphragm, it can cause devitalization of heart yang and disquieting of heart qì that manifests in the form of heart palpitations and hasty breathing. This is what is known as water qì intimidating the heart. The chief signs are heart palpitations, panting with inability to lie flat, generalized puffy swelling, and a bright white facial complexion. Other signs include flusteredness, lassitude of spirit and fatigue, fear of cold and cold limbs, and short voidings of scant clear urine.

6.3.2. 肺的证候 Lung Patterns

752. 肺气不宣〔肺氣不宣〕*fèi qì bù xuān,* **nondiffusion of lung qì** [ˌnɑndɪˈfjuʃən əv lʌŋ tʃi]: Obstruction of lung qì due to contraction of wind-cold, characterized by cough and nasal congestion.

753. **肺失肃降** 〔肺失肅降〕 *fèi shī sù jiàng,* **impaired depurative down-bearing of the lung** [ɪmˈpɛrd dɪˈpjurətɪv ˈdɑʊnˌbɛrɪŋ əv ðə lʌŋ]: A path-omechanism that involves a disturbance of the lung's functions of governing depurative downbearing and regulation of the waterways. The lung governs the qì of the whole body. If, for any reason, lung qì is inhibited, there may be signs such as cough, nasal congestion, and qì counterflow; if the movement and distribution of water is affected, there may be signs such as inhibited urination, puffy swelling, and panting and cough.

754. **肺气不利** 〔肺氣不利〕 *fèi qì bù lì,* **inhibition of lung qì** [ˌɪnhɪˈbɪʃən əv lʌŋ tʃi]: Any disturbance of depurative downbearing of lung qì and the lung's governing of the waterways. The lung governs the qì of the whole body and governs the regulation of the waterways. The appearance of cough or nasal congestion on the one hand, or inhibited urination or water swelling on the other, are signs of inhibition of lung qì.

755. **肺气虚** 〔肺氣虛〕 *fèi qì xū,* **lung qì vacuity** [lʌŋ tʃi vəˈkjuətɪ]: A disease pattern most commonly attributable to repeated impairment of lung qì diffusion and downbearing over a long period of time, although it may also be caused by general qì vacuity. The chief signs are forceless cough and panting, as well as shortness of breath. Other signs include a pale white or bright white facial complexion, fatigue and lack of strength, rapid breathing on exertion, spontaneous sweating, susceptibility to the common cold, laziness to speak, and low timid voice.

756. **肺阴虚** 〔肺陰虛〕 *fèi yīn xū,* **lung yīn vacuity** [lʌŋ jɪn vəˈkjuətɪ]: A disease pattern of lung vacuity with heat signs. Lung yīn vacuity is mostly the result of damage caused by long-lingering lung heat, which frequently develops in patients suffering from either general debilitation due to an enduring illness or from impaired lung downbearing. It sometimes arises as a result of invasion of the lung by dryness evil. The chief signs are cough without phlegm or with scant sticky phlegm, and tidal heat [effusion]. Other signs include emaciation, dry throat and mouth, postmeridian tidal heat [effusion], vexing heat in the five hearts, and night sweating. Sometimes the phlegm is flecked with blood or the voice is hoarse. The tongue is red with little liquid. The pulse is rapid and fine. Lung yīn vacuity frequently affects kidney yīn, resulting in lung-kidney yīn vacuity.

757. **肺肾阴虚** 〔肺腎陰虛〕 *fèi shèn yīn xū,* **lung-kidney yīn vacuity** [lʌŋ ˈkɪdnɪ jɪn vəˈkjuətɪ]: See kidney yīn vacuity.

6.3.3. 脾、胃和肠的证候 Spleen, Stomach, and Intestinal Patterns

758. **脾虚**〔脾虛〕*pí xū,* **spleen vacuity** [splin vəˈkjuətɪ]: Any disease pattern of spleen yīn or spleen yáng vacuity or of qì-blood insufficiency, usually stemming from dietary irregularities, exposure to excessive cold or warmth, anxiety and thought, taxation fatigue (overwork, etc.), or damage to the spleen through enduring sickness. Signs include emaciation with yellow face, lack of strength in the limbs, reduced food intake, nontransformation of food, abdominal pain, rumbling intestines, sloppy stool or diarrhea, puffy swelling, bloody stool, or flooding and spotting.

759. **脾气虚**〔脾氣虛〕*pí qì xū,* **spleen qì vacuity** [splin tʃi vəˈkjuətɪ]: A condition that occurs when irregular eating or anxiety, thought, or taxation fatigue damage the spleen and stomach. It may take different forms depending on the aspect of spleen function affected: The spleen failing to move and transform (脾失健运 *pí shī jiàn yùn*) is a disturbance of the spleen's governing of movement and transformation and the upbearing of the clear. It is characterized by abdominal distention, torpid intake, rumbling intestines, diarrhea, and other signs of poor digestion. Spleen failing to move and transform and causing damp obstruction (with signs including reduced food intake, fullness and oppression in the stomach duct, sloppy diarrhea, cumbersome fatigued limbs that may be swollen, thick slimy tongue fur, and a moderate pulse) is called spleen vacuity damp encumbrance (脾虚湿困 *pí xū shī kùn*). Insufficiency of center qì (中气不足 *zhōng qì bù zú*) is a general disturbance of the spleen and stomach function characterized by yellow face with little luster, pale or dark lips, poor appetite, abdominal distention after eating, dizziness, low voice, shortness of breath, fatigue and lack of strength, sloppy stool, tender-soft tongue with thick tongue fur, and a vacuous pulse. If there is stomach pain, it is relieved by pressure. *The Magic Pivot* (*Líng Shū, kǒu wèn*) states, "When center qì is insufficient, there are changes in stool and urine, and the intestines rumble." Center qì fall (中气下陷 *zhōng qì xià xiàn*) is failure of the spleen's governing of upbearing, which manifests in sinking effects such as prolapse of the rectum, enduring diarrhea, prolapse of the uterus, or, in infants, depressed fontanel gate. The spleen failing to control the blood (脾不统血 *pí bù tǒng xuè*) is a disturbance of the spleen's function of managing the blood that results in bleeding.

760. **脾失健运**〔脾失健運〕*pí shī jiàn yùn,* **spleen failing to move and transform** [splin ˈfelɪŋ tə muv ənd trænsˈfɔrm]: See spleen qì vacuity.

761. 脾虚湿困〔脾虛濕困〕*pí xū shī kùn,* **spleen vacuity damp encumbrance** [splin vəˈkjuətɪ dæmp ɪnˈkʌmbrəns]: See spleen qì vacuity.

762. 中气不足〔中氣不足〕*zhōng qì bù zú,* **insufficiency of center qì** [ˌɪnsəˈfɪʃənsɪ əv ˈsɛntɚ tʃi]: See spleen qì vacuity.

763. 脾不统血〔脾不統血〕*pí bù tǒng xuè,* **spleen failing to control the blood** [splin ˈfelɪŋ tə kənˈtrol ðə blʌd]: See spleen qì vacuity.

764. 脾阴虚〔脾陰虛〕*pí yīn xū,* **spleen yīn vacuity** [splin jɪn vəˈkjuətɪ]: The manifestation of the spleen failing to distribute essence. The spleen and stomach are the root of later heaven. The whole of the body relies on the spleen's function of distributing essence. Since essence is distributed by splenic movement and transformation, spleen yīn vacuity is actually dual vacuity of spleen qì and yīn. It most often results from enduring illness or from wear on the yīn humor of the stomach and spleen in febrile disease. The nondistribution of essence is reflected in emaciation. Spleen qì vacuity due to the spleen failing to move and transform may be reflected on the one hand in fatigue and lack of strength, and on the other in abdominal distention and sloppy stool. Insufficiency of stomach yīn, which may be a cause or result of spleen yīn vacuity, leads to failure of harmony and downbearing and, in severe cases, to stomach qì ascending counterflow; hence there is hunger with no desire for food and drink, torpid intake, or dry retching and hiccup. In spleen yīn vacuity, yīn may fail to restrain yáng, causing vacuity heat signs such as dry mouth and tongue, and red tongue with scant fur.

765. 脾阳虚〔脾陽虛〕*pí yáng xū,* **spleen yáng vacuity** [splin jæŋ/jɑŋ vəˈkjuətɪ]: Also called *devitalized spleen yáng.* A further development of spleen qì vacuity. Spleen yáng vacuity presents with pronounced cold signs in addition to spleen qì vacuity signs. It may thus be differentiated from spleen qì vacuity by the presence of a bright white facial complexion, fatigued spirit, physical cold, abdominal pain relieved by warmth and pressure, and diarrhea containing untransformed food. The pulse is sunken and weak, while the tongue is pale with white fur. It is often accompanied by signs of kidney yáng debilitation.

766. 脾阳不振〔脾陽不振〕*pí yáng bù zhèn,* **devitalized spleen yáng** [diˈvaɪtəlaɪzd splin jæŋ/jɑŋ]: spleen yáng vacuity.

767. 脾肺两虚〔脾肺兩虛〕*pí fèi liǎng xū,* **dual vacuity of the spleen and lung** [ˈduəl vəˈkjuətɪ əv ðə splin ənd lʌŋ]: Also called *spleen-lung qì vacuity.* Vacuity of both spleen and lung with signs of spleen vacuity such as reduced food intake, sloppy stool, and abdominal distention and signs of lung vacuity such as shortness of breath, cough, copious phlegm, and spontaneous sweating.

768. 脾肺气虚〔脾肺氣虛〕*pí fèi qì xū,* **spleen-lung qì vacuity** [splin lʌŋˈtʃi-vəˌkjuətɪ]: dual vacuity of the spleen and lung.

769. 心脾两虚〔心脾兩虛〕*xīn pí liǎng xū,* **dual vacuity of the heart and spleen** [ˈd(j)uəl vəˈkjuətɪ əv ðə hɑrt ənd splin]: A disease pattern characterized by signs of heart blood vacuity and spleen qì vacuity. Dual vacuity of the heart and spleen arises through excessive thought and anxiety, excessive taxation damage (overwork), enduring illness and improper nourishment, and loss of blood. The chief signs are heart palpitations or fearful throbbing, insomnia and forgetfulness, reduced eating, fatigue, abdominal distention, and sloppy stool. Other signs include withered-yellow facial complexion and dizzy and flowery vision. In some cases, there may be purple macules under the skin. In women, there may be menstrual irregularities, menstrual block, or flooding and spotting. The tongue is pale and tender. The pulse is fine and forceless. The heart and spleen are closely related. The spleen is the source of qì and blood formation, and it also manages the blood. When spleen qì is weak, blood production is insufficient, or blood management breaks down and blood spills out of the vessels. Either case may cause heart blood depletion. The heart governs the blood and vessels. When the blood is abundant, qì is plentiful; when blood is vacuous, qì becomes weak. When heart blood is insufficient and the means to produce qì are lacking, then spleen qì also becomes vacuous. Insufficiency of heart blood deprives the heart of nourishment and causes heart palpitations or fearful throbbing. When the heart spirit is disquieted and fails to keep to its abode, there is insomnia and profuse dreaming. Insufficiency of the blood depriving the head and eyes of nourishment causes dizziness and forgetfulness; when depriving the skin of nourishment, the facial complexion becomes withered-yellow and lusterless. Spleen qì vacuity with impaired movement and transformation causes poor appetite, abdominal distention, and sloppy stool. Qì vacuity with a generalized reduction in physiological function causes lack of strength and lassitude of spirit. Spleen qì vacuity with no power to contain the blood causes chronic bleeding. Insufficiency of qì and blood causes a pale tender tongue and a weak fine pulse.

770. 胃气虚寒〔胃氣虛寒〕*wèi qì xū hán,* **stomach qì vacuity cold** [ˈstʌmək tʃi vəˈkjuətɪ kold]: Also called *stomach vacuity cold.* A disease pattern characterized by stomach signs such as stomach pain and vomiting and by vacuity cold signs. It can be the result of damage to stomach qì from excessive consumption of raw and cold foods or other dietary irregularities. It may also occur when constrained emotions cause liver qì to invade the stomach and, in time, damages its qì. The stomach

pain usually occurs on an empty stomach and is relieved by eating or by pressure. Vomiting of clear cold sour fluid is sometimes observed. General signs include lusterless complexion, aversion to cold, lack of warmth in the extremities, and a pale enlarged tongue. The pulse is soggy, but may become stringlike or tight during pain attacks. Vacuity cold gives rise to signs of stomach qì disharmony such as belching and acid upflow. Stomach qì vacuity cold is characterized by stomach duct pain that may be exacerbated by contraction of external cold. It differs, however, from fulminant strike by cold evil (from catching cold or from excessive consumption of raw or cold foods), as it is less sudden and violent in onset, of longer duration, and characterized by a prominence of vacuity signs. Fulminant strike by cold evil is associated with pronounced cold signs, less pronounced vacuity signs, and a more sudden onset.

771. 胃虚寒〔胃虛寒〕 *wèi xū hán,* **stomach vacuity cold** ['stʌmək və'kjuə-tɪ kold]: stomach qì vacuity cold.

772. 胃阴虚〔胃陰虛〕 *wèi yīn xū,* **stomach yīn vacuity** ['stʌmək jɪn və'kjuətɪ]: The manifestation of insufficiency of stomach yīn (stomach yīn depletion), i.e., insufficiency of the yīn humor of the stomach; attributed to intense stomach heat, spleen-stomach damp-heat, or damage to liquid in externally contracted febrile (heat disease); characterized by dry lips and mouth, desire for fluids, reduced food intake, dry stool, short voidings of scant urine, and, in severe cases, dry retching or hiccup, a dry crimson area in the center of the tongue, and a rapid fine pulse.

773. 胃阴不足〔胃陰不足〕 *wèi yīn bù zú,* **insufficiency of stomach yīn** [ˌɪnsə'fɪʃənsɪ əv 'stʌmək jɪn]: See stomach yīn vacuity.

774. 胃热〔胃熱〕 *wèi rè,* **stomach heat** ['stʌmək hit]: Any heat pattern of the stomach. It arises when evil heat enters the interior (see externally contracted heat (febrile) disease pattern identification), when the stomach is damaged by excessive consumption of fried or otherwise rich fatty foods or hot spicy food, or when liver fire invades the stomach. Most cases of stomach heat are repletion heat. For stomach vacuity heat, see stomach yīn vacuity. Stomach heat can take a number of forms: (1) Affecting the stomach's function of intake, it can manifest in swift digestion and rapid hungering. (2) Affecting the downbearing of the stomach, it manifests as pain or burning sensation in the stomach duct, vomiting, clamoring stomach, and hard stool. (3) The upper body can manifest signs such as bad breath, painful swollen gums, gaping gums, or bleeding gums. In such cases, it is referred to as "stomach fire."

Whatever form stomach heat takes, it is invariably attended by a bitter taste in the mouth, dry mouth, red tongue with yellow fur, and a rapid slippery pulse.

775. 胃火〔胃火〕*wèi huǒ,* **stomach fire** ['stʌmək faɪr]: See stomach heat.

776. 胃气上逆〔胃氣上逆〕*wèi qì shàng nì,* **counterflow ascent of stomach qì** ['kaʊntɚflo əˌsɛnt əv 'stʌmək tʃi]: The chief manifestation of impaired harmonious downbearing of the stomach that causes nausea, vomiting, belching, or hiccup and that results from a number of causes including cold, heat, phlegm, foul turbidity, food stagnation, and gastrointestinal qì stagnation. Stomach qì ascending counterflow is a pattern that can occur in any stomach disease. Counterflow occurring in a cold pattern is usually characterized by a pale tongue, white face, vomiting of clear fluid, or vomiting in the evening of food ingested in the morning. Where heat is present, signs include red tongue with yellow fur, vomiting of sour or bitter fluid, and immediate vomiting of ingested food. If phlegm is the cause, a slimy tongue fur, repeated ejection of phlegm-drool, and occasionally dizziness are observed. Stomach qì ascending counterflow due to foul turbidity usually occurs in hot weather, is sudden in onset, and is characterized by abdominal pain, ungratified desire to vomit, and agonizing distention and oppression in the stomach duct. Where stomach qì ascending counterflow is a result of food stagnation, there is usually a history of food damage, and signs such as sour, putrid vomitus, with improvement brought by vomiting. Finally, stomach qì ascending counterflow owing to gastrointestinal qì stagnation is characterized by glomus in the chest, abdominal pain, and belching.

777. 大肠液亏〔大腸液虧〕*dà cháng yè kuī,* **large intestinal humor depletion** [lardʒ ɪn'tɛstɪnl̩ 'hjumɚ dɪ'pliʃən]: Also called *intestinal humor depletion*. A disease pattern of the large intestine caused by general lack of liquid and blood in the body. Large intestinal humor depletion is observed in postpartum blood vacuity, liquid depletion in the aged, and in enduring and severe diseases. It may also occur in externally contracted heat (febrile) disease prior to replenishment of the fluids. Signs comprise dry hard stool and difficult defecation. Generally, no pronounced abdominal distention or pain is observed. The patient is in a weak state of health.

778. 肠液亏耗〔腸液虧耗〕*cháng yè kuī hào,* **intestinal humor depletion** [ɪn'tɛstɪnl̩ 'hjumɚ dɪ'pliʃən]: large intestinal humor depletion.

779. 心肾阴虚〔心腎陰虛〕*xīn shèn yīn xū,* **heart-kidney yīn vacuity** ['hɑrt 'kɪdnɪ jɪn vəkjuətɪ]: See heart yīn vacuity.

780. 心脾血虚〔心脾血虛〕*xīn pí xuè xū,* **heart-spleen blood vacuity** [hɑrt splin blʌd vəˈkjuətɪ]: See heart yīn vacuity.

6.3.4. 肝与胆的证候 Liver and Gallbladder Patterns

781. 肝气郁结〔肝氣鬱結〕*gān qì yù jié,* **binding depression of liver qì** [ˈbɑɪndɪŋ dɪˈprɛʃən əv ˈlɪvɚ tʃi]: Also called *liver depression.* Stagnation in the liver and liver channel resulting from impairment of the liver's function of free coursing. It arises when affect-mind frustration leads to depression and anger that damage the liver and impair free coursing. Other factors include invasion of external damp-heat and insufficiency of yīn-blood depriving the liver of nourishment. The chief signs are affect-mind depression, vexation, agitation, and irascibility. There is also distention and pain in the rib-side, oppression in the chest, and sighing. Other signs include distention and pain in the breasts before menstruation, distention and pain in the lesser abdomen, menstrual irregularities, plum-pit qì, goiter, accumulations and gatherings under the rib-side, jaundice, and epilepsy. The tongue body may be normal. The tongue fur is thin and white. The pulse is stringlike.

782. 肝郁〔肝鬱〕*gān yù,* **liver depression** [ˈlɪvɚ–dɪˌprɛʃən]: binding depression of liver qì.

783. 肝郁化火〔肝鬱化火〕*gān yù huà huǒ,* **liver depression transforming into fire** [ˈlɪvɚ–dɪˌprɛʃən trænsˈfɔrmɪŋ ɪntə fɑɪr]: Also called depressed wood transforming into fire. Depressed liver qì giving rise to fire signs such as red face, red eyes, headache, dizziness, vomiting and retching, coughing of blood, and, in severe cases, mania.

784. 肝火上炎〔肝火上炎〕*gān huǒ shàng yán,* **liver fire flaming upward** [ˈlɪvɚ–ˌfɑɪr ˈflemɪŋ ˈʌpwɚd]: Liver fire characterized by pronounced upper body signs. Liver fire flaming upward is attributed to liver qì depression transforming into fire, to depressed internal damp-heat evils, or to excessive consumption of sweet and fatty foods or warming and supplementing medicinals. Liver fire flaming upward is characterized by qì and fire rising to the head and by pronounced heat signs. The main signs are red face, red eyes, bitter taste in the mouth, and dry mouth, as well as vexation, agitation, and irascibility. Other signs include scorching pain in the rib-side, headache, dizziness, tinnitus, deafness, insomnia and profuse dreaming, reddish urine, and constipation. In some cases, there is blood ejection or spontaneous external bleeding. The tongue is red with yellow fur. The pulse is stringlike and rapid.

785. 肝阳上亢〔肝陽上亢〕*gān yáng shàng kàng,* **ascendant hyperactivity of liver yáng; ascendant liver yáng** [əˈsɛndənt ˌhɑɪpəræk'tɪvəti əv

ˈlɪvɚ jæŋ/jɑŋ]: An imbalance of the liver's yīn and yáng aspects occurring when vacuity of liver-kidney yīn lets liver yáng get out of control
and stir upward excessively. This pathomechanism may be exacerbated
when depression, anger, or anxiety impair free coursing, since when
free coursing is impaired, depressed qì transforms into fire, fire damages yīn-blood, and yīn has no power to restrain yáng. Ascendant liver
yáng is identifiable by signs of upper body exuberance and by signs
of insufficiency of yīn-blood from which this condition stems. The
main signs are dizziness, tinnitus, distention and pain in the head, and
red face with baking heat due to upbearing fire. Other signs include insomnia and profuse dreaming, heart vexation, agitation and irascibility,
heavy head and light feet, limp aching lumbus and knees, and dry throat
and mouth. In some cases, there is sudden clouding collapse and unconsciousness. The pulse is stringlike and may also be fine. The tongue is
red. Predominance of ascendant yáng and yīn vacuity signs varies from
case to case. In some cases, both are equally pronounced.

786. 肝血虚〔肝血虛〕 *gān xuè xū,* **liver blood vacuity** [ˈlɪvɚ blʌd vəˈkjua-
tɪ]: The manifestation of insufficiency of liver blood. Liver blood vacuity is attributed to either or both of two causes: a) damage to yīn-blood
in the course of enduring illness, which deprives the liver of blood for
storage and for adequate nourishment; and b) continual expectoration
of blood, nosebleed, or profuse menstruation due to blood storage failure. In addition to general blood vacuity signs, liver blood vacuity is
associated with a variety of patterns: blood failing to nourish the liver,
blood failing to nourish the sinews or eyes, and thoroughfare (*chōng*)
and controlling (*rèn*) vessel diseases. Signs include dizziness, insomnia, profuse dreaming, flowery vision, blurred vision, inhibited sinew
movement, lusterless nails, reduced menstrual flow, or alternating menstrual block and flooding and spotting. In severe cases, the kidney may
be affected, resulting in liver-kidney essence-blood depletion and consequently in signs such as lumbar pain, seminal emission, sterility, menstrual block, emaciation, and tidal heat [effusion], in addition to the
above-mentioned signs.

787. 肝风内动〔肝風內動〕 *gān fēng nèi dòng,* **liver wind stirring internally** [ˈlɪvɚ wɪnd ˈstɝɪŋ ɪnˈtɝnəlɪ]: Liver disease that manifests in
spasm. *A Clinical Guide with Case Histories* (*Lín Zhèng Zhǐ Nán Yī
Àn*) states, "Internal wind is movement of the body's yáng qì," and is
the result of "depleted stocks of yīn in the viscera." Liver wind arises
from extreme yīn-yáng and qì-blood imbalance. Ascendant liver yáng,
liver fire flaming upward, and insufficiency of liver yīn and/or blood
may all, in extreme cases, stir liver wind. The chief signs of liver wind

stirring internally are severe dizziness, headache with pulling sensation (iron-band headache), tension and stiffness in the neck, tingling or
numbness in the limbs, and twitching of the sinews and flesh. In severe
cases, there may be pulling of the face and eyes, trembling lips, tongue,
and fingers, inhibited speech, or unsteady gait. In more severe cases,
there may be convulsions or tetanic reversal. *Elementary Questions (Sù
Wèn)* states, "All wind with shaking and [visual] dizziness is ascribed to
liver." Usually, the pulse is stringlike, the tongue is red, and the tongue
fur is dry. Liver wind stirring internally includes liver yáng transforming into wind, extreme heat engendering wind, and blood vacuity
engendering wind.

788. 肝阳化风〔肝陽化風〕*gān yáng huà fēng,* **liver yáng transforming
into wind** [ˈlɪvɚ jæŋ/jɑŋ trænsˈfɔrmɪŋ ˈɪntə wɪnd]: A further development of ascendant liver yáng that occurs when liver-kidney yīn depletion makes yīn unable to constrain yáng, so that liver yáng becomes
hyperactive and stirs wind. The main signs are dizziness that upsets
balance, shaking head and trembling of the limbs, and sluggish speech
or stiff tongue preventing speech. There may be sudden collapse and
unconsciousness leaving the patient with hemiplegia. Secondary signs
include headache, rigidity of the neck, numbness of the extremities, and
unsteady gait. The tongue is red with white or slimy tongue fur. The
pulse is stringlike and forceful.

789. 热极生风〔熱極生風〕*rè jí shēng fēng,* **extreme heat engendering
wind** [ɪksˈtrim hit ɪnˈdʒɛndərɪŋ wɪnd]: A pattern resulting from contraction of warm heat disease evil or one or more of the six excesses
when the evil becomes depressed, transforms into heat, damages construction-blood and the fluids, scorches the liver channel, and deprives
the sinews of nourishment. Occurring in children, this pattern is called
fright wind and is observed, for example, in what Western medicine
calls encephalitis B. The main signs are high fever with thirst, red face
and eyes, convulsions, hypertonicity, upward staring eyes, rigidity of
the neck and back, and clenched jaw. Other signs include upward-
staring eyes, arched-back rigidity, clenched jaw, short inhibited voidings of urine, constipation, and, in severe cases, clouded spirit and
delirious speech. The tongue is red or crimson. The pulse is stringlike
and rapid.

790. 血虚生风〔血虛生風〕*xuè xū shēng fēng,* **blood vacuity engendering wind** [blʌd vəˈkjuətɪ ɪnˈdʒɛndərɪŋ wɪnd]: Insufficiency of liver
blood depriving the sinews of nourishment and giving rise to spasm.
The chief signs are numbness of the limbs, hypertonicity of the sinews,

jerking sinews and twitching flesh, and clouded flowery vision. Other signs include somber white complexion, pale lips and nails, brittle dry nails, and dull rib-side pain. The tongue is pale and the pulse is stringlike and fine.

791. 肝经湿热〔肝經濕熱〕*gān jīng shī rè,* **liver channel damp-heat** [ˈlɪvɚ ˈtʃænl̩ ˈdæmp-hit]: A disease pattern that arises when enduring liver depression transforms into heat and invades the spleen causing dampness to gather, whereupon the dampness and heat then bind together and pour down to the lower burner. General signs include dizziness, bitter taste in the mouth, dry pharynx, and yellow urine. In women, it can cause thick malodorous yellow or mixed red and white vaginal discharge. In men, it can cause impotence or premature ejaculation.

792. 肝胆湿热〔肝膽濕熱〕*gān dǎn shī rè,* **liver-gallbladder damp-heat** [ˈlɪvɚ ˈgɔlblædɚ ˈdæmp-hit]: A disease pattern that occurs when the liver's free coursing is impaired owing either to internal damp-heat stemming from excessive consumption of fatty or sweet foods, or to externally contracted damp-heat. The chief signs are alternating [aversion to] cold and heat [effusion], bitter taste in the mouth, rib-side pain, abdominal pain, nausea and vomiting, abdominal distention, aversion to food, yellowing of the skin, and yellow or reddish urine. Stool tends to be dry if heat is more pronounced than dampness and sloppy if dampness is more pronounced than heat. The tongue fur is yellow and slimy. The pulse is rapid and stringlike.

793. 肝气犯胃〔肝氣犯胃〕*gān qì fàn wèi,* **liver qì invading the stomach** [ˈlɪvɚ tʃi ɪnˈvedɪŋ ðə ˈstʌmək]: Excessive free coursing of liver qì affecting the stomach. Liver qì invading the stomach manifests in stomach signs, such as stomach duct pain, vomiting of sour fluid, torpid stomach intake, aversion to food, abdominal distention, and diarrhea, in addition to liver signs, such as dizziness, rib-side pain, irascibility, smaller-abdominal distention, and a stringlike pulse. If the condition persists, it may develop into liver-spleen disharmony. Liver qì invading the stomach differs from liver qì invading the spleen by a predominance of stomach signs such as vomiting of sour fluid and torpid intake.

794. 肝气犯脾〔肝氣犯脾〕*gān qì fàn pí,* **liver qì invading the spleen** [ˈlɪvɚ tʃi ɪnˈvedɪŋ ðə splin]: A form of liver-spleen disharmony in which liver free coursing is excessive and liver qì moves cross counterflow and affects the spleen. Liver qì invading the spleen is characterized by headache, irascibility, bitter taste in the mouth, oppression in the chest and rib-side, glomus and fullness after eating, sloppy diarrhea, and a moderate stringlike pulse. This pattern differs from liver qì invading

the stomach by a predominance of spleen signs such as distention and diarrhea.

795. 胆热〔膽熱〕*dǎn rè,* **gallbladder heat** [ˈgɔlblædə hit]: Also called gallbladder fire. Heat in the gallbladder that arises when evil heat invades the gallbladder channel and causes depression of channel qì. The main signs of gallbladder heat are headache on both sides of the head, pain in the canthi, dizziness, tinnitus, bitter taste in the mouth, dry throat, fullness and pain in the chest and rib-side, and alternating heat [effusion] and [aversion to] cold. Other signs include vomiting of bitter water, vexation and agitation, and irascibility, as well as insomnia. In some cases, there is jaundice. The tongue is red with yellow fur. The pulse is stringlike, rapid, and forceful.

796. 胆火〔膽火〕*dǎn huǒ,* **gallbladder fire** [ˈgɔlblædə faɪr]: gallbladder heat.

797. 胆虚〔膽虛〕*dǎn xū,* **gallbladder vacuity** [ˈgɔlblædə vəˈkjuətɪ]: Also called *gallbladder vacuity and qì timidity* and *insufficiency of gallbladder qì*. A disease pattern of gallbladder vacuity and failure of the decision-making capacity. The chief signs are anxiety and indecision, clouded vision, tinnitus and poor hearing, dizzy head, "timid gallbladder" (lack of courage), and susceptibility to fright. Other signs include lassitude of spirit, insomnia, sighing, distention and fullness under the rib-side, and sloppy diarrhea. The tongue fur is thin, white, and glossy. The pulse is stringlike, fine, and slow.

798. 胆虚气怯〔膽虛氣怯〕*dǎn xū qì qiè,* **gallbladder vacuity and qì timidity** [ˈgɔlblædə vəˈkjuətɪ ənd tʃi tɪˈmɪdɪtɪ]: gallbladder vacuity.

799. 胆气不足〔膽氣不足〕*dǎn qì bù zú,* **insufficiency of gallbladder qì** [ˌɪnsəˈfɪʃənsɪ əv ˈgɔlblædə tʃi]: gallbladder vacuity.

800. 心虚胆怯〔心虛膽怯〕*xīn xū dǎn qiè,* **heart vacuity and gallbladder timidity** [hɑrt vəkjuətɪ ənd ˈgɔlblædə tɪˈmɪdɪtɪ]: Also called *heart-gallbladder vacuity timidity.* A feeling of emptiness in the heart and susceptibility to fright and fear. Vacuous heart and timid gallbladder usually occurs in insufficiency of heart blood and heart qì debilitation, and is partly related to mental factors.

801. 心胆虚怯〔心膽虛怯〕*xīn dǎn xū qiè,* **heart-gallbladder vacuity timidity** [hɑrt–ˈgɔlblædə vəkjuətɪ tɪˈmɪdɪtɪ]: heart vacuity and gallbladder timidity.

6.3.5. 肾的证候 Kidney Patterns

802. 肾阴虚〔腎陰虛〕*shèn yīn xū,* **kidney yīn vacuity** [ˈkɪdnɪ jɪn vəˈkjuətɪ]: The manifestation of insufficiency of kidney yīn. Kidney yīn is

the root of all yīn of the body. It is most closely related to the heart, liver, and lung. Thus, kidney yīn depletion frequently leads to vacuity of heart, liver, or lung yīn. Conversely, persistent yīn vacuity in these three related viscera may culminate in depletion of kidney yīn. Hence, in clinical practice, kidney yīn vacuity most commonly occurs in dual vacuity patterns. Kidney yīn vacuity is characterized by vacuity and heat signs and varies greatly in severity. Mild cases are characterized by dizziness, tinnitus, dry pharynx, dry mouth, tidal heat [effusion], lumbar pain, seminal emission, night sweating, and in some cases bleeding gums. The pulse is fine and rapid, and the tongue is distinctly red in color. Severe cases are marked by shedding of flesh and loss of bulk (severe emaciation) and by a red mirror tongue. The dual patterns are identified by additional signs. Liver-kidney yīn vacuity is characterized by headache, blurred or flowery vision, and loss of visual acuity, as well as menstrual irregularities and sterility. Heart-kidney yīn vacuity is characterized by signs such as insomnia, heart palpitations, forgetfulness, and profuse dreaming. Cough, expectoration of blood, and steaming bone tidal heat [effusion] are observed in lung-kidney yīn vacuity.

803. 肾阴枯涸〔腎陰枯涸〕 *shèn yīn kū hé*, **desiccation of kidney yīn** [ˌdɛsɪˈkeʃən əv ˈkɪdnɪ jɪn]: Severe insufficiency of kidney yīn manifesting in teeth dry as desiccated bones.

804. 肾阳虚〔腎陽虛〕 *shèn yáng xū*, **kidney yáng vacuity** [ˈkɪdnɪ jæŋ/jɑŋ vəˈkjuətɪ]: The manifestation of debilitation of kidney yáng (variously referred to as *debilitation of kidney yáng, insufficiency of true yáng, insufficiency of the true origin, exhaustion of the lower origin,* and *debilitation of the life gate fire*). Kidney yáng is the root of the yáng of the entire body and is most closely related to the yáng qì of the spleen and heart. Kidney yáng vacuity may cause, or be caused by, vacuity of the yáng qì of these two related viscera. Kidney yáng vacuity is characterized by both vacuity and cold signs, such as bright white facial complexion, torpor of essence-spirit, aversion to cold, lack of warmth in the extremities, dizziness, tinnitus, limp aching lumbus and knees, and an enlarged pale tongue. Where the reproductive function is affected, seminal efflux, impotence, sterility or infertility, and menstrual irregularities may be observed. Where the transformative function of kidney qì is impaired, there may be either signs of increased urination such as long voidings of clear urine and profuse urination at night, or signs of insufficient urination such as scant urine, urinary block, and water swelling. In severe cases, water-rheum may flood upward, intimidating the heart and shooting into the lung. Such cases are characterized by heart palpitations, rapid panting, and inability to assume

a lying posture. Spleen-kidney yáng vacuity is characterized by pronounced water swelling or enduring diarrhea, clear-grain diarrhea, or by fifth-watch diarrhea. Qì absorption failure, which generally stems from lung qì vacuity, is characterized by rapid breathing at the slightest exertion. Heart-kidney yáng debilitation is identified by the presence of heart palpitations, panting, water swelling, and, in severe cases, by reversal cold of the limbs, putting forth of oily sweat, and other critical signs.

805. 肾阳虚衰〔腎陽虛衰〕*shèn yáng xū shuāi*, **debilitation of kidney yáng** [dəˌbɪlɪˈteʃən of ˈkɪdnɪ jæŋ/jɑŋ]: kidney yáng vacuity.

806. 真阳不足〔眞陽不足〕*zhēn yáng bù zú*, **insufficiency of true yáng** [ˌɪnsɑˈfɪʃənsɪ əv tru jæŋ/jɑŋ]: kidney yáng vacuity.

807. 真元不足〔眞元不足〕*zhēn yuán bù zú*, **insufficiency of the true origin** [ˌɪnsɑˈfɪʃənsɪ əv ðə tru ˈɔrədʒɪn]: kidney yáng vacuity.

808. 下元虚惫〔下元虛憊〕*xià yuán xū bèi*, **exhaustion of the lower origin** [ɛgˈzɔstʃən əv ðə ˈloəˈɔrədʒɪn]: kidney yáng vacuity.

809. 阳虚水泛〔陽虛水泛〕*yáng xū shuǐ fàn*, **yáng vacuity water flood** [jæŋ/jɑŋ vəˈkjuətɪ wˈɔtəˈ flʌd]: Also called *kidney vacuity water flood*. Water swelling or phlegm-rheum that occurs when in spleen-kidney yáng vacuity, or especially kidney yáng (life gate fire) vacuity, yáng qì fails in its warming and moving function and causes water to accumulate.

810. 肾虚水泛〔腎虛水泛〕*shèn xū shuǐ fàn*, **kidney vacuity water flood** [ˈkɪdnɪ vəˈkjuətɪ wˈɔtəˈ flʌd]: yáng vacuity water flood.

811. 命门火衰〔命門火衰〕*mìng mén huǒ shuāi*, **debilitation of the life gate fire** [dɪˌbɪlɪˈteʃən əv ðə lɑɪf get faɪr]: Severe kidney yáng vacuity.

812. 肾精不足〔腎精不足〕*shèn jīng bù zú*, **insufficiency of kidney essence** [ˌɪnsəˈfɪʃənsɪ əv ˈkɪdnɪ ˈɛsəns]: A disease pattern resulting from enduring illness or improper development during the fetal stage. Insufficiency of kidney essence differs from kidney yīn and yáng vacuity in that vacuity signs are accompanied by neither cold nor heat signs of any marked degree. The kidney governs the bones and engenders marrow, and the brain is the sea of marrow. Only when kidney essential qì is abundant can the bone, marrow, and brain fulfill their functions. Insufficiency of kidney essence may thus lead to signs of essence-marrow depletion and sea-of-marrow vacuity, such as impairment of intellectual function, weak bones, and deficiency of the reproductive function. Insufficiency of kidney essence is generally characterized by dizziness, tinnitus, limp aching lumbus and knees, deficient reproductive function, loss of head hair, and loosening of the teeth. Insufficiency of

essence-marrow or sea-of-marrow vacuity manifests in different ways according to age. In children, it can result in retarded growth and development, short stature, sluggishness of physical movement, low intelligence, weak bones, or retarded closure of the fontanel gate. In adults it may lead to premature senility or weakness in the legs, difficulty in walking, dullness of essence-spirit, and slowness of physical movement.

813. 髓海空虚〔髓海空虚〕*suǐ hǎi kōng xū*, **emptiness of the sea of marrow** [ˈɛmptɪnɪs əv ðə si əv ˈmæro]: A kidney vacuity pattern in which the kidney's function of engendering marrow is affected; it is characterized by dizziness, slowness of thought, forgetfulness, etc.

814. 肾不纳气〔腎不納氣〕*shèn bù nà qì*, **kidney failing to absorb qì** [ˈkɪdnɪ ˈfelɪŋ tu əbˈzɔrb tʃi]: Kidney qì vacuity preventing the absorption of lung qì (air breathed in). The kidney failing to absorb qì is characterized by shortness of breath, panting, rapid breathing at the slightest movement, spontaneous sweating, and a forceless fine pulse or a vacuous floating pulse without root. This condition corresponds to chronic cardiopulmonary failure in Western medicine.

815. 肾气虚〔腎氣虚〕*shèn qì xū*, **kidney qì vacuity** [ˈkɪdnɪ tʃi vəˈkjuətɪ]: Debility of original qì in the kidney due to insufficiency of earlier heaven (congenital factors), debilitation of kidney qì in old age, excessive sexual activity, excessive childbirth, or enduring illness affecting the kidney. It is characterized by limp aching lumbus and knees and devitalized essence-spirit exacerbated by overexertion. Other signs include dizziness, lack of strength, deafness, tinnitus, heel pain, loose teeth, and hair loss. When the securing function of the kidney is affected, the condition is called insecurity of kidney qì, which is characterized by signs such as seminal efflux, premature ejaculation, vaginal discharge, or flooding and spotting. In kidney qì vacuity, the tongue is pale and enlarged; the pulse is fine and weak, especially at the cubit.

816. 肾气不固〔腎氣不固〕*shèn qì bù gù*, **insecurity of kidney qì** [ˌɪnsəˈkjurətɪ əv ˈkɪdnɪ tʃi]: Failure of the kidney's governing of opening and closing or its storing of essence that manifests in urinary disturbances, such as frequent and long voidings of clear urine, incontinence, enuresis, and dribbling urination, or disturbances of the reproductive function, such as seminal emission, seminal efflux, and premature ejaculation. Insecurity of kidney qì results from debilitation of kidney qì in old age or maldevelopment of kidney qì in youth, or from damage through sexual intemperance or early marriage (early commencement of sexual activity). It is usually, therefore, accompanied by signs of

general kidney vacuity such as fatigued spirit, lumbar back pain, limpness of the knees, a tongue that tends to be pale, and a fine weak pulse. Mild cold signs are also observed. Furthermore, stirring fetus due to kidney vacuity may also be considered as a manifestation of insecurity of kidney qì (see stirring fetus).

817. 肾虚〔腎虛〕*shèn xū,* **kidney vacuity** [ˈkɪdnɪ vəˈkjuətɪ]: Any vacuity pattern of the kidney (kidney yīn vacuity, kidney yáng vacuity, insecurity of kidney qì, etc.).

818. 心肾不交〔心腎不交〕*xīn shèn bù jiāo,* **noninteraction of the heart and kidney** [ˌnɑnɪntərˈækʃən əv ðə hɑrt ənd ˈkɪdnɪ]: A disturbance of the normal relationship between heart yáng and kidney yīn. Insufficiency of kidney yīn or stirring of heart fire may be the cause of the disturbance. Signs include heart vexation, insomnia, profuse dreaming, heart palpitations or fearful throbbing, and seminal emission. See heart fire flaming upward.

819. 心肾阳虚〔心腎陽虛〕*xīn shèn yáng xū,* **heart-kidney yáng vacuity** [hɑrt ˈkɪdnɪ jæŋ/jɑŋ vəˈkjuətɪ]: See heart yáng vacuity.

820. 脾肾阳虚〔脾腎陽虛〕*pí shèn yáng xū,* **spleen-kidney yáng vacuity** [splin ˈkɪdnɪ jæŋ/jɑŋ vəˈkjuətɪ]: See kidney yáng vacuity.

821. 肝肾阴亏〔肝腎陰虧〕*gān shèn yīn kuī,* **liver-kidney yīn depletion** [lɪvɚˈkɪdnɪ jɪn dɪˈpliʃən]: A disease pattern that comprises signs of both liver yīn vacuity and kidney yīn vacuity and that may be caused by insufficiency of either liver or kidney yīn. Liver-kidney yīn vacuity is characterized by dizziness, distention in the head, unclear vision, tinnitus, dry pharynx and dry mouth, vexing heat in the five hearts, seminal emission, insomnia, aching lumbus and knee, red tongue with little fur, and a forceless fine stringlike pulse.

6.4. 病邪辨证
Disease Evil Pattern Identification

6.4.1. 风 Wind

822. 外感风邪〔外感風邪〕*wài gǎn fēng xié,* **external contraction of wind evil** [ɪksˈtɜnl̩ kənˈtrækʃən əv ˈwɪnd–ivl̩]: Wind evil invading the body through the fleshy exterior, mouth, or nose, causing heat effusion (fever), aversion to wind, and headache, and in some cases cough, itchy throat, and expectoration of flesh. In severe cases, there may be signs of nondiffusion of lung qì such as rapid breathing.

823. **风寒**〔風寒〕*fēng hán,* **wind-cold** ['wɪnd–kold]: Wind-cold that causes an exterior pattern. The term "wind-cold" denotes not only a combination of evils, but also the patterns this combination gives rise to. The main signs are headache, generalized pain, and aversion to wind. Other signs include absence of sweating, absence of thirst, cough with expectoration of clear thin phlegm, glossy white tongue fur, and a tight floating pulse. This pattern is one form a common cold can take.

824. **风热**〔風熱〕*fēng rè,* **wind-heat** ['wɪnd–hit]: Wind-heat that causes an exterior pattern. The term "wind-heat" denotes not only a combination of evils, but also the patterns this combination gives rise to. The main signs are cough with sticky (sometimes yellow) phlegm, sore throat, dry mouth, red tongue, and rapid floating pulse. Other signs include heat effusion (fever), aversion to wind, headache, absence of sweating, and inhibited sweating.

825. **风热犯肺**〔風熱犯肺〕*fēng rè fàn fèi,* **wind-heat invading the lung** ['wɪnd–hit ɪn'vedɪŋ ðə lʌŋ]: Wind-heat that causes cough and thick yellow phlegm, in addition to exterior signs. See wind-heat.

826. **风寒束肺**〔風寒束肺〕*fēng hán shù fèi,* **wind-cold fettering the lung** ['wɪnd–kold 'fɛtərɪŋ ðə lʌŋ]: Wind-cold causing cough with expectoration of clear thin phlegm as well as other wind-cold signs. See wind-cold.

827. **风邪入经**〔風邪入經〕*fēng xié rù jīng,* **wind evil entering the channels** ['wɪnd–ivl̩ 'ɛntərɪŋ ðə 'tʃænlz]: Wind evil invading the channels and sinews causes obstruction of the channels and inhibited movement of the sinews. It can manifest as: a) deviated eyes and mouth, facial paralysis, or other local paralysis; b) rigidity of the neck and back, clenched jaw, and convulsion of the limbs, as in lockjaw; or c) general or localized pain in the muscles and joints, numbness, and restricted physical movement, as in impediment patterns.

6.4.2. 寒 Cold

828. **外感寒邪**〔外感寒邪〕*wài gǎn hán xié,* **external contraction of cold evil** [ɪks'tɜ·nl̩ kəntræbkʃən əv 'kold–ivl̩]: See wind-cold.

829. **寒痹**〔寒痹〕*hán bì,* **cold impediment** [kold ɪm'pɛdɪmənt]: Also called *painful impediment.* An impediment pattern understood to occur when wind-cold-damp, with a prevalence of cold, invades the joints and channels and causes acute pain in the joints that is exacerbated by exposure to cold and relieved by warmth. There may also be hypertonicity of the extremities.

830. **寒疝**〔寒疝〕*hán shàn,* **cold mounting** [kold ˈmɑuntɪŋ]: Accumulation of cold evil in the abdomen stemming from repeated wind-cold contractions that in turn stem either from vacuity cold in the spleen and stomach or from postpartum blood vacuity. Cold mounting is characterized by cold in the umbilical region, cold sweating, and counterflow cold in the limbs. The pulse is sunken and tight. In severe cases there is generalized cold in the body and numbness in the limbs. In blood vacuity patients, the abdominal pain stretches up the rib-side and is accompanied by cramping in the lower abdomen.

831. **寒气凝滞**〔寒氣凝滯〕*hán qì níng zhì,* **congealing cold and stagnant qì** [kəndʒilɪŋkold ənd ˈstægnənt tʃi]: Cold that gives rise to qì stagnation. Cold tends to congeal and obstruct qì transformation. It is a yīn evil that causes congealing and stagnation, contracture and tautness, and easily damages yáng qì. *Elementary Questions (Sù Wèn, Jǔ Tòng Lùn)* states, "When cold qì enters the channels, there is a slowing down, congealing, and nonmovement. When it settles outside the vessels, then blood is scant; when it settles inside the vessels, qì is blocked and there is sudden pain." Thus, when cold causes illness, there is pain, abdominal distention, swelling of the lower leg, hypertonicity, paralysis, and reversal cold.

832. **阴盛内寒**〔陰盛內寒〕*yīn shèng nèi hán,* **exuberant internal yīn cold** [ɪgˈzjubərənt ɪnˈtɜˑnḷ jɪn kold]: Exuberant yīn evil causes debilitation of yáng and the appearance of internal cold signs such as reverse-flow, phlegm-rheum, and water qì. *Elementary Questions (Sù Wèn, Tiáo Jīng Lùn)* states, "when yīn is exuberant, there is internal cold."

833. **寒滞肝脉**〔寒滯肝脈〕*hán zhì gān mài,* **cold stagnating in the liver vessel** [kold stægnˈetɪŋ ɪn ðə lɪvɚ ˈvɛsḷ]: Cold evil (usually externally contracted) congealing in the liver channel causing liver channel qì and blood to stagnate. The chief signs is lesser-abdominal pain that may stretch into the testicles and that may be associated with retracted scrotum. Secondary signs include bright white facial complexion, physical cold and cold limbs, green-blue or purple lips, long voidings of clear urine, and sloppy stool. The tongue is pale with a glossy white fur. The pulse is sunken and stringlike, and possibly slow.

6.4.3. 热、火、暑 Heat, Fire, Summerheat

834. **实热**〔實熱〕*shí rè,* **repletion heat** [rɪˈpliʃən hit]: A pattern marked by signs that include high fever, vexation and thirst with intake of fluid, constipation sometimes with abdominal pain that refuses pressure, yellow or reddish urine, dry yellow tongue fur, and a surging rapid pulse.

835. **虚热**〔虚熱〕*xū rè*, **vacuity heat** [vəˈkjuətɪ hit]: Also called vacuity fire. Heat due to insufficiency of yīn humor. Vacuity heat is characterized by vexing heat in the five hearts, insomnia, steaming bone tidal heat [effusion], dry throat and mouth, smooth bare red tongue, and a rapid fine pulse.

836. **虚火**〔虚火〕*xū huǒ*, **vacuity fire** [vəˈkjuətɪ fɑɪr]: See vacuity heat.

837. **阴虚火旺**〔陰虚火旺〕*yīn xū huǒ wàng*, **effulgent yīn vacuity fire** [ɪˈfʌldʒənt jɪn vəˈkjuətɪ fɑɪr]: See vacuity heat.

838. **暑热**〔暑熱〕*shǔ rè*, **summerheat-heat** [ˈsʌmɚhit hit]: A disease caused by summerheat, referred to as summerheat-heat by contradistinction to summerheat-damp. Summerheat-heat occurs mainly in the hot season and is characterized by pronounced heat signs such as high fever, thirst, scant urine, and heart vexation. In severe cases, there may be clouding of the spirit and tetanic reversal. Other signs include either absence of sweating or great sweating and a large rapid surging pulse. High fever poses the danger of damage to fluids and original qì, which is characterized by signs such as shortage of qì, fatigue and lack of strength, dry tongue fur, and a thin and rapid or large and vacuous pulse.

839. **暑湿**〔暑濕〕*shǔ shī*, **summerheat-damp** [ˈsʌmɚhit dæmp]: Disease occurring in hot, damp weather and caused by a combination of summerheat and dampness. Summerheat-damp is characterized by enduring low fever, fatigued and cumbersome limbs, poor appetite, oppression in the chest, and nausea and vomiting. There is frequently sloppy diarrhea with ungratifying defecation and short voidings of reddish urine. The pulse is soggy, and the tongue fur thick and slimy.

6.4.4. 湿 Dampness

840. **湿阻**〔濕阻〕*shī zǔ*, **damp obstruction** [dæmp əbˈstrʌkʃən]: A frequently observed disease in which the spleen and stomach are obstructed by dampness evil. It mainly occurs in summer and is characterized by impaired spleen-stomach movement and transformation. Signs include oppression in the chest, no thought of food and drink, and a bland or sweet taste or slimy sensation in the mouth. The tongue fur is thick and slimy; the pulse is soggy. Voidings are short with scant urine; the limbs are cumbersome and fatigued, and sometimes a low fever is observed.

841. **寒湿**〔寒濕〕*hán shī*, **cold-damp** [ˈkold–dæmp]: **1.** Cold and dampness combining to create stagnation of yáng qì and to inhibit the flow of blood, causing cold in the flesh and inhibited bending and stretching.

2. A disease pattern in which dampness encumbers the stomach and spleen and damages spleen yáng or in which water-rheum collects as a result of spleen-kidney yáng vacuity. It is characterized by cold limbs, abdominal distention, diarrhea, and in some cases water swelling.

842. 湿热〔濕熱〕 *shī rè,* **damp-heat** ['dæmp–hit]: A combination of dampness and heat.

843. 湿遏热伏〔濕遏熱伏〕 *shī è rè fú,* **dampness trapping hidden (deep-lying) heat** ['dæmpnıs 'træpıŋ 'hıdən ('dip–laıŋ) hit]: A condition in which the dampness prevents heat from effusing. Dampness trapping hidden heat is characterized by unsurfaced heat that arises in the afternoon to bring about sweating that fails to abate heat effusion. Other signs include lassitude of spirit, heavy-headedness, oppression in the chest and abdominal distention, aversion to food, yellow or reddish urine, white or yellow slimy tongue fur, and a rapid soggy pulse.

844. 湿热留恋气分〔濕熱留戀氣分〕 *shī rè liú liàn qì fèn,* **damp-heat lodged in the qì aspect** ['dæmp–hit lɑdʒd ın ðə 'tʃi–æspɛkt]: An externally contracted heat (febrile) disease pattern characterized by persistent low or remittent fever, fatigued limbs, and oppression in the chest. Thirst without appreciable intake of fluid is accompanied by a bland, bitter taste or slimy sensation in the mouth. Voidings are short with reddish urine. The tongue fur is yellow and slimy. Summerheat-damp and damp obstruction may also be characterized by such signs.

845. 湿热阻滞脾胃〔濕熱阻滯脾胃〕 *shī rè zǔ zhì pí wèi,* **damp-heat obstructing the spleen and stomach** ['dæmp–hit əb'strʌktıŋ ðə splin ənd 'stʌmək]: A disease pattern that results when damp-heat arising in the center burner or that is externally contracted brews in the spleen and disturbs normal movement and transformation. Spleen-stomach damp-heat is characterized by glomus and oppression in the stomach duct, torpid intake, nausea, sloppy stool, yellow urine, and heavy cumbersome limbs. Other possible signs include: yellowing of the skin (the color of tangerines) and fluctuating heat effusion (fever) unabated by sweating. The tongue is red with yellow slimy fur, and the pulse is soggy.

846. 湿热蕴结肝胆〔濕熱蘊結肝膽〕 *shī rè yùn jié gān dǎn,* **damp-heat brewing in the liver and gallbladder** ['dæmp–hit 'bruıŋ ın ðə 'lıvɚ ənd 'gɔlbædɚ]: A disease pattern that occurs when the liver's free coursing is impaired owing either to internal damp-heat stemming from excessive consumption of fatty or sweet foods, or to externally contracted damp-heat. The chief signs are alternating [aversion to] cold and heat [effusion], bitter taste in the mouth, rib-side pain, abdominal pain, nausea and vomiting, abdominal distention, aversion to food, yellowing of the

skin, and yellow or reddish urine. The stool tends to be dry if heat is more pronounced than dampness, and sloppy if dampness is more pronounced than heat. The tongue fur is yellow and slimy. The pulse is rapid and stringlike.

847. 湿热下注大肠〔濕熱下注大腸〕*shī rè xià zhù dà cháng,* **damp-heat pouring down into the large intestine** [ˈdæmp–hit ˈpɔrɪŋ dɑʊn ˈɪntə ðə lɑrdʒ ɪnˈtɛstin]: Also called large intestinal damp-heat. A disease pattern generally characterized by abdominal pain and diarrhea with ungratifying defecation and foul-smelling stool. An alternative pattern is dysentery, which is characterized by frequent defecation with blood and pus in the stool, abdominal pain, tenesmus, and a burning sensation in the rectum. In both cases, general signs include heat effusion (fever), bitter taste in the mouth, and a slimy yellow tongue fur.

848. 大肠湿热〔大腸濕熱〕*dà cháng shī rè,* **large intestinal damp-heat** [lɑrdʒ ɪnˈtɛstinl ˈdæmp–hit]: damp-heat pouring down into the large intestine.

849. 湿热下注膀胱〔濕熱下注膀胱〕*shī rè xià zhù páng guāng,* **damp-heat pouring down into the bladder** [ˈdæmp–hit ˈpɔrɪŋ dɑʊn ˈɪntə ðə ˈblædɚ]: Also called *bladder damp-heat.* A disease pattern occurring when damp-heat causes inhibited bladder qì transformation and that manifests in frequent urination, urinary urgency, inhibited urination, painful urination, red or yellow murky urine, or bloody urine. Other signs of bladder damp-heat include heat effusion (fever), lumbar pain, and sand or stones in the urine. The tongue is red with slimy yellow fur. The pulse is rapid and slippery.

850. 膀胱湿热〔膀胱濕熱〕*páng guāng shī rè,* **bladder damp-heat** [ˈblædɚˈdæmp–hit]: damp-heat pouring down into the bladder.

6.4.5. 燥 Dryness

851. 感受燥邪〔感受燥邪〕*gǎn shòu zào xié,* **contraction of dryness evil** [kənˈtrækʃən əv ˈdrɑɪnɪs–ˌivl]: Contraction of dryness evil is related to dry weather and, thus, most commonly occurs in autumn or in dry regions. The main signs are dry cough with either scant phlegm or thick, sticky phlegm that is difficult to expectorate, as well as dry throat, lips, tongue, and nostrils. Nosebleed may indicate dryness. Since all these signs are related to the respiratory tract, such patterns are sometimes described as "dryness evil invading the lung" (燥邪犯肺 *zào xié fàn fèi*). Further, since the lung is connected with the surface skin and [body] hair and since it stands in interior-exterior relationship with the large intestine, other signs include dry, cracked skin and dry, bound stool.

852. **伤津**〔傷津〕*shāng jīn,* **damage to liquid** [ˈdæmɪdʒ tə ˈlɪkwɪd]: A disease pattern that results from major depletion of fluids following high fever, excessive sweating in externally contracted heat (febrile) disease, or severe vomiting and diarrhea. Signs include thirst with desire to drink, dry throat, lips, tongue, nose, and skin, and a dry red tongue.

853. **伤阴**〔傷陰〕*shāng yīn,* **damage to yīn** [ˈdɑmɪdʒ tə jɪn]: Loss of fluids more severe than damage to liquid, generally occurring in the later stages of externally contracted heat (febrile) diseases when the patient's general condition is poor and characterized by a desiccated, peeling, or mirror tongue that is dull crimson in color. The throat, mouth, lips, nose, and skin are dry, although the thirst is not pronounced. There are also signs such as dry bound stool and short voidings of scant urine. In severe cases, there may be clouded spirit and tetanic reversal.

6.4.6. 食积 Food Accumulations

854. **伤食**〔傷食〕*shāng shí,* **food damage** [ˈfud–dæmɪdʒ]: Any disease pattern of damage to stomach and spleen by food. Food damage is caused by voracious eating and drinking or spleen-stomach vacuity. *Elementary Questions (Sù Wèn)* states, "Overeating causes damage to the stomach and intestines." It is characterized by aversion to food, nausea and vomiting, putrid belching, putrid-smelling vomitus, swallowing of upflowing acid, painful bloating of the abdomen, diarrhea or constipation, foul-smelling stool and flatus, and relief from pain and distention after defecation or passing of flatus. The tongue fur is slimy and either thick or yellow. In food damage, when food accumulation remains untransformed for days, the resulting condition is called abiding food.

855. **宿食**〔宿食〕*sù shí,* **abiding food** [əˈbɑɪdɪŋ fud]: See food damage.

856. **肠胃积滞**〔腸胃積滯〕*cháng wèi jī zhì,* **gastrointestinal accumulation** [ˌgæstroɪnˈtɛstɪnl̩ əˌkjumjəˈleʃən]: Accumulation of food in the stomach and intestines. Gastrointestinal accumulation shares the basic characteristics of food damage (aversion to food, nausea, vomiting or belching with putrid smelling vomitus or gas, diarrhea or constipation, foul-smelling stool and flatus, relief from pain and distention after defecation or the passing of flatus). However, gastrointestinal accumulation is usually more severe than most cases of food damage, especially with the addition of palpable accumulation lumps in the abdomen, painful distention that refuses pressure, diarrhea with ungratifying defecation, or tenesmus. Causes include excessive consumption of food, especially of cold, raw, fried, rich, or fatty foods, and ingestion of unclean foodstuffs.

857. **脾虚夹食**〔脾虚夾食〕*pí xū jiā shí*, **spleen vacuity with food damage** [splin və'kjuətɪ wɪð fud 'dæmɪdʒ]: Nontransformation of ingested food attributable to spleen-stomach vacuity. It is characterized by bloating after eating and by sloppy stool containing untransformed food. In general, there is no abdominal pain and the tongue fur may be completely normal. Signs such as no thought of food and drink and no pleasure in eating indicate prominence of stomach vacuity, while nontransformation of ingested food indicates prominence of spleen vacuity. Yellow face, emaciation, and rapacious eating with nonmovement of ingested food indicate a strong stomach and weak spleen.

858. **伤酒**〔傷酒〕*shāng jiǔ*, **liquor damage** ['lɪkɚ—ˌdæmɪdʒ]: Dizziness, headache, nausea, retching and vomiting, agitation and rashness, or clouding sleep attributable to excessive liquor consumption. Liquor is hot in nature and toxic, and tends to cause heat signs.

6.4.7. 痰 Phlegm

859. **湿痰**〔濕痰〕*shī tán*, **damp phlegm** [dæmp flɛm]: A pattern that is characterized by cough and copious white phlegm and that is attributable to the spleen failing to move and transform. It may be accompanied by glomus in the chest, retching and nausea, and fatigued cumbersome limbs. The pulse is slippery and the tongue fur is thick and slimy. This pattern is observed in diseases classified in Western medicine as chronic forms of respiratory tract inflammation such as chronic bronchitis.

860. **寒痰**〔寒痰〕*hán tán*, **cold phlegm** [kold flɛm]: Cold phlegm is characterized by cough, clear thin white phlegm, and a moist white tongue fur. The pulse is generally slightly stringlike. Patterns may also include physical cold and cold limbs. Cold phlegm may also be observed in diseases classified by Western medicine as chronic forms of respiratory tract inflammation such as chronic bronchitis and asthma.

861. **热痰**〔熱痰〕*rè tán*, **heat phlegm** [hit flɛm]: Heat phlegm is characterized by cough and rapid breathing with thick yellow or gluey white phlegm that is difficult to expectorate. General signs include fever, dry mouth, red tongue with yellow fur, and a slippery rapid pulse, all of which indicate heat. In Western medicine, heat phlegm roughly corresponds to acute inflammatory respiratory diseases (or acute attacks in chronic conditions).

862. **痰浊上扰**〔痰濁上擾〕*tán zhuó shàng rǎo*, **phlegm turbidity harassing the upper body** [flɛm tɝ'bɪdətɪ hə'ræsɪŋ ðə 'ʌpɚ—ˌbɑdɪ]: Dizziness is the main feature of phlegm turbidity harassing the upper body.

Hence it is said, "Where no phlegm is present, dizziness does not arise." Disturbance of vision may be so severe as to prevent the patient from sitting up. Milder cases present as dizzy head, distention in the head, and heavy-headedness. Other signs include insomnia, oppression in the chest, retching and nausea, little thought of food and drink, or nontransformation of ingested food. The tongue fur is slimy in texture and either white or yellow in color. The pulse is slippery and may also be stringlike. Where there is a heat complication (挟热 *jiā rè*), vexation and a bitter taste in the mouth may also be observed. These signs indicate disturbance of clear yáng in the upper body due to phlegm turbidity causing obstruction in the chest. This may develop when dampness gathers and transforms into phlegm as a result of the spleen failing to move and transform. Phlegm turbidity harassment of the upper body may be observed in diseases described in Western medicine as otogenic vertigo and hypertension.

863. 痰迷心窍〔痰迷心竅〕*tán mí xīn qiào,* **phlegm confounding the orifices of the heart** [flɛm kən'faʊndɪŋ ði 'ɔrəfɪsɪz əv ðə hɑrt]: Also called *phlegm turbidity clouding the pericardium.* A disease pattern that occurs when phlegm turbidity causes disturbance of the heart spirit. Phlegm confounding the orifices of the heart occurs in several different diseases. The main signs are: a) mental depression and dementia (withdrawal disease); b) clouded spirit-mind seeming conscious yet unconscious (damp warmth); c) sudden clouding collapse, unconsciousness, phlegm-drool foaming at the mouth, and convulsions of the limbs (epilepsy). Other signs include dull stagnant complexion, no thought of food and drink, soliloquy (talking alone), indifferent expression, irregular behavior, oppression in the chest and copious phlegm, and phlegm rale in the throat.

864. 痰浊蒙蔽心包〔痰濁蒙蔽心包〕*tán zhuó méng bì xīn bāo.* **phlegm turbidity clouding the pericardium** [flɛm tɝ'bɪdəti 'klaʊdɪŋ ðə ˌpɛrɪ'kɑrdɪəm]: phlegm confounding the orifices of the heart.

865. 痰火〔痰火〕*tán huǒ,* **phlegm-fire** [flɛm–faɪr]: **1.** Phlegm in the lung that is sticky and lumpy owing to the action of fire. Phlegm-fire is not usually manifest in overt signs, but external contractions and damage by food and drink can bring on episodes of wheezing and panting, with phlegm that is difficult to expectorate, heat vexation and pain in the chest, and dry mouth and lips. **2.** A phlegm node behind the ears or under the armpit having the appearance of rosary beads and being hard and of fixed location. A phlegm-fire is accompanied by a red tongue

with yellow fur and a rapid stringlike pulse. It is the result of liver fire and depressed phlegm.

866. 痰热〔痰熱〕*tán rè,* **phlegm-heat** [flɛm–hit]: Phlegm and heat that arise when external evils invade and transform into heat, which then combines with existing phlegm or damages liquid and condenses it into phlegm.

867. 痰火扰心〔痰火擾心〕*tán huǒ rǎo xīn,* **phlegm-fire harassing the heart** [flɛm–faɪr hə'ræsɪŋ ðə hɑrt]: A disease pattern arising when mental frustration causes qi depression that transforms into fire, which in turn condenses humor into phlegm, and the phlegm and fire bind together and harass the heart spirit. The chief signs are heart palpitations, vexation and sleeplessness or affect-mind abnormalities or manic agitation, or clouded spirit and delirious speech, vigorous heat [effusion], and phlegm rale. Other signs include red face and rough breathing, thirst with liking for cold drinks, oppression in the chest and copious phlegm, coughing of thick yellow phlegm, reddish urine and constipation, incoherent speech, abnormal crying and laughing, beating people and smashing objects, chiding and cursing regardless of who is present, dizziness, and profuse dreaming. The tongue is red with slimy yellow fur. The pulse is slippery and rapid.

868. 痰留经络〔痰留經絡〕*tán liú jīng luò,* **phlegm lodged in the channels** [flɛm lɑdʒd ɪn ðə 'tʃænlz]: Phlegm in the channels giving rise to goiter, phlegm nodes, and scrofula, all of which are relatively soft to the touch. Phlegm lodged in the limbs is characterized by numbness and pain in the upper or lower limbs or in one limb. It is not accompanied by any signs of blood vacuity or wind-cold-damp impediment. The tongue fur is white and slimy, and the pulse is slippery.

869. 痰饮〔痰飲〕*tán yǐn,* **phlegm-rheum** ['flɛm–rum]: Accumulation of fluid in the body. "Phlegm" denotes thick pathological fluids, whereas "rheum" denotes thinner pathological fluids. In practice, the term phlegm-rheum has two specific meanings: (1) Rheum (i.e., thin fluid) due to lung, spleen, or kidney disturbances that prevent the normal transportation and transformation of fluid and that is treated by warming and supplementing the spleen and kidney to secure the root and by disinhibiting water and expelling rheum to address the tip. It includes: "suspended rheum" (悬饮 *xuán yǐn*); "propping rheum" (支饮 *zhī yǐn*); "spillage rheum" (溢饮 *yì yǐn*); "lodged rheum" (留饮 *liú yǐn*); "deep-lying rheum" (伏饮 *fú yǐn*); "flowing rheum" (流饮 *liú yǐn*). (2) In a narrow sense, rheum lodged in the stomach and intestines; also called "flowing rheum." Phlegm-rheum is characterized by sloppy stool, poor

appetite, ejection of foamy drool, and emaciation occurring in obese people. In some cases there may be heart palpitations and shortness of breath.

870. 痰湿〔痰濕〕*tán shī*, **phlegm-damp** ['flɛm–dæmp]: Conditions that arise when dampness gathers to form phlegm and that are characterized by signs of both phlegm and dampness.

871. 痰浊〔痰濁〕*tán zhuó*, **phlegm turbidity** ['flɛm–tɜˑ'bɪdɪtɪ]: Phlegm as a turbid entity that is obstructive to the clear yáng qì of the body. Phlegm turbidity is often said to specifically refer to phlegm-damp or phlegm-rheum. However, phlegm turbidity often implies that the phlegm is thick and sticky, while phlegm-damp often implies that the phlegm is thin.

872. 风痰〔風痰〕*fēng tán*, **wind-phlegm** ['wɪnd-flɛm]: Wind-phlegm manifests in both wind and phlegm signs such as sudden collapse and loss of consciousness, foaming at the mouth, and convulsions. Wind-phlegm is most commonly seen in epilepsy.

6.5. 外感热病辨证
Externally Contracted Heat Disease Pattern Identification

873. 外感热病〔外感熱病〕*wài gǎn rè bìng*, **externally contracted heat (febrile) disease** [ɪks'tɜˑnəlɪ kən'træktɪd hit ('fɛbraɪl) dɪ'ziz]: Disease due to external evils such as the six excesses (wind, cold, summerheat, dampness, dryness, and fire) and broadly characterized by heat (effusion) (fever).

6.5.1. 六经辨证 Six-Channel Pattern Identification

874. 六经辨证〔六經辨證〕*liù jīng biàn zhèng*, **six-channel pattern identification** [sɪks 'tʃænl'pætən aɪˌdɛntɪfɪ'keʃən]: Six-channel pattern identification was first mentioned in *The Inner Canon* (*Nèi Jīng*) and subsequently refined in *On Cold Damage* (*Shāng Hán Lùn*). The latter presents a systematic synthesis of pre-Hàn experience and theory concerning external heat (febrile) diseases, and elaborated on the six-channel patterns discussed in *Elementary Questions* (*Sù Wèn*), in which observable signs and disease shifts are explained in terms of greater yáng (*tài yáng*), yáng brightness (*yáng míng*), and lesser yáng (*shào*

yáng) diseases (collectively known as the three yáng channel diseases), and greater yīn (*tài yīn*), lesser yīn (*shào yīn*), and reverting yīn (*jué yīn*) diseases (collectively known as the three yīn channel diseases). It describes the principal patterns, the methods, and formulas used to treat them, as well as combined and transmuted patterns and sequences of channel passage. *On Cold Damage (Shāng Hán Lùn)* is considered the basis of identification and treatment of external heat (febrile) disease patterns; the pathology, methods of treatment, formulas, and medicinals it discusses are used as a guide for miscellaneous internal damage disease as well.

875. 太阳病〔太陽病〕*tài yáng bìng*, **greater yáng disease** [ˈgretɚ jæŋ/jɑŋ dɪˈziz]: Any of a number of diseases affecting greater yáng (*tài yáng*). a) Greater yáng channel disease: Disease of the greater yáng (*tài yáng*) channels that forms Cinnamon Twig Decoction (*guì zhī tāng*) or Ephedra Decoction (*má huáng tāng*) patterns. Greater yáng disease patterns are exterior patterns that are observed before the evil passes into the interior. Thus, urine and stool are generally not affected, and there is no thirst. b) Greater yáng bowel patterns: These patterns arise when evil enters the bladder or bladder region. They include greater yáng water amassment (太阳蓄水 *tài yáng xù shuǐ*) and greater yáng blood amassment (太阳蓄血 *tài yáng xù xuè*). Water amassment is characterized by a floating pulse, heat effusion (fever), thirst with inhibited urination, lesser-abdominal fullness, and in some cases immediate vomiting of ingested fluids, the principal feature being inhibited urination. Blood amassment is characterized by smaller-abdominal pain and distention, and manic states. It is distinguished from water amassment by uninhibited urination.

876. 阳明病〔陽明病〕*yáng míng bìng*, **yáng brightness disease** [jæŋ/jɑŋ ˈbraɪtnɪs dɪˈziz]: A disease that occurs when externally contracted evil enters the yáng brightness (*yáng míng*) channel and exterior signs such as aversion to wind and cold give way to pronounced heat signs. Yáng brightness disease is characterized by generalized heat [effusion], sweating and aversion to heat, agitation, and thirst, or, in more severe cases, abdominal fullness and pain, constipation, and, in the most severe cases, delirious mania. The tongue fur is usually dry and old yellow in color. The pulse is generally surging and large, slippery and rapid, or sunken, replete, and forceful. Yáng brightness disease occurs in the exuberant heat stage of externally contracted heat (febrile) diseases, and manifests, in terms of the eight principles, as interior heat or interior repletion. Yáng brightness disease can be divided into channel and bowel patterns depending on the presence of constipation. In yáng brightness

channel patterns, the stomach liquid is damaged by exuberant heat, although there is no heat bind in the yáng brightness bowels (the stomach and large intestine). Yáng brightness bowel patterns are so named because they occur when an evil binds with food accumulation or dry waste in the stomach or intestines, causing repletion heat.

877. 少阳病〔少陽病〕*shào yáng bìng,* **lesser yáng disease** [ˈlɛsɚ jæŋ/jɑŋ dɪˈziz]: Disease of the hand lesser yáng (*shào yáng*) triple burner and the foot lesser yáng (*shào yáng*) gallbladder channels. Because the lesser yáng is located between the greater yáng (*tài yáng*) and yáng brightness (*yáng míng*), lesser yáng disease is often referred to as a "half-exterior half-interior pattern" (or "midstage pattern"). The essential signs are alternating [aversion to] cold and heat [effusion], chest and rib-side pain and fullness, bitter taste in the mouth, and vomiting. Other signs include no desire for food and drink, heart vexation, desire to vomit, dizzy vision, painful hard glomus under the rib-side, and a stringlike pulse. Lesser yáng disease occurs when, owing to debilitation of right qì, an evil invades the body through the interstices and binds in the gallbladder, impeding qì dynamic and disrupting upbearing and downbearing. Fullness in the chest and rib-side is explained by the lesser yáng gallbladder channel that traverses this area. Alternating [aversion to] cold and heat [effusion] are explained by the struggle between the evil and right. Heart vexation, bitter taste in the mouth, dry pharynx, and dizzy vision, as well as vomiting and no desire for food and drink, are the result of gallbladder heat rising counterflow up the channel that disturbs the harmony and downbearing of stomach qì. A stringlike pulse is classically associated with the gallbladder. Lesser yáng disease is different from greater yáng disease and yáng brightness disease, since the lesser yáng lies midway between the two other yáng channels. Greater yáng disease can pass to both yáng brightness and lesser yáng. Lesser yáng disease may resolve in an exterior pattern through a constant sweat or may also pass to the yáng brightness to form an interior pattern. It may pass to the yīn channels, causing vacuity patterns. Consequently, lesser yáng disease is commonly termed a midstage pattern. However, it may occur in combination with an exterior pattern characterized by heat effusion (fever), aversion to cold, and vexing pain in the joints of the limbs, or with a yáng brightness interior pattern characterized by abdominal fullness and constipation.

878. 太阴病〔太陰病〕*tài yīn bìng,* **greater yīn disease** [ˈgretɚ jɪn dɪˈziz]: Greater yīn disease is characterized by abdominal fullness with periodic pain, vomiting, diarrhea, nonmovement of ingested food, absence of thirst, and a weak moderate pulse. The pathomechanism of greater

yīn disease is failure of movement and transformation of food that results from devitalized spleen yáng and manifests as vomiting and diarrhea. The abdominal distention is explained by spleen vacuity qì stagnation, whereas the abdominal pain results from vacuity cold. Although it rarely occurs naturally in the progression of externally contracted heat (febrile) diseases, it may arise when incorrect treatment of yáng diseases damages spleen yáng, such as inappropriate precipitation in greater yáng (*tài yáng*) and lesser yáng (*shào yáng*) disease, or excessive use of cold and cool freeing precipitants in yáng brightness (*yáng míng*) disease. Cold evil can also directly enter the greater yīn as a result of underlying spleen vacuity. It may also occur when, owing to a regular spleen qì vacuity, cold evil enters the greater yīn directly. This is known as a direct strike on greater yīn. Like the yáng brightness bowel pattern, greater yīn disease is a digestive tract disease, but presents as vacuity rather than as repletion. It is characterized by vomiting, diarrhea, absence of thirst, vacuity fullness and pain, and a weak moderate pulse, whereas yáng brightness bowel patterns are identified by the presence of constipation, thirst, great repletion and fullness, and a sunken replete pulse. It is said, "Greater yīn disease is associated with vacuity, and yáng brightness disease is associated with repletion."

879. 少阴病 〔 少陰病 〕 *shào yīn bìng*, **lesser yīn disease** [ˈlɛsɚ jɪn dɪˈziz]: Disease of the foot lesser yīn (*shào yīn*) kidney channel and the hand lesser yīn (*shào yīn*) heart channel. Lesser yīn disease occurs when the heart and kidney are vacuous and when there is a marked drop in resistance to disease. It takes two different forms, vacuity cold and vacuity heat. (1) Vacuity cold: Cold evil damages yáng qì, and the main form of lesser yīn disease is a vacuity cold pattern that manifests as aversion to cold, curled-up lying posture, somnolence, reversal cold of the limbs, and faint fine pulse. Clear-grain diarrhea may occur in some cases. Generally there is no heat effusion (fever), and in severe cases the limbs may suffer a drop in temperature, indicating yáng collapse vacuity desertion. In *On Cold Damage* (*Shāng Hán Lùn*), the section on lesser yīn disease is headed with the statement, "The patient has a faint fine pulse and desires only to sleep." A faint fine pulse indicates vacuity of qì and blood, and desire only for sleep indicates debilitation of the spirit. These are both signs of general vacuity. Wherever a faint fine pulse occurs, whether in disease of recent onset or enduring disease, thought should be given to the possibility of lesser yīn disease. Absence of heat effusion (fever), aversion to cold, curled-up lying posture, and reversal cold of the limbs occurring with such a pulse indicate the presence of exuberant internal cold and the inability of debilitated yáng to

warm and nourish the skin and muscles and to fully permeate the limbs, thereby confirming the presence of lesser yīn disease. Clear-grain diarrhea is explained by kidney vacuity affecting the spleen (spleen-kidney yáng vacuity) and causing failure to move and transform food. Great sweating, reversal cold in the limbs, and a faint pulse verging on expiration indicate fulminant desertion of yáng qì. (2) Vacuity heat: Rarely, a lesser yīn transmuted pattern of vacuity heat may be observed. Insufficiency of kidney yīn and heart fire flaming upward cause signs such as heart vexation, insomnia, and dry pharynx and mouth.

880. 厥阴病〔厥陰病〕*jué yīn bìng,* **reverting yīn disease** [rɪ'vɝtɪŋ jɪn dɪ'ziz]: In the classical sequence, the reverting yīn is the last of the three yīn channels. Hence, it should theoretically be associated with the most severe diseases. *Elementary Questions (Sù Wèn)* states, "The reverting yīn channel skirts around the genitals and connects with the liver, so that its diseases include vexation and fullness, and retracted scrotum." The same chapter also mentions, among the signs of reverting yīn disease, "deafness, retraction of the scrotum, inability to ingest [even] liquid foods, and unconsciousness." *Elementary Questions (Sù Wèn)* enumerates signs but prescribes no formulas. Because the reverting yīn patterns described in *On Cold Damage (Shāng Hán Lùn)* are less severe, the real nature of reverting yīn disease is still in question, and further research is required to clarify the matter fully. Reverting yīn disease as described in *On Cold Damage (Shāng Hán Lùn)* is characterized by upper body heat and lower body cold, and may take the form of dispersion-thirst, qì surging up into the heart [region], pain and heat in the heart [region], hunger with no desire to eat, or vomiting of roundworm. Reversal cold of the limbs is also observed in some cases. Pathomechanically, upper body heat and lower body cold is explained as a cold-heat complex resulting from interior vacuity. Dispersion-thirst (消渴 *xiāo kě,* here meaning simply thirst), qì surging up into the heart [region], pain and heat in the heart [region], and clamoring stomach discomfort are the manifestations of upper body heat (heat in the area just above the diaphragm). No desire for food and vomiting of roundworm reflect lower body cold (in the intestines). This impairs movement and transformation of food, which disquiets the roundworm and causes it to rise counterflow. The reversal cold of the limbs indicates failure of yáng qì to reach the periphery of the body, which occurs when a cold-heat complex disturbs qì dynamic.

6.5.2. 卫气营血辨证 Four-Aspect Pattern Identification

881. 卫分证〔衛分證〕*wèi fēn zhèng*, **defense-aspect pattern** [dɪˈfɛns–æspɛkt–ˌpætən]: Warm disease principally characterized by heat effusion (fever), slight aversion to cold, presence or absence of sweating, and dry mouth. The tongue is distinctly red, and the pulse is floating and rapid. In some cases there may also be headache, cough, and sore red pharynx, and in others, distention in the head, clouded head, oppression in the chest, and upflow nausea. Defense-aspect patterns include signs common to the initial stage of all external heat diseases. Of these signs, heat effusion (fever) with slight aversion to wind and cold is the main indicator of defense-aspect disease. Like greater yáng (*tài yáng*) disease of the doctrine of cold damage, defense-aspect disease is seen as an exterior pattern in terms of the eight principles. However, whereas greater yáng disease may generally be classified as caused by cold, defense-aspect disease is classified as caused by heat. Warm evil enters the body through the nose and mouth, invariably invading the lung first. The lung is connected with the [surface] skin and [body] hair; it governs the exterior and defense. Thus, when it is invaded by an external evil, the defensive exterior is thwarted, and this causes heat effusion (fever) and slight aversion to cold. This is the fundamental law applied to defense-aspect disease. Warm evil is hot in nature, so that defense-aspect patterns include heat signs, and as such differ from greater yáng exterior patterns, which tend to be marked by cold signs. Once a defense-aspect pattern has been identified, it is usually necessary to determine whether warm evil is accompanied by wind or dampness. Wind warmth patterns are generally characterized by signs of lung heat such as cough, sore pharynx, and distinctly red tongue. Damp warmth patterns are characterized by signs of damp turbidity obstructing the center, such as heavy body, oppression in the chest, upflow nausea, dry throat with no desire for fluid, and a distinctly slimy tongue. Defense-aspect patterns are chiefly treated by the method of resolving the exterior with cool and acrid medicinals that discharge warm evil from the defense aspect.

882. 气分证〔氣分證〕*qì fēn zhèng*, **qì-aspect pattern** [ˈtʃi–æspɛkt–ˌpætən]: Any warm disease pattern of heat effusion (fever), aversion to heat rather than cold, thirst, bitter taste in the mouth, and yellow or reddish urine, a rapid pulse, and a yellow or yellow and white tongue fur. Qì-aspect disease is broad in scope and includes a large variety of exuberant-heat-stage externally contracted febrile diseases. These may be divided as follows: a) Initial-stage qì-aspect heat, which is characterized by generalized heat [effusion], thirst, heart vexation, burning

sensation in the heart [region], and mixed yellow and white tongue fur. b) Exuberant lung-stomach heat characterized by the classic signs of wind warmth, such as high fever, cough, rapid breathing, thirst, and yellow tongue fur. c) Great heat in the qì aspect, which is equivalent to yáng brightness (*yáng míng*) channel disease. d) Gastrointestinal heat bind, which is Equivalent to the yáng brightness bowel pattern. e) Damp-heat lodged in the triple burner, which is characterized by the classic signs of damp warmth: persistent remittent heat effusion (fever), oppression in the chest, thirst without great intake of fluids, upflow nausea, abdominal distention, short voidings of scant urine, a slimy tongue fur that is either white or slightly yellow in color, and a soggy rapid pulse. Also observable at this stage is brewing damp-heat steaming the stomach and intestines, characterized either by oppression in the chest and hard stool or by foul-smelling diarrhea, a slimy yellow tongue fur, and a slippery rapid pulse. These five patterns show marked differences between wind warmth and damp warmth in the qì aspect. Wind warmth may take the form of initial-stage qì-aspect heat, great heat in the qì aspect, gastrointestinal heat bind, or exuberant heat in the lung and stomach (which is characterized by four main signs of exuberant heat: heat effusion (fever), thirst, cough, and panting). Damp warmth presents differently. It is marked by unsurfaced heat and steaming of the stomach by brewing damp-heat. It develops slowly over a relatively long period of time.

883. 营分证 〔 營分證 〕 *yíng fēn zhèng,* **construction-aspect pattern** [kən-ˈstrʌkʃən–ˌæspɛkt ˈpætərn]: Warm disease one stage more advanced than a qì-aspect pattern, characterized by red or crimson tongue, a rapid pulse, generalized heat [effusion], heart vexation, and unquiet sleep. The essential characteristic of construction-aspect patterns is a red or crimson tongue, which indicates that evil heat has entered the construction aspect. Identification of construction-aspect patterns poses two requirements. a) It is important to determine whether the evil entering the construction aspect is warm-heat, wind-heat, or damp-heat. Warm heat and wind-heat evils entering the construction aspect are characterized by a red or crimson tongue with either no fur or a very thin fur. Damp-heat evil entering construction is characterized by a red or crimson tongue with a thick slimy or turbid tongue fur (indicating that the dampness evil has not transformed dryness) or by a parched black tongue fur (indicating that dryness formation has occurred). b) It is essential to determine the degree to which the construction aspect has been penetrated. Initial-stage construction-aspect patterns invariably include qì-aspect signs, such as red to crimson (deep red) tongue with a yellow, or mixed yellow-and-white tongue fur. Deep penetration

of the construction aspect is characterized by a dry deep red tongue, as well as signs such as clouded spirit-mind (see pericardiac pattern) and stirring wind and tetanic reversal.

884. **血分证**〔血分證〕 *xuè fèn zhèng,* **blood-aspect pattern** [ˈblʌd–æs-pɛkt–ˌpætən]: Any warm disease pattern that occurs when an evil enters the blood aspect. Signs include a deep crimson tongue and signs of frenetic movement of hot blood such as bleeding and purple maculopapular eruptions. The tongue may, in addition to being crimson, be bare and smooth like a mirror, indicating damage to yīn and fluid desertion. Such a condition may include signs of vacuity stirring internal wind such as convulsions of the limbs or tetanic reversal. These latter signs are nevertheless differentiated from the tetanic reversal and convulsions associated with extreme heat engendering wind. The accent in blood-aspect patterns may be on repletion signs such as frenetic blood movement; or it may be on vacuity of right with a lodged evil, where signs such as desiccated tongue and teeth, dry pharynx and mouth, heart vexation, and a rapid fine pulse indicate that although the heat has abated, the evil is still present and yīn humor is severely damaged.

885. **热入营血**〔熱入營血〕 *rè rù yíng xuè,* **heat entering construction-blood** [hit ˈenterɪŋ kənˈstrʌkʃən-blʌd]: See preceeding two items.

886. **心包证**〔心包證〕 *xīn bāo zhèng,* **pericardiac patterns** [ˌpɛrɪkɑr-dɪæk–ˌpætənz]: Warm disease patterns that occur when warm evils invade the pericardium and give rise to signs such as clouded spirit, delirious speech and manic agitation, and in severe cases coma. Portending signs are agitation, somnolence, and trembling of the tip of the tongue. Warm evils usually, though not invariably, pass to the construction aspect before gradually falling inward to the pericardium. In some cases, such as what Western medicine calls infectious encephalitis B, the evil falls inward directly from the defense aspect without passing through the construction aspect. This is known as "abnormal passage to the pericardium" (逆传心包 *nì chuán xīn bāo*). Two main patterns are identified. One is known as heat entering the pericardium, which is characterized by heat signs such as red to crimson tongue and, in most cases, a burnt-yellow tongue fur. The other is a phlegm-damp pattern referred to as phlegm clouding the pericardium, which is marked by a grimy sticky slimy fur that covers what may or may not be a red or crimson tongue.

887. **热入心包**〔熱入心包〕 *rè rù xīn bāo,* **heat entering the pericardium** [hit ˈentərɪŋ ðə ˌpɛrɪkɑrdɪəm]: See pericardiac patterns.

888. 痰蒙心包〔痰蒙心包〕*tán méng xīn bāo,* **phlegm clouding the peri-cardium** [flɛm ˈklaʊdɪŋ ðə ˌpɛrɪkɑrdɪəm]: See pericardiac patterns.

889. 风温〔風溫〕*fēng wēn,* **wind warmth** [wɪnd wɔrmθ]: A warm disease due to the contraction of wind warmth evil. Wind warmth usually occurs in winter or spring. At onset, the disease is in the lung and defense, and signs include generalized heat [effusion], cough, heart vexation, and thirst, but it easily makes an abnormal passage to the pericardium and causes clouded spirit, delirious speech, and tetanic reversal with convulsions.

890. 湿温〔濕溫〕*shī wēn,* **damp warmth** [dæmp wɔrmθ]: A febrile disease occurring in the summer or autumn that is attributed to damp-heat and characterized by persistent heat effusion, heavy-headedness, generalized pain, glomus and oppression in the chest and stomach duct, white or yellow slimy tongue fur, and a soggy pulse.

891. 气阴两虚〔氣陰兩虛〕*qì yīn liǎng xū,* **dual vacuity of qì and yīn** [ˈd(j)uəl vəˈkjuətɪ əv tʃi ənd jɪn]: A pattern of both qì vacuity and yīn vacuity commonly occurring in febrile disease. It includes qì vacuity signs, such as fatigued spirit and lack of strength, faint low voice, sweating, shortness of breath, torpid intake, and sloppy stool, and yīn vacuity signs, such as dry mouth, sore throat, vexing heat in the five hearts, postmeridian tidal heat [effusion], and night sweating. It occurs in the following circumstances: (1) Warm-heat disease that causes wear on the fluids and gives rise to a vacuity desertion trend characterized by great sweating, hasty panting, vexation and thirst, pale red or dry crimson tongue, and a large diffuse or fine rapid pulse. (2) Advanced-stage warm heat disease and miscellaneous internal damage disease in which depletion of true yīn and major damage to original qì causes lassitude of spirit and physical fatigue, shortage of qì and laziness to speak, dry mouth and pharynx, low fever or tidal heat [effusion] or vexing heat in the five hearts, spontaneous sweating, night sweating, red tongue with scant fur, and a large vacuous or rapid vacuous pulse. (3) Evil lodged in the qì aspect in warm disease causing unthorough sweating that eventually damages qì and humor and gives rise to the appearance of white miliaria that is dry, white, and sheenless. In addition, dual vacuity of qì and yīn is also observed in certain consumptive diseases.

习题
Questions

Answer the following questions in English:

621. In eight-principle pattern identification, what does the sudden onset of heat effusion (fever) with aversion to cold indicate? ....

622. What liver disease pattern does distention and pain in the breasts indicate? ....

623. What are the different forms of liver wind stirring internally? ....

624. Would a child with fever and arched-back rigidity, diagnosed in Western medicine as having encephalitis B, be said to be suffering from a) extreme heat engendering wind or b) liver-gallbladder damp-heat? ....

625. What stomach signs accompany liver qì invading the stomach? ....

626. What spleen signs arise with liver qì invading the spleen? ....

627. To what is improper development in the fetal stage ascribed? ....

628. List the general signs of qì vacuity. ....

629. What are the characteristic signs of qì stagnation? ....

630. In what way does the pain associated with blood stasis differ from that of qì stagnation? ....

631. Which viscera and bowels are susceptible to qì counterflow? ....

632. What complexion is associated with blood vacuity? ....

633. What are the main signs of blood heat? ....

634. In what pattern are great dripping sweat and faint pulse on the verge of expiration observed? ....

635. In what way does yáng vacuity differ from qì vacuity? ....

636. A patient with heart palpitations, heart vexation, insomnia and profuse dreaming, vexing heat in the five hearts, and night sweating is diagnosed as having what heart disease pattern? ....

637. Dull pain and stifling oppression in the chest indicate what heart pattern? ....

638. In eight-principle pattern identification, what does alternating [aversion to] cold and heat [effusion] indicate? ....

639. What pathology of the lung is indicated by cough and nasal congestion? ....

640. What does a forceless cough, panting, and shortness of breath indicate? ....

641. Spleen qi vacuity can take several forms. What are they?
....

642. What is the main sign of spleen failing to control the blood?
....

643. Irascibility, distention and pain in the rib-side, oppression in the chest, and sighing are commonly observed in what liver disease pattern? ....

644. If a patient has dizziness, tinnitus, distention and pain in the head, and red face with baking heat due to upbearing fire, what pattern does he/she display? ....

645. How would you diagnose a patient with signs such as dizziness, insomnia, profuse dreaming, flowery vision, inhibited sinew movement, and lusterless nails? ....

646. In eight-principle pattern identification, what does marked aversion to cold with a pulse that is floating and tight indicate? ....

647. To what is lumbar pain (or aching lumbus) not due to external injury attributed? ....

648. When the main signs a patient displays are frequent and long voidings of clear urine, incontinence, enuresis, or dribbling urination on the one hand or seminal loss or premature ejaculation on the other, what kidney disease pattern should the patient be diagnosed as displaying? ....

649. What pattern is attributed to liver qi depression forming into fire?
....

650. What does anemia classically correspond to in Chinese medicine? ....

651. What is the pattern called that is qi desertion developing from heavy blood loss? ....

652. What heart patterns is insomnia observed in? ....

653. In what heart patterns do heart palpitations occur? ....

654. What is the combined pattern of heart yīn vacuity and kidney yīn vacuity called? ....

655. Which pattern is seen in illness of rapid onset, nondiffusion of lung qì, or impaired depurative downbearing of the lung? ....

Give the Pīnyīn and English for the following Chinese terms:

656. 阴虚火旺 ....

657. 湿热下注大肠 ....

658. 伤食 ....

659. 脾肾阳虚 ....

660. 下元虚惫 ....

661. 营分证 ....

662. 阳虚水泛 ....

663. 半表半里 ....

664. 热入心包 ....

665. 肺气不利 ....

666. 肝阳上亢 ....

667. 肾气不固 ....

668. 风寒 ....

669. 痰浊上扰 ....

670. 表实 ....

671. 气血俱虚 ....

672. 脾肺两虚 ....

673. 湿阻 ....

674. 寒疝 ....

675. 卫分证 ....

Supply the Chinese and English for the following:

676. *Rè jí shēng fēng.* ....

677. *Gān qì yù jié.* ....

678. *Mìng mén huǒ shuāi.* ....

679. *Shèn jīng bù zú.* ....

680. *Wài gǎn hán xié.* ....

681. *Shī rè liú liàn qì fèn.* ....

682. *Tài yáng bìng.* ....

683. *Tán yǐn.* ....

684. *Tán méng xīn bāo.* ....

685. *Xuè rè wàng xíng.* ....

686. *Qì bì.* ....

687. *Tán zhuó méng bì xīn bāo.* ....

688. *Wèi fèn zhèng.* ....

689. *Qì nì.* ....

690. *Zhōng qì xià xiàn.* ....

691. *Wáng xuè.* ....

692. *Lǐ zhèng.* ....

693. *Qì zhì.* ....

694. *Qì suí xuè tuō.* ....

695. *Gān huǒ shàng yán.* ....

Give the Chinese and Pīnyīn for the following:

696. Gastrointestinal accumulation. ....

697. Damage to liquid. ....

698. Phlegm confounding the orifices of the heart. ....

699. Greater yáng disease. ....

700. Cold pattern. ....

701. Vacuity pattern. ....

702. Pattern identification. ....

703. Qì stagnation and blood stasis. ....

704. Heart qì vacuity. ....

第七章 治则与治法
Principles and Methods of Treatment

In this chapter, the names of medicinals and formulas are given in Chinese, Pīnyīn, and English. The names of medicinals are followed by a Latin pharmaceutical name in parentheses. Note that some of the Latin names of medicinals use in previous publications have been changed to conform with the *Chinese Pharmacopoeia* (2000). This has also led to changes in English names of medicinals and formulas.

7.1. 治则
Principles of Treatment

892. **实则泻之**〔實則瀉之〕*shí zé xiè zhī,* **repletion is treated by draining** [rɪˈpliʃən ɪz ˈtritɪd baɪ ˈdrenɪŋ]: Disease patterns that arise when evil qì is exuberant and right qì is not debilitated (e.g., external contractions, phlegm-rheum, static blood, food stagnation, and cold accumulation patterns) are treated by methods that remove the evil qì (e.g., resolving the exterior, dispelling phlegm, quickening the blood and transforming stasis, softening hardness, draining precipitation, and abductive dispersion).

893. **虚则补之**〔虛則補之〕*xū zé bǔ zhī,* **vacuity is treated by supplementing** [vəˈkjuətɪ ɪz ˈtritɪd baɪ ˈsʌplɪˌmɛntɪŋ]: The principle that weakness, i.e., vacuity, is treated by supplementing. Different vacuity patterns, such as qì vacuity, blood vacuity, yīn vacuity, and yáng vacuity, are treated by different forms of supplementation (supplementing qì, supplementing blood, supplementing yīn, supplementing yáng, etc.).

894. **治本**〔治本〕*zhì běn,* **treating the root** [tritɪŋ ðə rut]: Treating the main aspect of a condition. The phrase, "disease should be treated from the root" (治病必求于本 *zhì bìng bì qiú yú běn*) has been the major guiding principle of pattern identification and treatment for millennia. The word "root" is used in opposition to "tip," the two terms being of

varying significance depending on the context. For example, root frequently refers to the essential nature of the disease, while tip refers to symptoms; root can also refer to the cause of disease, while tip refers to the clinically observable changes in the human body; root can also denote right qì, in which case tip refers to the evil; finally, in other contexts, the primary condition may be described as the root in contradistinction to the resulting secondary conditions that are the tip. The principle of treating disease from the root, or radical treatment, applies to most diseases and is divided into two forms: straight treatment and paradoxical treatment.

895. 治标〔治標〕 *zhì biāo,* **treating the tip** [trɪtɪŋ ðə tɪp]: See treating the root.

896. 正治〔正治〕 *zhèng zhì,* **straight treatment** ['stret–trɪtmɛnt]: The most commonly applied principle of treatment whereby the nature and pathomechanism are directly counteracted, as when a cold pattern is treated with hot medicinals and a heat pattern is treated with cold medicinals, or when vacuity patterns are treated by supplementing or repletion patterns are treated by draining.

897. 反治〔反治〕 *fǎn zhì,* **paradoxical treatment** [‚pærə'dɑksɪkl̩ trɪtmɛnt]: The principle of treating false signs with medicinals of the same nature, e.g., treating heat with heat, cold with cold, the stopped by stopping, and flow by promoting flow. Treating cold with cold, for example, means using heavy doses of heat-clearing toxin-resolving agents to treat exuberant heat in externally contracted heat disease that presents with false signs of cold such as aversion to cold or shivering, and cold of the limbs. Compare straight treatment.

7.2. 治法
Methods of Treatment

898. 八法〔八法〕 *bā fǎ,* **eight methods** [et 'mɛθədz]: A classification of medicinal treatment methods by Chéng Zhōng-Líng (程钟龄) of the Qīng Dynasty under the eight rubrics sweating (汗法 *hàn fǎ*), ejection (吐法 *tù fǎ*), precipitation (下法 *xià fǎ*), harmonization (和法 *hé fǎ*), warming (温法 *wēn fǎ*), clearing (清法 *qīng fǎ*), supplementation (补法 *bǔ fǎ*), and dispersion (消法 *xiāo fǎ*). This classification system has lost favor with medical scholars since it does not cover the full gamut of treatments. In the present chapter, methods of treatment

are classified according to a modern system, but references are made to the eight methods where clear correspondences exist.

7.2.1. 解表 Resolving the Exterior

899. **解表**〔解表〕*jiě biǎo,* **resolving the exterior** [rɪˈzɑlv-ɪŋ ði ɪksˈtɪrɪɚ]: A method of treatment used to eliminate evil from the fleshy exterior by effusing sweat. The two main methods are resolving the exterior with warmth and acridity and resolving the exterior with coolness and acridity. Resolving the exterior is called sweating in the eight methods.

900. **汗法**〔汗法〕*hàn fǎ,* **sweating** [ˈswɛtɪŋ]: One of the eight methods. Sweating corresponds to resolving the exterior.

901. **辛温解表**〔辛溫解表〕*xīn wēn jiě biǎo,* **resolving the exterior with warmth and acridity** [rɪˈzɑlvɪŋ ði ɪksˈtɪrɪɚ wɪð wɔrmθ ənd əˈkrɪdɪtɪ]: A method of treating exterior cold patterns marked by pronounced aversion to cold, pronounced headache and aching bones, high or low fever, moist white tongue fur, tight floating pulse, and absence of any heat signs such as red tongue, dry mouth, or red sore swollen tongue.

Medicinals:
麻黄 *má huáng,* ephedra (Ephedrae Herba)
桂枝 *guì zhī,* cinnamon twig (Cinnamomi Ramulus)
紫苏叶 *zǐ sū yè,* perilla leaf (Perillae Folium)
荆芥 *jīng jiè,* schizonepeta (Schizonepetae Herba)
生姜 *shēng jiāng,* fresh ginger (Zingiberis Rhizoma Recens)
防风 *fáng fēng,* saposhnikovia (Saposhnikoviae Radix)
羌活 *qiāng huó,* notopterygium (Notopterygii Rhizoma et Radix)
连须葱白 *lián xū cōng bái,* scallion white with root (Allii Fistulosi Bulbus cum Radice)

Formulas:
麻黄汤 *má huáng tāng,* Ephedra Decoction
桂枝汤 *guì zhī tāng,* Cinnamon Twig Decoction
荆防败毒散 *jīng fáng bài dú sǎn,* Schizonepeta and Saposhnikovia Toxin-Vanquishing Powder

902. **辛凉解表**〔辛涼解表〕*xīn liáng jiě biǎo,* **resolving the exterior with coolness and acridity** [rɪˈzɑlvɪŋ ði ɪksˈtɪrɪɚ wɪð ˈkulnɪs ənd əˈkrɪdɪtɪ]: A method of treatment used for exterior heat patterns with mild aversion to cold and pronounced heat signs, such as thirst, red sore pharynx, red tongue with dry thin white fur, and rapid floating pulse.

Medicinals:

薄荷 *bò hé*, mint (Menthae Herba)

桑叶 *sāng yè*, mulberry leaf (Mori Folium)

淡豆豉 *dàn dòu chǐ*, fermented soybean (Sojae Semen Praeparatum)

牛蒡子 *niú bàng zǐ*, arctium (Arctii Fructus)

葛根 *gé gēn*, pueraria (Puerariae Radix)

柽柳 *chēng liǔ*, tamarisk (Tamaricis Cacumen)

Formulas:

银翘散 *yín qiáo sǎn*, Lonicera and Forsythia Powder

桑菊饮 *sāng jú yǐn*, Mulberry Leaf and Chrysanthemum Beverage

羌蒡蒲薄汤 *qiāng bàng pú bò tāng*, Notopterygium, Arctium, Dandelion, and Mint Decoction

903. **疏表** 〔 疏表 〕 *shū biǎo*, **coursing the exterior** [ˈkɔrsɪŋ ði ɪksˈtɪrɪɚ]: A method of treatment used to free the exterior of evil without necessarily making the patient sweat. Medicinals used to course the exterior are mild exterior-resolving medicinals such as warm acrid perilla leaf (*zǐ sū yè*) and saposhnikovia (*fáng fēng*), and cool acrid mint (*bò hé*), mulberry leaf (*sāng yè*), and pueraria (*gé gēn*).

904. **疏风泄热** 〔 疏風泄熱 〕 *shū fēng xiè rè*, **coursing wind and discharging heat** [ˈkɔrsɪŋ wɪnd ənd dɪsˈtʃɑrdʒɪŋ hit]: A method of treatment used for exterior wind-heat with interior heat in colds and flu marked by sore throat, dry mouth, red tongue, and thin yellow fur.

Formulas:

桑菊饮 *sāng jú yǐn*, Mulberry Leaf and Chrysanthemum Beverage

银翘散 *yín qiáo sǎn*, Lonicera and Forsythia Powder

905. **滋阴解表** 〔 滋陰解表 〕 *zī yīn jiě biǎo*, **enriching yīn and resolving the exterior** [ɪnˈrɪtʃɪŋ jɪn ənd rɪˈzɑlvɪŋ ði ɪksˈtɪrɪɚ]: A method of treatment used to enrich yīn and promote sweating in order to resolve an exterior pattern in patients suffering from yīn vacuity. In such patterns, sweating therapy would be ruled out on the grounds that it would worsen the vacuity condition further. For this method, yīn-enriching medicinals such as dried/fresh rehmannia (*shēng dì huáng*), Solomon's seal (*yù zhú*), and ophiopogon (*mài mén dōng*) are combined with exterior-resolving medicinals such as fermented soybean (*dàn dòu chǐ*), pueraria (*gé gēn*), perilla leaf (*zǐ sū yè*), scallion white (*cōng bái*), and mint (*bò hé*).

Formula:

加减葳蕤汤 *jiā jiǎn wēi ruí tāng*, Solomon's Seal Variant Decoction

906. 助阳解表〔助陽解表〕*zhù yáng jiě biǎo*, **reinforcing yáng and resolving the exterior** [ˌrɪmˈfɔrsɪŋ jæŋ/jɑŋ ənd rɪˈzɑlvɪŋ ði ɪksˈtɪrɪɚ]: A method of treatment used for yáng qì vacuity when the patient also has an external contraction. Such conditions are characterized by signs such as pronounced aversion to cold with mild heat effusion, absence of sweating, lack of warmth in the extremities, desire to wrap up well to keep warm, fatigued essence-spirit, headache, somnolence, somber white facial complexion, faint low voice, white tongue fur, and a forceless sunken pulse.

Formula:

再造散 *zài zào sǎn*, Renewal Powder
黄芪 *huáng qí*, astragalus (Astragali Radix)
党参 *dǎng shēn*, codonopsis (Codonopsis Radix)
桂枝 *guì zhī*, cinnamon twig (Cinnamomi Ramulus)
甘草 *gān cǎo*, licorice (Glycyrrhizae Radix)
熟附子 *shú fù zǐ*, cooked aconite (Aconiti Radix Lateralis Conquita)
细辛 *xì xīn*, asarum (Asari Herba)
羌活 *qiāng huó*, notopterygium (Notopterygii Rhizoma et Radix)
防风 *fáng fēng*, saposhnikovia (Saposhnikoviae Radix)
川芎 *chuān xiōng*, chuanxiong (Chuanxiong Rhizoma)
生姜 *shēng jiāng*, fresh ginger (Zingiberis Rhizoma Recens)
芍药 *sháo yào*, peony (Paeoniae Radix)
大枣 *dà zǎo*, jujube (Jujubae Fructus)

907. 益气解表〔益氣解表〕*yì qì jiě biǎo*, **boosting qì and resolving the exterior** [ˈbustɪŋ tʃi ənd rɪˈzɑlvɪŋ ði ɪksˈtɪrɪɚ]: A method of treatment used to address continual common colds and copious sweat from qì vacuity that increases vulnerability to external evils and reduces the body's ability to expel an evil once it has entered. In such cases, qì-boosting medicinals may be combined with exterior-resolving medicinals.

Formula:

参苏饮 *shēn sū yǐn*, Ginseng and Perilla Beverage
党参 *dǎng shēn*, codonopsis (Codonopsis Radix)
白苏叶 *bái sū yè*, white perilla leaf (Perillae Albae Folium)
葛根 *gé gēn*, pueraria (Puerariae Radix)
前胡 *qián hú*, peucedanum (Peucedani Radix)
姜半夏 *jiāng bàn xià*, ginger pinellia (Pinelliae Rhizoma cum Zingibere Praeparatum)
陈皮 *chén pí*, tangerine peel (Citri Reticulatae Pericarpium)
桔梗 *jié gěng*, platycodon (Platycodonis Radix)

茯苓 *fú líng*, poria (Poria)

木香 *mù xiāng*, costusroot (Aucklandiae Radix)

枳壳 *zhǐ qiào*, bitter orange (Aurantii Fructus)

甘草 *gān cǎo*, licorice (Glycyrrhizae Radix)

908. **表里双解**〔表裡雙解〕*biǎo lǐ shuāng jiě*, **resolving both the exterior and interior; exterior-interior resolution** [rɪˈzɑlvɪŋ boθ ði ɪksˈtɪrɪɚ ənd ɪnˈtɪriər; ɪksˈtɪrɪɚ ɪnˈtɪriər ˌrɛzəˈluʃən]: A method of treatment used to address interior and exterior patterns at the same time. There are two main forms: (1) Treating exterior evils in the outer body with repletion accumulation in the interior marked by aversion to cold, heat effusion, abdominal distention and pain, nausea and constipation, and a slippery floating pulse. A representative formula is Officinal Magnolia Bark Seven Agents Decoction (*hòu pò qī wù tāng*), which contains Cinnamon Twig Decoction (*guì zhī tāng*) minus peony (*sháo yào*) to resolve the exterior, and Officinal Magnolia Bark Three Agents Decoction (*hòu pò sān wù tāng*) to treat the interior. (2) Treating exuberant interior heat with a concurrent exterior pattern, marked by high fever without sweating, red face and eyes, generalized hypertonicity, dry nose, thirst, bitter taste in the mouth, vexation and agitation, delirious speech, dry tongue, and a rapid surging pulse. A representative formula is Three Yellows and Gypsum Decoction (*sān huáng shí gāo tāng*) in which ephedra (*má huáng*) and litsea (*dòu chǐ jiāng*) resolve the exterior, while gypsum (*shí gāo*), scutellaria (*huáng qín*), coptis (*huáng lián*), and gardenia (*shān zhī zǐ*) clear the interior.

7.2.2. 清法 Clearing

909. **清气分热**〔清氣分熱〕*qīng qì fēn rè*, **clearing qì-aspect heat** [ˈklɪrɪŋ ˈtʃi–æspɛkt hit]: A method of treatment used to address qì-aspect heat patterns, which are marked by vigorous heat effusion (fever), thirst, dry tongue, and surging pulse.

Medicinals:

石膏 *shí gāo*, gypsum (Gypsum Fibrosum)

知母 *zhī mǔ*, anemarrhena (Anemarrhenae Rhizoma)

山栀子 *shān zhī zǐ*, gardenia (Gardeniae Fructus)

Formulas:

白虎汤 *bái hǔ tāng*, White Tiger Decoction

栀子豉汤 *zhī zǐ chǐ tāng*, Gardenia and Fermented Soybean Decoction

910. **清营凉血**〔清營涼血〕*qīng yíng liáng xuè*, **clearing construction and cooling the blood** [ˈklɪrɪŋ kənˈstrʌkʃən ənd ˈkulɪŋ θə blʌd]: A

method of treatment used to address heat entering construction-blood in heat diseases with general signs such as high fever, clouded spirit, and crimson tongue, and specific signs of frenetic movement of hot blood (blood ejection, spontaneous external bleeding, bloody stool, or bloody urine). Also called cooling the blood.

Medicinals:

牡丹皮 *mǔ dān pí*, moutan (Moutan Cortex)

赤芍药 *chì sháo yào*, red peony (Paeoniae Radix Rubra)

犀角 *xī jiǎo*, rhinoceros horn (Rhinocerotis Cornu)

生地黄 *shēng dì huáng*, dried/fresh rehmannia (Rehmanniae Radix Exsiccata seu Recens)

紫草 *zǐ cǎo*, arnebia/lithospermum (Arnebiae/Lithospermi Radix)

Formula:

犀角地黄汤 *xī jiǎo dì huáng tāng*, Rhinoceros Horn and Rehmannia Decoction

911. 凉血〔凉血〕*liáng xuè,* **cooling the blood** ['kulɪŋ ðə blʌd]: See clearing construction and cooling the blood.

912. **清热解暑**〔清熱解暑〕*qīng rè jiě shǔ,* **clearing heat and resolving summerheat** ['klɪrɪŋ hit ənd rɪ'zɑlvɪŋ 'sʌməhit]: A method of treatment used to address externally contracted summerheat-heat characterized by headache, generalized heat [effusion], sweating, vexation and thirst, short voidings of reddish urine, thin yellow tongue fur, and a rapid floating pulse.

Medicinals:

鲜薄荷 *xiān bò hé*, fresh mint (Menthae Herba Recens)

扁豆花 *biǎn dòu huā*, lablab flower (Lablab Flos)

青蒿 *qīng hāo*, sweet wormwood (Artemisiae Annuae Herba)

香薷 *xiāng rú*, mosla (Moslae Herba)

金银花 *jīn yín huā*, lonicera (Lonicerae Flos)

连翘 *lián qiào*, forsythia (Forsythiae Fructus)

芦根 *lú gēn*, phragmites (Phragmitis Rhizoma)

黄连 *huáng lián*, coptis (Coptidis Rhizoma)

Formulas:

清络饮 *qīng luò yǐn*, Network-Clearing Beverage

王氏清暑益气汤 *wáng shì qīng shǔ yì qì tāng*, Wáng's Summerheat-Clearing Qì-Boosting Decoction

913. **清热解毒**〔清熱解毒〕*qīng rè jiě dú,* **clearing heat and resolving toxin** ['klɪrɪŋ hit ənd rɪ'zɑlvɪŋ 'tɑksɪn]: A method of treatment used to address any repletion pattern attributed to heat toxin, such as intense

heat toxin in externally contracted heat (febrile) disease, sores (yáng patterns), cinnabar toxin, maculopapular eruption, pulmonary welling-abscess, dysentery with blood and pus in the stool, and heat strangury with painful urination and reddish urine. Such patterns are characterized by scorching heat, heat effusion (fever), swelling and distention, pain, suppuration, and putrefaction.

Medicinals:

大青叶 *dà qīng yè*, isatis leaf (Isatidis Folium)

板蓝根 *bǎn lán gēn*, isatis root (Isatidis Radix)

蒲公英 *pú gōng yīng*, dandelion (Taraxaci Herba)

黄芩 *huáng qín*, scutellaria (Scutellariae Radix)

黄连 *huáng lián*, coptis (Coptidis Rhizoma)

黄柏 *huáng bǎi*, phellodendron (Phellodendri Cortex)

金银花 *jīn yín huā*, lonicera (Lonicerae Flos)

连翘 *lián qiào*, forsythia (Forsythiae Fructus)

生甘草 *shēng gān cǎo*, raw licorice (Glycyrrhizae Radix Cruda)

山栀子 *shān zhī zǐ*, gardenia (Gardeniae Fructus)

紫花地丁 *zǐ huā dì dīng*, violet (Violae Herba)

青黛 *qīng dài*, indigo (Indigo Naturalis)

鱼腥草 *yú xīng cǎo*, houttuynia (Houttuyniae Herba)

射干 *shè gān*, belamcanda (Belamcandae Rhizoma)

山豆根 *shān dòu gēn*, bushy sophora (Sophorae Tonkinensis Radix)

马勃 *mǎ bó*, puffball (Lasiosphaera seu Calvatia)

土茯苓 *tǔ fú líng*, smooth greenbrier (Smilacis Glabrae Rhizoma)

Formulas:

黄连解毒汤 *huáng lián jiě dú tāng*, Coptis Toxin-Resolving Decoction

普济消毒饮 *pǔ jì xiāo dú yǐn*, Universal Salvation Toxin-Dispersing Beverage

914. **清脏腑热**〔清臟腑熱〕*qīng zàng fǔ rè*, **clearing bowel and visceral heat** [ˈklɪrɪŋ ˈbɑʊəl ənd ˈvɪsərəl hit]: Any method of dispelling heat or fire from any of the bowels and viscera, e.g., draining the heart (*xiè xīn*), clearing the heart and opening the orifices (*qīng xīn kāi qiào*), draining the lung (*xiè fèi*), clearing and depurating lung qì (*qīng sù fèi qì*), clearing the lung and moistening dryness (*qīng fèi rùn zào*).

915. **清虚热**〔清虛熱〕*qīng xū rè*, **clearing vacuity heat** [ˈklɪrɪŋ vəˈkjuəti hit]: A method of treatment used to address advanced-stage externally contracted heat (febrile) diseases or chronic diseases, such as pulmonary consumption, that manifest in steaming bone or tidal heat [effusion], night sweating, persistent low fever, reddening of the cheeks,

emaciation, and red or crimson tongue with little fur, which indicate that yīn humor is damaged and evil heat is lodged in the yīn aspect.

Medicinals:

鳖甲 *biē jiǎ*, turtle shell (Trionycis Carapax)

青蒿 *qīng hāo*, sweet wormwood (Artemisiae Annuae Herba)

地骨皮 *dì gǔ pí*, lycium bark (Lycii Cortex)

银柴胡 *yín chái hú*, stellaria (Stellariae Radix)

秦艽 *qín jiāo*, large gentian (Gentianae Macrophyllae Radix)

白薇 *bái wēi*, black swallowwort (Cynanchi Atrati Radix)

Formulas:

青蒿鳖甲汤 *qīng hāo biē jiǎ tāng*, Sweet Wormwood and Turtle Shell Decoction

清骨散 *qīng gǔ sǎn*, Bone-Clearing Powder

7.2.3. 下法 Precipitation[1]

916. **寒下**〔寒下〕*hán xià,* **cold precipitation** [kold prə͵sɪpɪ'teʃən]: A method of treating interior heat repletion patterns characterized by constipation (often called heat bind, 热结 *rè jié*) with abdominal fullness, tidal heat [effusion], dry mouth and thirst, parched yellow tongue fur, and a forceful slippery rapid pulse; also treats food and water accumulations.

Medicinals:

大黄 *dà huáng*, rhubarb (Rhei Radix et Rhizoma)

芒硝 *máng xiāo*, mirabilite (Natrii Sulfas)

Formulas:

大承气汤 *dà chéng qì tāng*, Major Qì-Coordinating Decoction

小承气汤 *xiǎo chéng qì tāng*, Minor Qì-Coordinating Decoction

调胃承气汤 *tiáo wèi chéng qì tāng*, Stomach-Regulating Qì-Coordinating Decoction

917. **温下**〔溫下〕*wēn xià,* **warm precipitation** [wɔrm prə͵sɪpɪ'teʃən]: A method of precipitation applied to cold-natured accumulation and stagnation that form interior repletion patterns often referred to as "cold bind" (寒结 *hán jié*) or "cold constipation" and characterized by constipation with abdominal fullness, cold extremities, white slimy tongue fur, and sunken stringlike or slow sunken pulse.

---

[1] The word "precipitation" has been chosen in preference to the English "purgation" since it conveys the idea of downward movement that the English "purgation" (= cleaning) does not.

Medicinals:

巴豆 *bā dòu*, croton (Crotonis Fructus)

大黄 *dà huáng*, rhubarb (Rhei Radix et Rhizoma) (a cold precipitating medicinal that can be combined with the following two hot medicinals)

附子 *fù zǐ*, aconite (Aconiti Radix Lateralis Praeparata)

细辛 *xì xīn*, asarum (Asari Herba)

Formulas:

三物备急丸 *sān wù bèi jí wán*, Three Agents Emergency Pill

大黄附子汤 *dà huáng fù zǐ tāng*, Rhubarb and Aconite Decoction

918. 润下〔潤下〕*rùn xià*, **moist precipitation** [mɔɪst prəˌsɪpɪˈteʃən]: Also called humor-increasing moist precipitation. Treating constipation with moist medicinals. Using moist and oily medicinals such as cannabis fruit (*huǒ má rén*) and honey (*mì*) to treat dry stool in the elderly, habitual constipation, constipation in pregnancy, and postpartum constipation.

Medicinals:

火麻仁 *huǒ má rén*, cannabis fruit (Cannabis Fructus)

杏仁 *xìng rén*, apricot kernel (Armeniacae Semen)

栝楼子 *guā lóu zǐ*, trichosanthes seed (Trichosanthis Semen)

郁李仁 *yù lǐ rén*, bush cherry kernel (Pruni Semen)

蜜 *mì*, honey (Mel)

Formulas:

麻子仁丸 *má zǐ rén wán*, Cannabis Fruit Pill

润肠丸 *rùn cháng wán*, Intestine-Moistening Pill

五仁丸 *wǔ rén wán*, Five Kernels Pill

"Moist precipitation" also denotes a method of treating intestinal heat bind and desiccated fluid constipation using fluid-enriching medicinals such as scrophularia (*xuán shēn*), ophiopogon (*mài mén dōng*) (with the hearts left in), and dried/fresh rehmannia (*shēng dì huáng*). This method is also called humor-increasing moist precipitation.

919. 增液润下〔增液潤下〕*zēng yè rùn xià*, **humor-increasing moist precipitation** [ˈhjumər–ɪnˈkrisɪŋ mɔɪst prəˌsɪpɪˈteʃən]: See moist precipitation.

920. 逐水〔逐水〕*zhú shuǐ*, **expelling water** [ɪkˈspɛlɪŋ ˈwɔtər]: A method of treatment used to eliminate yáng water repletion patterns by precipitation. Such patterns include hydrothorax and ascites, which are characterized by urinary and fecal stoppage, abdominothoracic fullness that inhibits respiration, and a forceful replete pulse. This method may be

used where the evil is strong, and right qì is still resilient enough to withstand attack. In modern clinical practice, it is mainly used to treat what Western medicine identifies as ascites due to cirrhosis of the liver. Commonly used water-expelling medicinals are kansui (*gān suì*), genkwa (*yuán huā*), euphorbia/knoxia (*dà jǐ*), and morning glory (*qiān niú zǐ*). Ten Jujubes Decoction (*shí zǎo tāng*) and Boats and Carts Pill (*zhōu chē (jū) wán*) drain abdominal water, whereas Drool-Controlling Elixir (*kòng xián dān*) is used to drain hydrothorax.

7.2.4. 和法 Harmonization

921. **和解少阳**〔和解少陽〕*hé jiě shào yáng*, **harmonizing (and resolving) the lesser yáng** [ˈhɑrmə,naɪzɪŋ (ənd rɪˈzɔlvɪŋ) ðə ˈlɛsɚ jæŋ/jɑŋ)]: A method of treatment used to resolve the exterior and harmonize the interior in order to treat lesser yáng (*shào yáng*) midstage patterns in externally contracted heat (febrile) diseases. These are characterized by alternating [aversion to] cold and heat [effusion], oppression and fullness in the chest and rib-side region, bitter taste in the mouth and dry pharynx, and nausea and vomiting.

Medicinals:
> 柴胡 *chái hú*, bupleurum (Bupleuri Radix)
> 青蒿 *qīng hāo*, sweet wormwood (Artemisiae Annuae Herba)

To clear interior heat:
> 黄芩 *huáng qín*, scutellaria (Scutellariae Radix)

To harmonize the center:
> 半夏 *bàn xià*, pinellia (Pinelliae Rhizoma)
> 生姜 *shēng jiāng*, fresh ginger (Zingiberis Rhizoma Recens)
> 甘草 *gān cǎo*, licorice (Glycyrrhizae Radix)
> 大枣 *dà zǎo*, jujube (Jujubae Fructus)

Formulas:
> 小柴胡汤 *xiǎo chái hú tāng*, Minor Bupleurum Decoction

922. **和解半表半里**〔和解半表半裡〕*hé jiě bàn biǎo bàn lǐ*, **harmonizing (and resolving) midstage patterns; harmonizing (and resolving) half-exterior half-interior patterns** [ˈhɑrmə,naɪzɪŋ (ənd rɪˈzɔlvɪŋ)) ˈmɪdstedʒ ˈpætɚnz; hæf ɪksˈtɪrɪɚ hæf ɪnˈtɪrɪɚ ˈpætɚnz]: See harmonizing the lesser yáng.

923. **调和肝脾**〔調和肝脾〕*tiáo hé gān pí*, **harmonizing the liver and spleen** [ˈhɑrmə,naɪzɪŋ ðə ˈlɪvɚ ənd splin]: A method of treatment used to address liver-spleen disharmony that is attributed to liver qì depression and the spleen failing to move and transform and that is marked

by signs such as abdominal distention, abdominal pain, rumbling intestines, and diarrhea, which occur in episodes associated with emotional depression.

To course the liver:

柴胡 *chái hú*, bupleurum (Bupleuri Radix)

白芍药 *bái sháo yào*, white peony (Paeoniae Radix Alba)

To fortify the spleen:

白术 *bái zhú*, white atractylodes (Atractylodis Macrocephalae Rhizoma)

茯苓 *fú líng*, poria (Poria)

陈皮 *chén pí*, tangerine peel (Citri Reticulatae Pericarpium)

Formulas:

痛泻要方 *tòng xiè yào fāng*, Pain and Diarrhea Formula

逍遥散 *xiāo yáo sǎn*, Free Wanderer Powder

924. 调和肝胃〔調和肝胃〕 *tiáo hé gān wèi*, **harmonizing the liver and stomach** [ˈhɑrməˌnɑɪzɪŋ ðə ˈlɪvɚ ənd ˈstʌmək]: A method of treatment used to address liver-stomach disharmony from impaired free coursing of liver qì and impaired downbearing of stomach qì, characterized by the classic liver sign of distending pain in the chest and rib-side and by stomach signs such as pain, fullness, and distention in the stomach duct, poor appetite, belching, vomiting of sour matter, or retching and nausea.

To course the liver:

吴茱萸 *wú zhū yú*, evodia (Evodiae Fructus)

紫苏 *zǐ sū*, perilla (Perillae Folium, Caulis, et Calyx)

To harmonize the stomach:

半夏 *bàn xià*, pinellia (Pinelliae Rhizoma)

生姜 *shēng jiāng*, fresh ginger (Zingiberis Rhizoma Recens)

To clear stomach heat:

黄连 *huáng lián*, coptis (Coptidis Rhizoma)

竹茹 *zhú rú*, bamboo shavings (Bumbusae Caulis in Taenia)

Formula:

柴胡疏肝散 *chái hú shū gān sǎn*, Bupleurum Liver-Coursing Powder

925. 调和肠胃〔調和腸胃〕 *tiáo hé cháng wèi*, **harmonizing the stomach and intestines** [ˈhɑrməˌnɑɪzɪŋ ðə ˈstʌmək ənd ɪnˈtɛstɪnz]: A method of treatment used to address gastrointestinal disharmony with disrupted upbearing and downbearing and cold-heat complexes presenting with glomus and fullness below the heart, vomiting, rumbling intestines, and diarrhea.

Cold bitter medicinals:

黄连 *huáng lián*, coptis (Coptidis Rhizoma)

黄芩 *huáng qín*, scutellaria (Scutellariae Radix)

Warm acrid medicinals:

干姜 *gān jiāng*, dried ginger (Zingiberis Rhizoma)

半夏 *bàn xià*, pinellia (Pinelliae Rhizoma)

Formula:

半夏泻心汤 *bàn xià xiè xīn tāng*, Pinellia Heart-Draining Decoction

7.2.5. 祛湿 Dispelling Dampness

926. 祛湿〔祛濕〕*qū shī*, **dispelling dampness** [dɪˈspɛlɪŋ ˈdæmpnɪs]: Any method of treatment used to eliminate dampness. It includes: transforming dampness (eliminating upper burner dampness), drying dampness (eliminating center burner dampness), and disinhibiting dampness (eliminating lower burner dampness). Dispelling dampness is often combined with treatment to fortify the spleen since the spleen governs movement and transformation of water-damp. *NB:* The term "transforming dampness" is used in the general sense of dispelling dampness and in the specific sense of removing dampness from the upper burner.

927. 燥湿和胃〔燥濕和胃〕*zào shī hé wèi*, **drying dampness and harmonizing the stomach** [ˈdraɪɪŋ ˈdæmpnɪs ənd ˈhɑrməˌnaɪzɪŋ ðə ˈstʌmək]: A method of treatment used to treat damp turbidity obstructing the spleen giving rise to spleen-stomach disharmony that manifests in glomus and fullness in the stomach duct and abdomen, belching and swallowing of upflowing acid, vomiting and diarrhea, reduced eating and fatigue, a bland taste in the mouth, and thick slimy tongue fur. Drying dampness and harmonizing the center makes use of warm acrid dampness-drying, aromatic turbidity-transforming, and heat-clearing dampness-transforming medicinals such as atractylodes (*cāng zhú*), officinal magnolia bark (*hòu pò*), agastache (*huò xiāng*), and cardamom (*bái dòu kòu*).

Formulas:

平胃散 *píng wèi sǎn*, Stomach-Calming Powder

藿香正气散 *huò xiāng zhèng qì sǎn*, Agastache Qì-Righting Powder

928. 清热祛湿〔清熱祛濕〕*qīng rè qū shī*, **clearing heat and dispelling dampness** [ˈklɪrɪŋ hit ənd dɪsˈpɛlɪŋ ˈdæmpnɪs]: Any method of treatment used to treat damp-heat. Clearing heat and dispelling dampness is applied to damp warmth, jaundice, cholera, heat strangury, and

wilting or impediment due to damp-heat external contractions, exuberant internal damp-heat, or damp-heat pouring downward.

Medicinals:

茵陈蒿 *yīn chén hāo*, virgate wormwood (Artemisiae Scopariae Herba)

薏苡仁 *yì yǐ rén*, coix (Coicis Semen)

滑石 *huá shí*, talcum (Talcum)

山栀子 *shān zhī zǐ*, gardenia (Gardeniae Fructus)

Formulas:

三仁汤 *sān rén tāng*, Three Kernels Decoction

茵陈蒿汤 *yīn chén hāo tāng*, Virgate Wormwood Decoction

甘露消毒丹 *gān lù xiāo dú dān*, Sweet Dew Toxin-Dispersing Elixir

929. **清利湿热**〔清利濕熱〕*qīng lì shī rè*, **clearing heat and disinhibiting dampness** [ˈklɪrɪŋ hit ənd ˌdɪsɪnˈhɪbɪtɪŋ ˈdæmpnɪs]: A method of treatment used to address lower burner damp-heat characterized by urgency and distention of the smaller abdomen, murky reddish urine, pain on urination, dribbling urination, and yellow slimy tongue fur.

Formulas:

八正散 *bā zhèng sǎn*, Eight Corrections Powder

石苇散 *shí wéi sǎn*, Pyrrosia Powder

930. **利水渗湿**〔利水滲濕〕*lì shuǐ shèn shī*, **disinhibiting water and percolating dampness** [ˌdɪsɪnˈhɪbɪtɪŋ ˈwɔtɚ ənd ˈpɚkəˌletɪŋ ˈdæmpnɪs]: To eliminate dampness by freeing urination in the treatment of stranguryturbidity, water swelling, and diarrhea due to water-damp congesting in the lower burner. Disinhibiting water and percolating dampness makes use of sweet and bland water-disinhibiting medicinals such as poria (*fú líng*), alisma (*zé xiè*), and polyporus (*zhū líng*). Representative formulas include Poria Five Powder (*wǔ líng sǎn*) and Five-Peel Powder (*wǔ pí sǎn*).

931. **温化水湿**〔溫化水濕〕*wēn huà shuǐ shī*, **warming and transforming water-damp** [ˈwɔrmɪŋ ənd trænsˈfɔrmɪŋ ˈwɔtɚ-dæmp]: A method of treating phlegm-rheum, water swelling, impediment patterns and leg qì that arise when vacuous yáng fails to transform water and dampness forms with cold. Warming and transforming water-damp uses hot acrid medicinals that warm and free yáng qì, such as cinnamon twig (*guì zhī*) and aconite (*fù zǐ*), combined with an appropriate amount of dampness-disinhibiting medicinals, such as poria (*fú líng*) and white atractylodes (*bái zhú*), to eliminate water-damp.

Formulas:

萆薢分清饮 *bì xiè fēn qīng yǐn*, Fish Poison Yam Clear-Turbid Separation Beverage

苓桂术甘汤 *líng guì zhú gān tāng*, Poria, Cinnamon Twig, White Atractylodes, and Licorice Decoction

甘草干姜茯苓白术汤 *gān cǎo gān jiāng fú líng bái zhú tāng*, Licorice, Dried Ginger, Poria, and White Atractylodes Decoction

实脾饮 *shí pí yǐn*, Spleen-Firming Beverage

真武汤 *zhēn wǔ tāng*, True Warrior Decoction

932. 祛风胜湿〔祛風勝濕〕*qū fēng shèng shī*, **dispelling wind and overcoming dampness** [dɪsˈpɛlɪŋ wɪnd ənd ˌovɚˈkʌmɪŋ ˈdæmpnɪs]: A method of treatment used to address wind-damp lodged in the channels and network vessels, the flesh, and the joints that causes wandering pain.

Medicinals:

独活 *dú huó*, pubescent angelica (Angelicae Pubescentis Radix)

羌活 *qiāng huó*, notopterygium (Notopterygii Rhizoma et Radix)

防风 *fáng fēng*, saposhnikovia (Saposhnikoviae Radix)

秦艽 *qín jiāo*, large gentian (Gentianae Macrophyllae Radix)

威灵仙 *wēi líng xiān*, clematis (Clematidis Radix)

桑枝 *sāng zhī*, mulberry twig (Mori Ramulus)

五加皮 *wǔ jiā pí*, acanthopanax (Acanthopanacis Cortex)

933. 健脾利水〔健脾利水〕*jiàn pí lì shuǐ*, **fortifying the spleen and disinhibiting water** [ˈfɔrtɪˌfaɪŋ ðə splin ənd ˌdɪsɪnˈhɪbɪtɪŋ ˈwɔtɚ]: A method of treatment that addresses water-damp from the spleen failing to dam water (脾布制水 *pí bù zhì shuǐ*), which manifests in generalized swelling, oppression in the stomach duct and reduced food intake, abdominal distention, and sloppy stool. A classic spleen-fortifying water-disinhibiting formula is Poria Five Powder (*wǔ líng sǎn*), among whose ingredients white atractylodes (*bái zhú*) and poria (*fú líng*) fortify the spleen, and polyporus (*zhū líng*) and alisma (*zé xiè*) disinhibit water.

934. 健脾利湿〔健脾利濕〕*jiàn pí lì shī*, **fortifying the spleen and disinhibiting dampness** [ˈfɔrtɪˌfaɪŋ ðə splin ənd ˌdɪsɪnˈhɪbɪtɪŋ ˈdæmpnɪs]: See fortifying the spleen and disinhibiting water.

7.2.6. 润燥 Moistening Dryness

935. 润燥〔潤燥〕*rùn zào*, **moistening dryness** [ˈmɔɪsnɪŋ ˈdraɪnɪs]: A method of treatment used to eliminate dryness-heat with moist enriching medicinals.

936. **轻宣润燥**〔輕宣潤燥〕*qīng xuān rùn zào*, **moistening dryness by light diffusion** ['maɪsnɪŋ 'draɪnɪs baɪ laɪt dɪ'fjuʒən]: A method of treatment used to address dryness-heat that damages the lung characterized by heat effusion, headache, dry cough with scant phlegm, qì counterflow panting in some cases, and a tongue that is dry and without fur (or dry thin white tongue fur) and that is red at the tip and margins.

Formula:

桑杏汤 *sāng xìng tāng*, Mulberry Leaf and Apricot Kernel Decoction

937. **滋阴润燥**〔滋陰潤燥〕*zī yīn rùn zào*, **enriching yīn and moistening dryness** [ɪn'rɪtʃɪŋ jɪn ənd 'maɪsnɪŋ 'draɪnɪs]: A method of treatment used to address damage to lung-stomach yīn by dryness, characterized by dry pharynx and thirst, postmeridian generalized heat [effusion], red tongue, a rapid fine pulse, and sometimes cough with scant phlegm, or constipation. A commonly used yīn-nourishing dryness-moistening formula is Adenophora/Glehnia and Ophiopogon Decoction (*shā shēn mài dōng tāng*). If there is constipation, Humor-Increasing Decoction (*zēng yè tāng*) may be used.

7.2.7. 温法 Warming

938. **温中散寒**〔溫中散寒〕*wēn zhōng sàn hán*, **warming the center and dissipating cold** ['wɔrmɪŋ ðə 'sɛntɚ ənd 'dɪsɪˌpetɪŋ kold]: A method of treatment used to treat cold in constitutional yáng vacuity, spleen-stomach vacuity cold, or external cold entering the interior, which are characterized by a moist white tongue fur, moderate soggy or slow sunken pulse, physical debilitation and fatigued spirit, aversion to cold, diarrhea, abdominal pain that likes pressure and heat, stomach pain, and vomiting of clear fluid.

To warm the center:

干姜 *gān jiāng*, dried ginger (Zingiberis Rhizoma)

炮姜 *páo jiāng*, blast-fried ginger (Zingiberis Rhizoma Praeparatum)

高良姜 *gāo liáng jiāng*, lesser galangal (Alpiniae Officinarum Rhizoma)

花椒 *huā jiāo*, zanthoxylum (Zanthoxyli Pericarpium)

To fortify the spleen and boost the stomach:

白术 *bái zhú*, white atractylodes (Atractylodis Macrocephalae Rhizoma)

茯苓 *fú líng*, poria (Poria)

甘草 *gān cǎo*, licorice (Glycyrrhizae Radix)

炙甘草 *zhì gān cǎo*, mix-fried licorice (Glycyrrhizae Radix cum Liquido Fricta)

For pronounced cold signs:

附子 *fù zǐ*, aconite (Aconiti Radix Lateralis Praeparata)

肉桂 *ròu guì*, cinnamon bark (Cinnamomi Cortex)

Formulas:

大顺散 *dà shùn sǎn*, Great Rectifying Powder

理中丸 *lǐ zhōng wán*, Center-Rectifying Pill

吴茱萸汤 *wú zhū yú tāng*, Evodia Decoction

939. 回阳救逆 〔回陽救逆〕 *huí yáng jiù nì*, **returning yáng and stemming counterflow** [rɪˈtɜˈnɪŋ jæŋ/jɑŋ ənd ˈstɛmɪŋ ˈkɑʊntəˈˌflo]: A method of treatment used to address great yáng collapse vacuity desertion, which is characterized by aversion to cold, curled-up lying posture, counterflow cold of the limbs, drop in both body temperature and blood pressure, cold sweats, a somber white complexion, and a faint fine pulse or vacuous rapid pulse.

To warm yáng:

附子 *fù zǐ*, aconite (Aconiti Radix Lateralis Praeparata)

干姜 *gān jiāng*, dried ginger (Zingiberis Rhizoma)

肉桂 *ròu guì*, cinnamon bark (Cinnamomi Cortex)

To boost qì:

甘草 *gān cǎo*, licorice (Glycyrrhizae Radix)

党参 *dǎng shēn*, codonopsis (Codonopsis Radix)

For severe cases:

人参 *rén shēn*, ginseng (Ginseng Radix)

To constrain sweat and stem desertion:

龙骨 *lóng gǔ*, dragon bone (Mastodi Ossis Fossilia)

牡蛎 *mǔ lì*, oyster shell (Ostreae Concha)

To constrain yīn and nourish humor:

五味子 *wǔ wèi zǐ*, schisandra (Schisandrae Fructus)

熟地黄 *shú dì huáng*, cooked rehmannia (Rehmanniae Radix Praeparata)

Formula:

四逆汤 *sì nì tāng*, Counterflow Cold Decoction

940. 温经散寒 〔溫經散寒〕 *wēn jīng sàn hán*, **warming the channels and dissipating cold** [ˈwɔrmɪŋ ðə ˈtʃænlz ənd ˈdɪsɪˌpetɪŋ kold]: A method of treatment used to address wind-cold-damp impediment with pronounced cold signs, such as pain in the joints relieved by warmth and inhibited bending and stretching.

To warm the channels:

川乌头 *chuān wū tóu*, aconite root (Aconiti Radix)

桂枝 *guì zhī*, cinnamon twig (Cinnamomi Ramulus)

全蝎 *quán xiē*, scorpion (Scorpio)

独活 *dú huó*, pubescent angelica (Angelicae Pubescentis Radix)

To nourish the blood and boost qì:

当归 *dāng guī*, Chinese angelica (Angelicae Sinensis Radix)

白芍药 *bái sháo yào*, white peony (Paeoniae Radix Alba)

黄芪 *huáng qí*, astragalus (Astragali Radix)

党参 *dǎng shēn*, codonopsis (Codonopsis Radix)

Formulas:

乌头汤 *wū tóu tāng*, Aconite Root Decoction

当归四逆汤 *dāng guī sì nì tāng*, Chinese Angelica Counterflow Cold Decoction

7.2.8. 理气 Rectifying Qì

941. **理气**〔理氣〕*lǐ qì*, **rectifying qì** [ˈrɛktɪˌfɑɪŋ tʃi]: Correction of any morbidity of qì (qì stagnation, qì counterflow, qì vacuity, qì fall), especially to treat qì stagnation or qì counterflow.

942. **行气**〔行氣〕*xíng qì*, **moving qì** [ˈmuvɪŋ tʃi]: A method of treatment that dissipates qì stagnation to address distention, oppression, and pain in the chest and abdomen. Moving qì is a form of rectifying qì and includes coursing depression and rectifying qì and harmonizing the stomach and rectifying qì.

943. **疏郁理气**〔疏鬱理氣〕*shū yù lǐ qì*, **coursing depression and rectifying qì** [ˈkɔrsɪŋ dɪˈprɛʃən ənd ˈrɛktɪˌfɑɪŋ tʃi]: A method of treatment used to address qì stagnation due to emotional depression characterized by glomus and oppression in the chest and diaphragm and by pain and distention in the rib-side and lesser abdomen.

Medicinals:

香附子 *xiāng fù zǐ*, cyperus (Cyperi Rhizoma)

佛手柑 *fó shǒu gān*, Buddha's hand (Citri Sarcodactylis Fructus)

乌药 *wū yào*, lindera (Linderae Radix)

砂仁 *shā rén*, amomum (Amomi Fructus)

944. **和胃理气**〔和胃理氣〕*hé wèi lǐ qì*, **harmonizing the stomach and rectifying qì** [ˈhɑrməˌnɑɪzɪŋ ðə ˈstʌmək ənd ˈrɛktɪˌfɑɪŋ tʃi]: A method of treatment used to address stomach qì disharmony characterized by distention and oppression in the stomach duct, belching, vomiting of sour fluid, and pale tongue with white fur.

Medicinals:

陈皮 *chén pí*, tangerine peel (Citri Reticulatae Pericarpium)
姜半夏 *jiāng bàn xià*, ginger pinellia (Pinelliae Rhizoma cum Zingibere Praeparatum)
木香 *mù xiāng*, costusroot (Aucklandiae Radix)
砂仁 *shā rén*, amomum (Amomi Fructus)

Formula:

平胃散 *píng wèi sǎn*, Stomach-Calming Powder

945. **降逆止呕** 〔降逆止嘔〕 *jiàng nì zhǐ ǒu*, **downbearing counterflow and checking vomiting** [ˈdaʊnˌbɛrɪŋ ˈkaʊntɚflo ənd ˈtʃɛkɪŋ ˈvɑmɪtɪŋ]: A method of treatment used to downbear counterflow and precipitate qì in order to treat stomach vacuity cold with vomiting, persistent hiccup, discomfort in the chest, and a slow pulse.

Formula:

丁香柿蒂汤 *dīng xiāng shì dì tāng*, Clove and Persimmon Decoction

946. **降气平喘** 〔降氣平喘〕 *jiàng qì píng chuǎn*, **downbearing qì and calming panting** [ˈdaʊnˌbɛrɪŋ tʃi ənd ˈkɑmɪŋ ˈpæntɪŋ]: A method of treatment used to downbear counterflow and precipitate qì in the treatment of wheezing and panting or rapid panting breathing, and copious phlegm. For repletion patterns, use Panting-Stabilizing Decoction (*dìng chuǎn tāng*); for repletion patterns, use Six Gentlemen Decoction (*liù jūn zǐ tāng*).

947. **破气** 〔破氣〕 *pò qì*, **breaking qì** [ˈbrekɪŋ tʃi]: Rectifying qì with drastic medicinals such as unripe tangerine peel (*qīng pí*) and unripe bitter orange (*zhǐ shí*), which dissipate binds and abduct stagnation.

7.2.9. 消导化积 Abductive Dispersion and Transforming Accumulations

948. **消导化积** 〔消導化積〕 *xiāo dǎo huà jī*, **abductive dispersion and transforming accumulations** [æbˈdʌktɪv dɪsˈpɝʒən ənd trænsˈfɔrmɪŋ əˈkjumjəˈleʃənz]: A group of therapeutic methods that treat food stagnation on the one hand and hard masses such as goiter, scrofula, concretions, conglomerations, accumulations, and gatherings on the other.

949. **消食导滞** 〔消食導滯〕 *xiāo shí dǎo zhì*, **dispersing food and abducting stagnation** [dɪsˈpɝsɪŋ fud ənd əbˈdʌktɪŋ stægˈneʃən]: A method of treatment used to disperse stagnant food and enable it to be carried through the digestive tract. Dispersing food and abducting stagnation, often called abductive dispersion, is employed in the treatment

of food stagnation causing oppression in the stomach duct and abdominal distention, poor appetite, putrid belching, swallowing of upflowing acid, nausea and upflow, abdominal pain, and constipation or diarrhea with ungratifying defecation. Commonly used abductive dispersion medicinals include crataegus (*shān zhā*), medicated leaven (*shén qū*), barley sprout (*mài yá*), gizzard lining (*jī nèi jīn*), and millet sprout (*gǔ yá*). Radish seed (*lái fú zǐ*), unripe bitter orange (*zhǐ shí*), and areca (*bīng láng*) may be added to break qì, precipitate phlegm, and free the stool. A formula used for this purpose is Harmony-Preserving Pill (*bǎo hé wán*), which includes crataegus (*shān zhā*), medicated leaven (*shén qū*), pinellia (*bàn xià*), poria (*fú líng*), tangerine peel (*chén pí*), forsythia (*lián qiào*), and radish seed (*lái fú zǐ*). Unripe Bitter Orange Stagnation-Abducting Pill (*zhǐ shí dǎo zhì wán*) has an additional precipitant action. When the food stagnation is due to spleen-stomach vacuity, abductive dispersing medicinals can be combined with supplementing medicinals, which enhance digestive system function, thereby reducing susceptibility to food accumulation in the long term. An example of such a formula is Spleen-Fortifying Pill (*jiàn pí wán*).

健脾丸 *jiàn pí wán*, Spleen-Fortifying Pill
   白术 *bái zhú*, white atractylodes (Atractylodis Macrocephalae Rhizoma)
   白茯苓 *bái fú líng*, white poria (Poria Alba)
   党参 *dǎng shēn*, codonopsis (Codonopsis Radix)
   甘草 *gān cǎo*, licorice (Glycyrrhizae Radix)
   木香 *mù xiāng*, costusroot (Aucklandiae Radix)
   连翘 *lián qiào*, forsythia (Forsythiae Fructus)
   黄连 *huáng lián*, coptis (Coptidis Rhizoma)
   神曲 *shén qū*, medicated leaven (Massa Medicata Fermentata)
   陈皮 *chén pí*, tangerine peel (Citri Reticulatae Pericarpium)
   麦芽 *mài yá*, barley sprout (Hordei Fructus Germinatus)
   砂仁 *shā rén*, amomum (Amomi Fructus)
   山楂 *shān zhā*, crataegus (Crataegi Fructus)
   肉豆蔻 *ròu dòu kòu*, nutmeg (Myristicae Semen)
   山药 *shān yào*, dioscorea (Dioscoreae Rhizoma)

950. 消食〔消食〕*xiāo shí*, **dispersing food** [dɪs'pɜ˞sɪŋ fud]: See dispersing food and abducting stagnation.

951. 消瘿瘰痰核〔消瘿瘰痰核〕*xiāo yǐng luó tán hé*, **dispersing goiter, scrofula, and phlegm nodes** [dɪs'pɜ˞sɪŋ gɔɪtə˞, 'skrɑfjələ, ənd 'flɛm-nodz]: Any method used to treat goiter, scrofula, and phlegm nodes.

Dispersing goiter, scrofula, and phlegm nodes makes use of phlegm-transforming, hardness-softening, bind-dispersing medicinals.

Medicinals:

海藻 *hǎi zǎo*, sargassum (Sargassum)
昆布 *kūn bù*, kelp (Laminariae/Eckloniae Thallus)
夏枯草 *xià kū cǎo*, prunella (Prunellae Spica)

Formulas:

内消瘰疬丸 *nèi xiāo luǒ lì wán*, Scrofula Internal Dispersion Pill
海藻玉壶汤 *hǎi zǎo yù hú tāng*, Sargassum Jade Flask Decoction

952. **消癥瘕积聚**〔消癥瘕積聚〕*xiāo zhēng jiǎ jī jù,* **dispersing concretions, conglomerations, accumulations, and gatherings** [dɪsˈpɝsɪŋ kənˈkriʃənz kənˌglɑməˈreʃənz əˌkjumjəˈleʃənz ənd ˈgæðərɪŋz]: The method of treating concretions, conglomerations, accumulations, and gatherings, i.e., any masses in the abdomen.

Medicinals:

桃仁 *táo rén*, peach kernel (Persicae Semen)
红花 *hóng huā*, carthamus (Carthami Flos)
牡丹皮 *mǔ dān pí*, moutan (Moutan Cortex)
赤芍药 *chì sháo yào*, red peony (Paeoniae Radix Rubra)
桂枝 *guì zhī*, cinnamon twig (Cinnamomi Ramulus)

Formulas:

桂枝茯苓丸 *guì zhī fú líng wán*, Cinnamon Twig and Poria Pill
鳖甲煎丸 *biē jiǎ jiān wán*, Turtle Shell Decocted Pill

953. **软坚**〔軟堅〕*ruǎn jiān,* **softening hardness** [ˈsɔfnɪŋ ˈhɑrdnɪs]: See preceding two items.

7.2.10. 驱虫 Expelling Worms

954. **驱虫**〔驅蟲〕*qū chóng,* **expelling worms** [ɪkˈspɛlɪŋ wɝmz]: A method of treatment used to cause the elimination of worms (especially in the intestines). Commonly used worm-expelling medicinals are listed below.

Medicinals:

使君子 *shǐ jūn zǐ*, quisqualis (Quisqualis Fructus)
苦楝皮 *kǔ liàn pí*, chinaberry bark (Meliae Cortex)
槟榔 *bīng láng*, areca (Arecae Semen)
大腹皮 *dà fù pí*, areca husk (Arecae Pericarpium)
南瓜子 *nán guā zǐ*, pumpkin seed (Cucurbitae Semen)
雷丸 *léi wán*, omphalia (Omphalia)

鹤虱 *hè shī*, carpesium seed (Carpesii Fructus)

榧子 *fěi zǐ*, torreya (Torreyae Semen)

芜荑 *wú yí*, elm cake (Ulmi Fructus Praeparatio)

贯众 *guàn zhòng*, aspidium (Aspidii Rhizoma)

7.2.11. 理血 Rectifying the Blood

955. 理血〔理血〕*lǐ xuè,* **rectifying the blood** [ˈrɛktɪˌfaɪɪŋ ðə blʌd]: Correction of any blood-aspect pathologies; includes supplementing the blood, cooling the blood, dispelling stasis and quickening the blood, and stanching bleeding. The first two of these are presented in other sections of this chapter. The latter two are presented below.

956. 祛瘀活血〔祛瘀活血〕*qū yū huó xuè,* **dispelling stasis and quickening the blood** [dɪsˈpɛlɪŋ ˈstesɪs ənd ˈkwɪkənɪŋ ðə blʌd]: A method of treatment used to restore normal movement of the blood by eliminating blood stasis. The power of action provides the basis for distinguishing quickening the blood, transforming stasis, and breaking blood.

To quicken the blood (mild action):

丹参 *dān shēn*, salvia (Salviae Miltiorrhizae Radix)

赤芍药 *chì sháo yào*, red peony (Paeoniae Radix Rubra)

川芎 *chuān xiōng*, chuanxiong (Chuanxiong Rhizoma)

牡丹皮 *mǔ dān pí*, moutan (Moutan Cortex)

鸡血藤 *jī xuè téng*, spatholobus (Spatholobi Caulis)

To transform stasis (stronger action):

桃仁 *táo rén*, peach kernel (Persicae Semen)

红花 *hóng huā*, carthamus (Carthami Flos)

没药 *mò yào*, myrrh (Myrrha)

乳香 *rǔ xiāng*, frankincense (Olibanum)

For women:

泽兰 *zé lán*, lycopus (Lycopi Herba)

益母草 *yì mǔ cǎo*, leonurus (Leonuri Herba)

蒲黄 *pú huáng*, typha pollen (Typhae Pollen)

五灵脂 *wǔ líng zhī*, squirrel's droppings (Trogopteri Faeces)

For pain:

延胡索 *yán hú suǒ*, corydalis (Corydalis Rhizoma)

乳香 *rǔ xiāng*, frankincense (Olibanum)

没药 *mò yào*, myrrh (Myrrha)

三七 *sān qī*, notoginseng (Notoginseng Radix)

For swelling from knocks and falls:

穿山甲 *chuān shān jiǎ*, pangolin scales (Manis Squama)

蒲黄 *pú huáng*, typha pollen (Typhae Pollen)

五灵脂 *wǔ líng zhī*, squirrel's droppings (Trogopteri Faeces)

刘寄奴 *liú jì nú*, anomalous artemisia (Artemisiae Anomalae Herba)

海桐皮 *hǎi tóng pí*, erythrina (Erythrinae Cortex)

To break blood (powerful action):

水蛭 *shuǐ zhì*, leech (Hirudo)

虻虫 *méng chóng*, tabanus (Tabanus)

蟅虫 *zhè chóng*, ground beetle (Eupolyphaga seu Steleophaga)

三棱 *sān léng*, sparganium (Sparganii Rhizoma)

莪术 *é zhú*, curcuma rhizome (Curcumae Rhizoma)

蜣螂 *qiāng láng*, dung beetle (Catharsius)

Formulas:

复元活血汤 *fù yuán huó xuè tāng*, Origin-Restorative Blood-Quickening Decoction

桃红四物汤 *táo hóng sì wù tāng*, Peach Kernel and Carthamus Four Agents Decoction

失笑散 *shī xiào sǎn*, Sudden Smile Powder

七厘散 *qī lí sǎn*, Seven Pinches Powder

鳖甲煎丸 *biē jiǎ jiān wán*, Turtle Shell Decocted Pill

身痛逐瘀汤 *shēn tòng zhú yū tāng*, Generalized Pain Stasis-Expelling Decoction

957. 活血化瘀〔活血化瘀〕*huó xuè huà yū*, **quickening the blood and transforming stasis** ['kwɪkənɪŋ ðə blʌd ənd træns'fɔrmɪŋ 'stesɪs]: See dispelling stasis and quickening the blood.

958. 破血〔破血〕*pò xuè*, **breaking blood** ['brekɪŋ blʌd]: See dispelling stasis and quickening the blood.

959. 止血〔止血〕*zhǐ xuè*, **stanching bleeding** ['stɔntʃɪŋ 'blidɪŋ]: Any of various methods of treatment used to address bleeding. Different medicinals are used depending on whether it occurs in cold or heat patterns.

Cool blood-stanching medicinals:

墨旱莲 *mò hàn lián*, eclipta (Ecliptae Herba)

侧柏叶 *cè bǎi yè*, arborvitae leaf (Platycladi Cacumen)

白茅根 *bái máo gēn*, imperata (Imperatae Rhizoma)

棕榈皮 *zōng lǘ pí*, trachycarpus (Trachycarpi Petiolus)

荷叶 *hé yè*, lotus leaf (Nelumbinis Folium)

小蓟 *xiǎo jì*, field thistle (Cirsii Herba)

槐花 *huái huā*, sophora flower (Sophorae Flos)

土大黄 *tǔ dà huáng*, Madaio dock root (Rumicis Madaio Radix)

Warm blood-stanching medicinals:

艾叶 *ài yè*, mugwort (Artemisiae Argyi Folium)

仙鹤草 *xiān hè cǎo*, agrimony (Agrimoniae Herba)

三七 *sān qī*, notoginseng (Notoginseng Radix)

炮姜 *páo jiāng*, blast-fried ginger (Zingiberis Rhizoma Praeparatum)

伏龙肝 *fú lóng gān*, oven earth (Terra Flava Usta)

For flooding and spotting:

艾叶 *ài yè*, mugwort (Artemisiae Argyi Folium)

牛角䚡 *niú jiǎo sāi*, ox horn bone (Bovis Cornus Os)

For bloody urine:

蒲黄 *pú huáng*, typha pollen (Typhae Pollen)

大蓟 *dà jì*, Japanese thistle (Cirsii Japonici Herba seu Radix)

小蓟 *xiǎo jì*, field thistle (Cirsii Herba)

For blood ejection:

白及 *bái jí*, bletilla (Bletillae Rhizoma)

白茅根 *bái máo gēn*, imperata (Imperatae Rhizoma)

For bloody stool:

地榆 *dì yú*, sanguisorba (Sanguisorbae Radix)

槐花 *huái huā*, sophora flower (Sophorae Flos)

伏龙肝 *fú lóng gān*, oven earth (Terra Flava Usta)

Securing astringents:

侧柏叶 *cè bǎi yè*, arborvitae leaf (Platycladi Cacumen)

棕榈皮 *zōng lǘ pí*, trachycarpus (Trachycarpi Petiolus)

荷叶 *hé yè*, lotus leaf (Nelumbinis Folium)

白及 *bái jí*, bletilla (Bletillae Rhizoma)

伏龙肝 *fú lóng gān*, oven earth (Terra Flava Usta)

Formulas:

十灰丸 *shí huī wán*, Ten Cinders Pill

7.2.12. 祛痰 Dispelling Phlegm

960. 祛痰〔袪痰〕 *qū tán*, **dispelling phlegm** [dɪsˈpɛlɪŋ flɛm]: Any method of treatment used to eliminate phlegm. The term "transforming phlegm" (化痰 *huà tán*) is the most common. The terms "dispersing phlegm" (消痰 *xiāo tán*), "flushing phlegm" (涤痰 *dí tán*), "expelling phlegm" (逐痰 *zhú tán*), "sweeping phlegm" (豁痰 *huò tán*), and "attacking phlegm" (攻痰 *gōng tán*) refer to more forceful actions. The term "transforming

phlegm," like "dispelling phlegm," is generic, but is also used in the specific sense of dispelling phlegm in the upper burner.

961. 燥湿化痰〔燥濕化痰〕 *zào shī huà tán,* **drying dampness and transforming phlegm** [ˈdraɪɪŋ ˈdæmpnɪs ənd trænsˈfɔrmɪŋ flɛm]: A method of treatment used to address damp phlegm that arises when devitalization of spleen yáng results in impairment of normal movement and transformation, characterized by white easily expectorated phlegm, oppression in the chest and nausea, slimy glossy white tongue, and in some cases dizziness and heart palpitations. Dampness-drying phlegm-transforming formulas include Two Matured Ingredients Decoction (*èr chén tāng*) plus white atractylodes (*bái zhú*) or atractylodes (*cāng zhú*), and Six Gentlemen Decoction (*liù jūn zǐ tāng*).

962. 宣肺化痰〔宣肺化痰〕 *xuān fèi huà tán,* **diffusing the lung and transforming phlegm** [dɪˈfjuzɪŋ ðə lʌŋ ənd trænsˈfɔrmɪŋ flɛm]: A method of treatment used to address inhibited lung qì with cough, panting, and copious phlegm.

Medicinals:
麻黄 *má huáng,* ephedra (Ephedrae Herba)
杏仁 *xìng rén,* apricot kernel (Armeniacae Semen)
桔梗 *jié gěng,* platycodon (Platycodonis Radix)
蝉蜕 *chán tuì,* cicada molting (Cicadae Periostracum)
紫苏 *zǐ sū,* perilla (Perillae Folium, Caulis, et Calyx)

963. 温肺化饮〔溫肺化飲〕 *wēn fèi huà yǐn,* **warming the lung and transforming rheum** [ˈwɑrmɪŋ ðə lʌŋ ənd trænsˈfɔrmɪŋ rum]: A method of treatment used to address cold rheum lying latent in the lung characterized by cough, counterflow panting with fullness that prevents the patient from lying down, copious foamy white phlegm, and swelling of the face and instep; these signs occur in episodes brought on by exposure to cold.

Formulas:
小青龙汤 *xiǎo qīng lóng tāng,* Minor Green-Blue Dragon Decoction.
苓甘五味姜辛汤 *líng gān wǔ wèi jiāng xīn tāng,* Poria, Licorice, Schisandra, Ginger, and Asarum Decoction
射干麻黄汤 *shè gān má huáng tāng,* Belamcanda and Ephedra Decoction
痰饮丸 *tán yǐn wán,* Phlegm-Rheum Pill

964. 润肺化痰〔潤肺化痰〕 *rùn fèi huà tán,* **moistening the lung and transforming phlegm** [ˈmɔɪsnɪŋ ðə lʌŋ ənd trænsˈfɔrmɪŋ flɛm]: A method of treatment used to address externally contracted warm dryness or lung yīn vacuity with scorching vacuity fire, giving rise to phlegm

that is difficult to expectorate, with dry throat, pain on swallowing, cough, and red tongue with dry yellow fur.

Medicinals:

贝母 *bèi mǔ*, fritillaria (Fritillariae Bulbus)

栝楼 *guā lóu*, trichosanthes (Trichosanthis Fructus)

沙参 *shā shēn*, adenophora/glehnia (Adenophorae seu Glehniae Radix)

麦门冬 *mài mén dōng*, ophiopogon (Ophiopogonis Radix)

梨皮 *lí pí*, pear peel (Pyri Exocarpium)

Formulas:

贝母瓜蒌散 *bèi mǔ guā lóu sǎn*, Fritillaria and Trichosanthes Powder

沙参麦冬汤 *shā shēn mài dōng tāng*, Adenophora/Glehnia and Ophiopogon Decoction

965. 治风化痰〔治風化痰〕*zhì fēng huà tán*, **controlling wind and transforming phlegm** [kənˈtrolɪŋ wɪnd ənd trænsˈfɔrmɪŋ flɛm]: A method of treatment that eliminates internal wind-phlegm. Phlegm may arise when damp turbidity fails to transform and congeals or when intense internal fire heat condenses humor. It may rise with wind and penetrate the channels and network vessels, causing, in mild cases, numbness or dizziness and headache with spinning head and black vision and, in severe cases, paralysis. It is for this condition that the method of controlling wind and transforming phlegm is used.

Formula:

半夏白术天麻汤 *bàn xià bái zhú tiān má tāng*, Pinellia, White Atractylodes, and Gastrodia Decoction

966. 顺气化痰〔順氣化痰〕*shùn qì huà tán*, **normalizing qì and transforming phlegm** [ˈnɔrməˌlɑɪzɪŋ tʃi ənd trænsˈfɔrmɪŋ flɛm]: A method of treatment used to address phlegm bind with fullness in the chest, counterflow qì cough, copious phlegm, and food stagnation.

Formulas:

三子养亲汤 *sān zǐ yǎng qīn tāng*, Three-Seed Filial Devotion Decoction

顺气导痰汤 *shùn qì dǎo tán tāng*, Qì-Normalizing Phlegm-Abducting Decoction

967. 攻痰〔攻痰〕*gōng tán*, **attacking phlegm** [əˈtækɪŋ flɛm]: A method of treatment used to address stagnant, binding phlegm such as occurs in epilepsy, mania and withdrawal, or child fright wind characterized by gurgling phlegm congesting the throat and convulsions of the limbs.

Medicinals:

礞石 *méng shí*, chlorite/mica (Chloriti seu Micae Lapis)

葶苈子 *tíng lì zǐ*, lepidium/descurainiae (Lepidii/Descurainiae Semen)

Formula:

礞石滚痰丸 *méng shí gǔn tán wán*, Chlorite/Mica Phlegm-Rolling Pill

7.2.13. 安神 Quieting the Spirit

968. **安神**〔安神〕*ān shén*, **quieting the spirit** ['kwaɪətɪŋ ðə 'spɪrɪt]: A method of treatment used to address disquieted spirit (heart palpitations, insomnia, agitation, mania). See nourishing the heart and quieting the spirit and quieting the spirit with heavy settlers.

969. **养心安神**〔養心安神〕*yǎng xīn ān shén*, **nourishing the heart and quieting the spirit** ['nɜˑɪʃɪŋ ðə hɑrt ənd 'kwaɪətɪŋ ðə 'spɪrɪt]: A method of treatment used to address disquieted heart spirit due to heart blood depletion characterized by heart palpitations, susceptibility to fright, forgetfulness, insomnia, abstraction, profuse dreaming and seminal emission, dry bound stool, mouth and tongue sores, red tongue with scant fur, and a rapid fine pulse.

Formula:

柏子养心丸 *bǎi zǐ yǎng xīn wán*, Arborvitae Seed Heart-Nourishing Pill

970. **重镇安神**〔重鎮安神〕*zhòng zhèn ān shén*, **quieting the spirit with heavy settlers** ['kwaɪətɪŋ ðə 'spɪrɪt wɪð 'hɛvɪ 'sɛtlɚz]: A method of treatment used to address disquieted heart spirit (heart palpitations, fearful throbbing, insomnia, fright mania) using heavy mineral and shell medicinals.

Formula:

安神丸 *ān shén wán*, Spirit-Quieting Pill

7.2.14. 祛风 Dispelling Wind

971. **祛风**〔祛風〕*qū fēng*, **dispelling wind** [dɪs'pɛlɪŋ wɪnd]: Any method of treatment used to eliminate wind.

972. **疏散外风**〔疏散外風〕*shū sàn wài fēng*, **coursing and dissipating external wind** ['kɔrsɪŋ ənd 'dɪsɪˌpetɪŋ ɪks'tɜˑnl̩ wɪnd]: Any of a number of methods of treatment using mainly acrid dissipating wind-coursing medicinals to treat external wind invading the channels, the flesh, the sinew and bone, and the joints. It includes: coursing wind and relieving pain to treat headache or dizziness due to wind invading the head; coursing wind and relieving itching, and clearing heat and eliminating

dampness to treat itching, wind papules, or eczema due to wind-heat or wind-damp becoming depressed in the skin and spreading through the blood vessels; dispelling wind and transforming phlegm to treat deviated eyes and mouth due to wind evil with phlegm obstructing the channels and network vessels of the face and head; dispelling wind and checking tetany to treat lockjaw that arises when "wind evil toxic qì" invades through a wound; dispelling wind and eliminating dampness, quickening the blood and freeing the network vessels to treat numbness of the extremities with inhibited bending and stretching due to wind, phlegm-damp, and static blood obstructing the network vessels. The main medicinals used are listed below.

Medicinals:

羌活 *qiāng huó*, notopterygium (Notopterygii Rhizoma et Radix)

独活 *dú huó*, pubescent angelica (Angelicae Pubescentis Radix)

防风 *fáng fēng*, saposhnikovia (Saposhnikoviae Radix)

白芷 *bái zhǐ*, Dahurian angelica (Angelicae Dahuricae Radix)

荆芥 *jīng jiè*, schizonepeta (Schizonepetae Herba)

川芎 *chuān xiōng*, chuanxiong (Chuanxiong Rhizoma)

973. 平息内风〔平息內風〕*píng xī nèi fēng*, **calming and extinguishing internal wind** [ˈkɑmɪŋ ənd ɪkˈstɪŋgwɪʃɪŋ ɪnˈtɜ˞nl̩ wɪnd]: Any method of treatment used to eliminate internal wind.

974. 平肝息风〔平肝息風〕*píng gān xī fēng*, **calming the liver and extinguishing wind** [ˈkɑmɪŋ ðə ˈlɪvɚ ənd ɪkˈstɪŋgwɪʃɪŋ wɪnd]: A method of treatment used to address ascendant liver yáng stirring internal wind with pulling pain in the head, dizziness, deviated eyes and mouth, numbness or tremor of the limbs, stiff tongue, deviated trembling tongue, unclear speech, red tongue with thin fur, a stringlike pulse, and, in severe cases, clouding collapse, hypertonicity or convulsions of the limbs.

Medicinals:

钩藤 *gōu téng*, uncaria (Uncariae Ramulus cum Uncis)

天麻 *tiān má*, gastrodia (Gastrodiae Rhizoma)

刺蒺藜 *cì jí lí*, tribulus (Tribuli Fructus)

菊花 *jú huā*, chrysanthemum (Chrysanthemi Flos)

地龙 *dì lóng*, earthworm (Pheretima)

珍珠母 *zhēn zhū mǔ*, mother-of-pearl (Concha Margaritifera)

牡蛎 *mǔ lì*, oyster shell (Ostreae Concha)

石决明 *shí jué míng*, abalone shell (Haliotidis Concha)

Formulas:

镇肝熄风汤 *zhèn gān xī fēng tāng*, Liver-Settling Wind-Extinguishing
Decoction

羚角钩藤汤 *líng jiǎo gōu téng tāng*, Antelope Horn and Uncaria Decoction

建瓴汤 *jiàn líng tāng*, Sweeping Down Decoction

975. **滋阴息风**〔滋陰息風〕*zī yīn xī fēng*, **enriching yīn and extinguish-ing wind** [ɪn'rɪtʃɪŋ jɪn ənd ɪk'stɪŋgwɪʃɪŋ wɪnd]: A method of treatment used to address wind stirring from yīn vacuity due to damage to true yīn by heat in febrile disease, characterized by unpronounced but per-sistent heat effusion, heat in the hearts of the soles and palms, red fa-cial complexion, vacuity vexation and insomnia, flusteredness and las-situde, tinnitus, wriggling movement or convulsions of the extremities, dry crimson tongue with little fur, and a rapid vacuous pulse.

Medicinals:

地黄 *dì huáng*, rehmannia (Rehmanniae Radix)

白芍药 *bái sháo yào*, white peony (Paeoniae Radix Alba)

麦门冬 *mài mén dōng*, ophiopogon (Ophiopogonis Radix)

鸡子黄 *jī zǐ huáng*, egg yolk (Galli Vitellus)

龟版 *guī bǎn*, tortoise shell (Testudinis Carapax et Plastrum)

鳖甲 *biē jiǎ*, turtle shell (Trionycis Carapax)

牡蛎 *mǔ lì*, oyster shell (Ostreae Concha)

钩藤 *gōu téng*, uncaria (Uncariae Ramulus cum Uncis)

Formula:

大定风珠 *dà dìng fēng zhū*, Major Wind-Stabilizing Pill

976. **祛风解痉**〔祛風解痙〕*qū fēng jiě jìng*, **dispelling wind and resolv-ing tetany** [dɪs'pɛlɪŋ wɪnd ənd rɪ'zɑlvɪŋ 'tɛtənɪ]: A method of treat-ment used to address tetany using wind-dispelling medicinals. Wind-dispelling tetany-resolving formulas include: True Jade Powder (*yù zhēn sǎn*) or Five-Tigers-Chasing-the-Wind Powder (*wǔ hǔ zhuī fēng sǎn*), which are used to treat lockjaw; Pull Aright Powder (*qiān zhèng sǎn*), which is used to treat facial paralysis; and Uncaria Beverage (*gōu téng yǐn*), which used to treat tetany (acute child fright wind) due to exuberant heat engendering wind.

7.2.15. 开窍法 Opening the Orifices

977. **清热开窍**〔清熱開竅〕*qīng rè kāi qiào*, **clearing heat and opening the orifices** ['klɪrɪŋ hit ənd 'opənɪŋ ði 'ɔrəfɪsɪz]: A method of treatment used to address externally contracted febrile disease patterns, such as heat entering the pericardium, that are characterized by high fever with

clouded spirit and delirious speech, vexation and agitation, parched lips and dry teeth, tetanic reversal, and convulsions, including child fright wind.

Formulas:

安宫牛黄丸 *ān gōng niú huáng wán*, Peaceful Palace Bovine Bezoar Pill
紫雪丹 *zǐ xuě dān*, Purple Snow Elixir
神犀丹 *shén xī dān*, Spirit-Like Rhinoceros Horn Elixir
至宝丹 *zhì bǎo dān*, Supreme Jewel Elixir

978. **清心开窍**〔清心開竅〕 *qīng xīn kāi qiào*, **clearing the heart and opening the orifices** ['klɪrɪŋ ðə hɑrt ənd 'opənɪŋ ði 'ɔrəfɪsɪz]: See clearing heat and opening the orifices.

979. **凉开**〔涼開〕 *liáng kāi*, **cool opening** [kul 'opənɪŋ]: See clearing heat and opening the orifices.

980. **逐寒开窍**〔逐寒開竅〕 *zhú hán kāi qiào*, **expelling cold and opening the orifices** [ɪks'pɛlɪŋ kold ənd 'opənɪŋ ði 'ɔrəfɪsɪz]: To treat coma due to cold-damp phlegm turbidity obstructing the pericardium by means of formulas such as Storax Pill (*sū hé xiāng wán*). This method is used, for example, in the treatment of wind stroke with clouding collapse, unconsciousness, green-blue or white complexion, cold limbs, and a sunken pulse.

981. **温开**〔溫開〕 *wēn kāi*, **warm opening** [wɔrm 'opənɪŋ]: See expelling cold and opening the orifices.

982. **化痰开窍**〔化痰開竅〕 *huà tán kāi qiào*, **transforming phlegm and opening the orifices** [træns'fɔrmɪŋ flɛm ənd 'opənɪŋ ði 'ɔrəfɪsɪz]: To treat clouded spirit in phlegm patterns. Distinction is made between heat phlegm and cold phlegm. Heat phlegm patterns are characterized by exuberant phlegm with rough breathing, clouded spirit and delirious speech, generalized heat [effusion], vexation and agitation, and a red tongue with yellow fur. Cold phlegm patterns are characterized by phlegm drool congestion, clouded spirit, green-blue or white face, cold extremities, and a sunken pulse.

For heat phlegm:

牛黄丸 *niú huáng wán*, Bovine Bezoar Pill
至宝丹 *zhì bǎo dān*, Supreme Jewel Elixir

For cold phlegm:

苏合香丸 *sū hé xiāng wán*, Storax Pill

983. **豁痰开窍**〔豁痰開竅〕 *huò tán kāi qiào*, **sweeping phlegm and opening the orifices** ['swipɪŋ flɛm ənd 'opənɪŋ ði 'ɔrəfɪsɪz] See transforming phlegm and opening the orifices.

7.2.16. 补法 Supplementation

984. 补气〔補氣〕*bǔ qì*, **supplementing qì** [ˈsʌpləˌmɛntɪŋ tʃi]: Also called *boosting qì*. A method of treatment used to address qì vacuity that presents with general physical weakness, shortness of breath, fatigue, spontaneous sweating, soft weak soggy pulse, prolapse of the rectum or uterus, general physical debilitation following illness, and qì deserting with the blood in cases of massive bleeding.

Medicinals:

黄芪 *huáng qí*, astragalus (Astragali Radix)

党参 *dǎng shēn*, codonopsis (Codonopsis Radix)

人参 *rén shēn*, ginseng (Ginseng Radix)

甘草 *gān cǎo*, licorice (Glycyrrhizae Radix)

Formulas:

四君子汤 *sì jūn zǐ tāng*, Four Gentlemen Decoction

补中益气汤 *bǔ zhōng yì qì tāng*, Center-Supplementing Qì-Boosting Decoction

985. 益气〔益氣〕*yì qì*, **boosting qì** [ˈbustɪŋ tʃi]: See supplementing qì.

986. 补血〔補血〕*bǔ xuè*, **supplementing the blood** [ˈsʌpləˌmɛntɪŋ ðə blʌd]: A method of treatment used to address conditions of blood vacuity characterized by a drawn, withered-yellow or pale white complexion, dizzy head, tinnitus, heart palpitations, pale scant menstrual flow, fine pulse, and pale tongue.

Medicinals:

生地黄 *shēng dì huáng*, dried/fresh rehmannia (Rehmanniae Radix Exsiccata seu Recens)

当归 *dāng guī*, Chinese angelica (Angelicae Sinensis Radix)

何首乌 *hé shǒu wū*, flowery knotweed (Polygoni Multiflori Radix)

枸杞子 *gǒu qǐ zǐ*, lycium berry (Lycii Fructus)

阿胶 *ē jiāo*, ass hide glue (Asini Corii Colla)

龙眼肉 *lóng yǎn ròu*, longan flesh (Longan Arillus)

Formulas:

四物汤 *sì wù tāng*, Four Agents Decoction

八珍汤 *bā zhēn tāng*, Eight-Gem Decoction

归脾汤 *guī pí tāng*, Spleen-Returning Decoction

987. 气血双补〔氣血雙補〕*qì xuè shuāng bǔ*, **supplementing both qì and blood; dual supplementation of qì and blood** [ˈsʌpləmɛntɪŋ boθ tʃi ənd blʌd; ˈduəl ˌsʌpləmenˈteʃən əv tʃi ənd blʌd]: A method of treatment used to address dual vacuity of qì and blood characterized by

somber white facial complexion, dizziness, heart palpitations, shortness of breath, lack of strength, a soft-red pale tongue, and a weak fine
pulse.

Formula:

八珍汤 *bā zhēn tāng*, Eight-Gem Decoction

988. 补阴〔補陰〕*bǔ yīn*, **supplementing yīn** ['sʌpləˌmɛntɪŋ jɪn]: Also
called *nourishing yīn*, *enriching yīn*, and *fostering yīn*. A method of
treatment used for yīn vacuity, which is characterized by emaciation,
vacuity heat, upbearing fire, night sweating, dry mouth, dry pharynx,
expectoration of blood, insomnia, vexation, heat in the hearts of the
palms and soles, red tongue with scant or peeling fur, and a fine rapid
pulse.

To supplement lung and stomach yīn:

北沙参 *běi shā shēn*, glehnia (Glehniae Radix)

麦门冬 *mài mén dōng*, ophiopogon (Ophiopogonis Radix)

石斛 *shí hú*, dendrobium (Dendrobii Herba)

玉竹 *yù zhú*, Solomon's seal (Polygonati Odorati Rhizoma)

To clear vacuity heat:

生地黄 *shēng dì huáng*, dried/fresh rehmannia (Rehmanniae Radix
    Exsiccata seu Recens)

石斛 *shí hú*, dendrobium (Dendrobii Herba)

玄参 *xuán shēn*, scrophularia (Scrophulariae Radix)

To supplement liver-kidney yīn:

生地黄 *shēng dì huáng*, dried/fresh rehmannia (Rehmanniae Radix
    Exsiccata seu Recens)

阿胶 *ē jiāo*, ass hide glue (Asini Corii Colla)

天门冬 *tiān mén dōng*, asparagus (Asparagi Radix)

龟版 *guī bǎn*, tortoise shell (Testudinis Carapax et Plastrum)

鳖甲 *biē jiǎ*, turtle shell (Trionycis Carapax)

To supplement liver-kidney yīn without clogging (不腻 *bù nì*):

女贞子 *nǚ zhēn zǐ*, ligustrum (Ligustri Lucidi Fructus)

墨旱莲 *mò hàn lián*, eclipta (Ecliptae Herba)

桑椹 *sāng shèn*, mulberry (Mori Fructus)

To nourish heart, lung, and kidney yīn:

麦门冬 *mài mén dōng*, ophiopogon (Ophiopogonis Radix)

百合 *bǎi hé*, lily bulb (Lilii Bulbus)

玄参 *xuán shēn*, scrophularia (Scrophulariae Radix)

柏子仁 *bǎi zǐ rén*, arborvitae seed (Platycladi Semen)

Formulas:

知柏地黄丸 *zhī bǎi dì huáng wán*, Anemarrhena, Phellodendron, and
    Rehmannia Pill

大补阴丸 *dà bǔ yīn wán*, Major Yīn Supplementation Pill

增液汤 *zēng yè tāng*, Humor-Increasing Decoction

养胃汤 *yǎng wèi tāng*, Stomach-Nourishing Decoction

989. **养阴**〔養陰〕*yǎng yīn*, **nourishing yīn** [ˈnɜˑɪʃɪŋ jɪn]: See supplementing yīn.

990. **滋阴**〔滋陰〕*zī yīn*, **enriching yīn** [ɪnˈrɪtʃɪŋ jɪn]: See supplementing yīn.

991. **育阴**〔育陰〕*yù yīn*, **fostering yīn** [ˈfɔstərɪŋ jɪn]: See supplementing yīn.

992. **补阳**〔補陽〕*bǔ yáng*, **supplementing yáng** [ˈsʌpləˌmɛntɪŋ jæŋ/jɑŋ]:
Also called *assisting yáng*. A method of treatment used to address yáng
vacuity, which is characterized by aversion to cold, cold extremities,
aching and limpness of the lumbus and knees, impotence, seminal efflux, long voidings of copious clear urine, a pale tongue, and a sunken
weak pulse.

Medicinals:

仙茅 *xiān máo*, curculigo (Curculiginis Rhizoma)

淫羊藿 *yín yáng huò*, epimedium (Epimedii Herba)

鹿角 *lù jiǎo*, deerhorn (Cervi Cornu)

肉苁蓉 *ròu cōng róng*, cistanche (Cistanches Herba)

附子 *fù zǐ*, aconite (Aconiti Radix Lateralis Praeparata)

肉桂 *ròu guì*, cinnamon bark (Cinnamomi Cortex)

Formulas:

桂附八味丸 *guì fù bā wèi wán*, Cinnamon Bark and Aconite
    Eight-Ingredient Pill

右归丸 *yòu guī wán*, Right-Restoring [Life Gate] Pill

993. **助阳**〔助陽〕*zhù yáng*, **assisting yáng** [əˈsɪstɪŋ jæŋ/jɑŋ]: See supplementing yáng.

7.2.17. 固涩法 Securing and Astriction

994. **固涩**〔固澀〕*gù sè*, **securing and astriction** [sɪˈkjurɪŋ ənd əˈstrɪkʃn]:
The method of treating efflux desertion patterns (i.e., enduring or critical discharge or loss of sweat, blood, semen, etc.).

995. **敛汗固表**〔斂汗固表〕*liǎn hàn gù biǎo,* **constraining sweat and securing the exterior** [kənˈstrenɪŋ swɛt ənd sɪˈkjurɪŋ ðə ɪksˈtɪrɪɚ]: A method of treatment used to address exterior vacuity with copious sweating. Exterior vacuity may take the form of qì vacuity or yīn vacuity. Qì vacuity patterns are characterized by spontaneous sweating, heart palpitations, susceptibility to fright, shortness of breath, heart vexation fatigue, and a large forceless pulse. Representative sweat-constraining exterior-securing formulas for qì vacuity include Oyster Shell Powder (*mǔ lì sǎn*) and Jade Wind-Barrier Powder (*yù píng fēng sǎn*). Yīn vacuity patterns are characterized by night sweating, postmeridian tidal heat [effusion], dry lips and mouth, red tongue, and a rapid fine pulse. Use formulas such as Chinese Angelica Six Yellows Decoction (*dāng guī liù huáng tāng*) and Six-Ingredient Rehmannia Decoction (*liù wèi dì huáng tāng*) plus oyster shell (*mǔ lì*), light wheat (*fú xiǎo mài*), and glutinous rice root (*nuò dào gēn xū*).

996. **涩肠固脱**〔澀腸固脫〕*sè cháng gù tuō,* **astringing the intestines and stemming desertion** [əˈstrɪndʒɪŋ ðə ɪnˈtɛstinz ənd ˈstɛmɪŋ dɪˈzɝˈʃən]: The method of treating enduring diarrhea and fecal incontinence or persistent pus and blood in the stool with dark red blood, conditions that culminate in efflux desertion and prolapse of the rectum, abdominal pain that likes warmth and pressure, and a weak slow pulse. Intestine astringing medicinals include ones that are warm and supplement the spleen and kidney combined with securing astringent medicinals to astringe the bowels and stem desertion.

Medicinals that are warm and supplement the spleen and kidney:

党参 *dǎng shēn,* codonopsis (Codonopsis Radix)
白术 *bái zhú,* white atractylodes (Atractylodis Macrocephalae Rhizoma)
附子 *fù zǐ,* aconite (Aconiti Radix Lateralis Praeparata)
桂枝 *guì zhī,* cinnamon twig (Cinnamomi Ramulus)
干姜 *gān jiāng,* dried ginger (Zingiberis Rhizoma)

Securing astringent medicinals:

补骨脂 *bǔ gǔ zhī,* psoralea (Psoraleae Fructus)
肉豆蔻 *ròu dòu kòu,* nutmeg (Myristicae Semen)
五味子 *wǔ wèi zǐ,* schisandra (Schisandrae Fructus)
罂粟壳 *yīng sù qiào,* poppy husk (Papaveris Pericarpium)
赤石脂 *chì shí zhī,* halloysite (Halloysitum Rubrum)
禹余粮 *yǔ yú liáng,* limonite (Limonitum)
山药 *shān yào,* dioscorea (Dioscoreae Rhizoma)
芡实 *qiàn shí,* euryale (Euryales Semen)
莲肉 *lián ròu,* lotus seed (Nelumbinis Semen)

Formula:

真人养脏汤 *zhēn rén yǎng zàng tāng*, True Man Viscus-Nourishing Decoction.

997. 涩精止遗〔澀精止遺〕*sè jīng zhǐ yí*, **astringing essence and checking (seminal) emission and enuresis** [əˈstrɪndʒɪŋ ˈɛsəns ənd ˈtʃɛkɪŋ (ˈsɛmɪnl̩) ɪˈmɪʃən ənd ɪˈnjurəsɪs]: A method of treatment that addresses seminal emission or seminal efflux attributed to kidney vacuity with insecurity of the essence gate or enuresis or frequent urination due to kidney vacuity with bladder retention failure. For kidney vacuity seminal emission, kidney-supplementing essence-astringing medicinals such as complanate astragalus seed (*shā yuàn zǐ*), dragon bone (*lóng gǔ*), oyster shell (*mǔ lì*), lotus stamen (*lián xū*), mantis egg-case (*sāng piāo xiāo*), euryale (*qiàn shí*), cornus (*shān zhū yú*), and Cherokee rose fruit (*jīn yīng zǐ*) are used. For enuresis or frequent urination, a similar range of medicinals are used: mantis egg-case (*sāng piāo xiāo*), rubus (*fù pén zǐ*), and alpinia (*yì zhì rén*). Representative formulas: Golden Lock Essence-Securing Pill (*jīn suǒ gù jīng wán*), designed for seminal emission, but also used for enuresis; Mantis Egg-Case Powder (*sāng piāo xiāo sǎn*), originally designed for enuresis, but also used for seminal emission; and Stream-Reducing Pill (*suō quán wán*), mainly used for enuresis, frequent urination, and child bedwetting.

998. 缩尿〔縮尿〕*suō niào*, **reducing urine** [rɪˈdjusɪŋ ˈjurɪn]: See preceding item.

999. 固崩止带〔固崩止帶〕*gù bēng zhǐ dài*, **stemming flooding and checking (vaginal) discharge** [ˈstɛmɪŋ ˈflʌdɪŋ ənd ˈtʃɛkɪŋ (ˈvædʒənl̩) ˈdɪstʃɑrdʒ]: A method of treatment used to address flooding and spotting, incessant menses, and vaginal discharge using astringent agents combined with spleen-fortifying kidney-supplementing medicinals, such as:

Astringent agents:

煅龙骨 *duàn lóng gǔ*, calcined dragon bone (Mastodi Ossis Fossilia Calcinata)

煅牡蛎 *mǔ lì*, calcined oyster shell (Ostreae Concha Calcinata)

樗根白皮 *shū gēn bái pí*, ailanthus root bark (Ailanthi Altissimae Radicis Cortex)

海螵蛸 *hǎi piāo xiāo*, cuttlefish bone (Sepiae Endoconcha)

茜草根 *qiàn cǎo gēn*, madder (Rubiae Radix)

五倍子 *wǔ bèi zǐ*, sumac gallnut (Galla Chinensis)

Spleen-fortifying kidney-supplementing medicinals:

黄芪 *huáng qí*, astragalus (Astragali Radix)

人参 *rén shēn*, ginseng (Ginseng Radix)

山药 *shān yào*, dioscorea (Dioscoreae Rhizoma)

菟丝子 *tù sī zǐ*, cuscuta (Cuscutae Semen)

杜仲炭 *dù zhòng tàn*, charred eucommia (Eucommiae Cortex Carbonisatus)

鹿角胶 *lù jiǎo jiāo*, deerhorn glue (Cervi Cornus Gelatinum)

For flooding and spotting or incessant menses due to yīn vacuity and blood heat, use Menses-Securing Pill (*gù jīng wán*). For dribbling vaginal discharge due to damp-heat, use Ailanthus Root Bark Pill (*shū shù pí wán*).

1000 敛肺止咳〔斂肺止咳〕*liǎn fèi zhǐ ké*, **constraining the lung and suppressing cough** [kən'strenɪŋ ðə lʌŋ ənd sə'prɛsɪŋ kɔf]: A method of treatment used to address enduring cough and lung vacuity characterized by scant phlegm, hasty breathing, spontaneous sweating, dry mouth and tongue, and vacuous rapid pulse. It uses lung-constraining cough-suppressing medicinals combined with general cough-suppressing medicinals.

Lung-constraining cough-suppressing medicinals:

五味子 *wǔ wèi zǐ*, schisandra (Schisandrae Fructus)

诃子 *hē zǐ*, chebule (Chebulae Fructus)

罂粟壳 *yīng sù qiào*, poppy husk (Papaveris Pericarpium)

General cough-suppressing medicinals:

百部 *bǎi bù*, stemona (Stemonae Radix)

紫菀 *zǐ wǎn*, aster (Asteris Radix)

马兜铃 *mǎ dōu líng*, aristolochia fruit (Aristolochiae Fructus)

枇杷叶 *pí pá yè*, loquat leaf (Eriobotryae Folium)

款冬花 *kuǎn dōng huā*, coltsfoot (Farfarae Flos)

Formulas:

五味子汤 *wǔ wèi zǐ tāng*, Schisandra Decoction

当归 *dāng guī*, Chinese angelica (Angelicae Sinensis Radix)

五味子 *wǔ wèi zǐ*, schisandra (Schisandrae Fructus)

麦门冬 *mài mén dōng*, ophiopogon (Ophiopogonis Radix)

杏仁 *xìng rén*, apricot kernel (Armeniacae Semen)

橘红 *jú hóng*, red tangerine peel (Citri Reticulatae Pericarpium Rubrum)

生姜 *shēng jiāng*, fresh ginger (Zingiberis Rhizoma Recens)

大枣 *dà zǎo*, jujube (Jujubae Fructus)

九仙散 *jiǔ xiān sǎn*, Nine Immortals Powder.

7.2.18. 涌吐 Ejection

1001涌吐〔湧吐〕*yǒng tù,* **ejection** [ɪˈdʒɛktʃən]: A method of treatment that involves induction of vomiting either by medicinals or by mechanical means (e.g., tickling the throat with a feather) in order to expel collected phlegm or lodged food. In clinical practice, ejection is used when phlegm-drool obstructs the throat and hampers breathing or when, after voracious eating, food stagnates in the stomach, causing distention, fullness, and pain. This method may also be used to treat poisoning, provided treatment is administered swiftly after ingestion of the toxic substance. It is generally contraindicated in pregnancy and must be used with care in weak patients.

Medicinals:

瓜蒂 *guā dì,* melon stalk (Melonis Pedicellus)
常山 *cháng shān,* dichroa (Dichroae Radix)
蜀漆 *shǔ qī,* dichroa leaf (Dichroae Folium)
胆矾 *dǎn fán,* chalcanthite (Chalcanthitum)
藜芦 *lí lú,* veratrum (Veratri Nigri Radix et Rhizoma)
人参芦 *rén shēn lú,* ginseng top (Ginseng Rhizoma)
皂荚 *zào jiá,* gleditsia (Gleditsiae Fructus)
盐 *yán,* salt (Sal)

Commonly used formulas include the powerful Melon Stalk Powder (*guā dì sǎn*) and less powerful Ginseng Tops Beverage (*shēn lú yǐn*).

习题
Questions

Answer the following questions in English:

721. What do we call the method used to eliminate upper burner dampness? ....

722. What method is used to treat enduring cough and lung vacuity characterized by scant phlegm, hasty breathing, spontaneous sweating, dry mouth and tongue, and vacuous rapid pulse? ....

723. By what term is "treating the cause of a disease as opposed to its symptoms" known? ....

724. Treating cold with cold is an example of what treatment principle?
....

725. What is the method of treatment used to free urination in strangury-turbidity, water swelling, and diarrhea due to water-damp congesting in the lower burner? ....

726. What is the method of treatment used to treat enduring diarrhea and fecal incontinence? ....

727. What is the method of treatment used to address enuresis and frequent long voidings of clear urine? ....

728. What method of treatment is used to address exterior heat patterns with mild aversion to cold and pronounced heat signs such as thirst, red sore pharynx, red tongue with dry thin white fur, and a rapid floating pulse? ....

729. What does "coursing the exterior" mean? ....

730. What method of treatment is used to address heat patterns characterized by scorching heat, heat effusion, swelling and distention, pain, suppuration, and putrefaction? ....

731. By what method is lower burner damp-heat treated?

....

732. What method of treatment is used for heat entering construction-blood in heat diseases with general signs such as high fever, clouded spirit, and crimson tongue? ....

733. What are the three major forms of precipitation? ....

734. What method of treatment is used to treat lesser yáng (*shào yáng*) midstage patterns in externally contracted heat diseases?

....

735. What are the three main forms of dispelling dampness?

....

736. What is the name of the general method used to address bleeding?

....

737. What method of treatment is used to treat ascendant hyperactivity of liver yáng? ....

738. What method of treatment is used to address dryness-heat damaging the lung characterized by heat effusion, headache, and dry cough with scant phlegm? ....

739. By what general method is yīn vacuity treated?

....

740. What is the method of treatment used to treat distending pain in the chest and rib-side with stomach signs such as pain, fullness, and distention in the stomach duct, poor appetite, belching, vomiting of sour matter, or retching and nausea? ....

741. By what method is great yáng collapse vacuity desertion treated? ....

742. What method of treatment is used to address stomach qì disharmony characterized by distention and oppression in the stomach duct, belching, and vomiting of sour fluid? ....

743. What is the general method of treating food stagnation? ....

744. What is the general method of treating scrofula, phlegm nodes, goiter, calculi, and abdominal concretions called? ....

745. What is the method of downbearing counterflow and precipitating qì used for wheezing and panting or rapid panting breathing with copious phlegm? ....

746. What do we call the method of treatment used to treat flooding and spotting? ....

747. What is the general method used to treat qì vacuity? ....

748. What is the difference between boosting qì and supplementing qì? ....

749. What method of treatment is used to address yáng vacuity that is characterized by aversion to cold, cold extremities, limp aching lumbus and knees, impotence, seminal efflux, long voidings of copious clear urine, a pale tongue, and a sunken weak pulse? ....

750. Name the method used to treat heart palpitations or fearful throbbing, insomnia, or fright mania. ....

Give the Pīnyīn and English for the following Chinese terms:

751. 缩尿 ....

752. 燥湿 ....

753. 育阴 ....

754. 祛湿 ....

755. 温经散寒 ....

756. 正治 ....

757. 降逆止呕 ....

758. 回阳救逆 ....

759. 调和肝脾 ....

760. 软坚 ....

761. 实则泻之 ....

762. 解表 ....

763. 破气 ....

764. 疏表 ....

765. 清法 ....

766. 消导 ....

767. 清热祛湿 ....

768. 助阳 ....

769. 温下 ....

770. 涩肠固脱 ....

Supply the Chinese and English for the following:

771. *Qīng qì fèn rè.* ....

772. *Qīng lì shī rè.* ....

773. *Hé fǎ.* ....

774. *Zhú shuǐ.* ....

775. *Zhòng zhèn ān shén.* ....

776. *Bǔ yīn.* ....

777. *Zī yīn jiě biǎo.* ....

778. *Zhì biāo.* ....

779. *Qū chóng.* ....

780. *Huò tán kāi qiào.* ....

781. *Lì shī.* ....

782. *Qīng xuè rè.* ....

783. *Zhù yáng.* ....

784. *Xuān fèi huà tán.* ....

785. *Tiáo hé cháng wèi.* ....

786. *Huó xuè huà yū.* ....

787. *Zhǐ xuè.* ....

788. *Liàn hàn gù biǎo.* ....

789. *Qīng rè kāi qiào.* ....

790. *Huà tán.* ....

Give the Chinese and Pīnyīn for the following:

791. Treating the root. ....

792. Harmonizing midstage patterns. ....

793. Transforming phlegm and suppressing cough. ....

794. Method of treatment. ....

795. Ejection. ....

796. Warming the lung and transforming rheum. ....

797. Principle of treatment. ....

798. Securing essence. ....

799. Drying dampness. ....

800. Clearing heat and disinhibiting dampness. ....

801. Assisting yáng. ....

802. Opening the orifices. ....

803. Harmonizing the liver and spleen. ....

804. Disinhibiting dampness. ....

805. Securing and astringing. ....

806. Moist precipitation. ....

807. Sweeping phlegm and opening the orifices. ....

808. Returning yáng and stemming counterflow. ....

809. Attacking phlegm. ....

810. Boosting qì. ....

第八章　中药学
Chinese Pharmaceutics

8.1. 性能
Characteristics

1002. 性味 [性味] *xìng wèi,* **nature and flavor** [ˈnetʃɚ ənd ˈflevɚ]: See four natures and five flavors.

1003. 四性 [四性] *sì xìng,* **four natures** [fɔr ˈnetʃɚz]: The four natures of medicinals: cold, heat, warmth, and coolness. Cold medicinals are ones effective in treating heat patterns, whereas hot medicinals are effective in treating cold patterns. Warm and cool medicinals are mildly hot or cold natures. In addition, there is also a balanced nature that is neither predominantly hot nor cold.

1004. 四气 [四氣] *sì qì,* **four qì** [fɔr tʃi]: See four natures.

1005. 五味 [五味] *wǔ wèi,* **five flavors** [fɑɪv ˈflevɚz]: Acridity, sourness, sweetness, bitterness, and saltiness. Medicinals or foodstuffs of different flavors have different actions. Acridity can dissipate and move; sourness can contract and astringe; sweetness can supplement and relax (i.e., relieve pain and tension); bitterness can drain and dry; saltiness can soften hardness and induce moist precipitation. These actions are explained by modern pharmacy as follows: Acrid medicinals contain volatile oils; sour medicinals contain organic acids; sweet medicinals contain sugars; bitter medicinals contain biological alkalis, glycosides, or bitter substances. In addition to the five flavors, there is a sixth, blandness (淡 *dàn*), which has a water-disinhibiting action. According to *Elementary Questions (Sù Wèn)*, the flavors can be classified as yīn and yáng: "Acrid and sweet effusing (i.e., diaphoretic) and dissipating medicinals are yáng; sour and bitter upwelling (i.e., emetic) and discharging (i.e., draining) medicinals are yīn; salty upwelling and discharging medicinals are yīn; bland percolating and discharging medicinals are yáng." According to *The Comprehensive*

Herbal Foundation (*Běn Cǎo Gāng Mù*), there is a relationship between flavor and bearing (upbearing, downbearing, floating, and sinking): "No sour or salty medicinals bear upward; no sweet or acrid ones bear downward. No cold medicinals float; no hot ones sink."

1006. 归经 [歸經] *guī jīng*, **channel entry** ['tʃænl‑ˌɛntri]: Action (of a medicinal) on a particular channel and the organ to which the channel homes. For example, platycodon (*jié gěng*) and coltsfoot (*kuǎn dōng huā*) treat cough and panting and are said to enter the lung channel; gastrodia (*tiān má*), scorpion (*quán xiē*), and antelope horn (*líng yáng jiǎo*) treat convulsions and are said to enter the liver channel. Some medicinals enter two channels or more, suggesting that they have a broad scope of action. For example, apricot kernel (*xìng rén*) enters the lung and the large intestine; it treats both cough and constipation. Alisma (*zé xiè*) enters the kidney, bladder, and triple burner channels and treats water-damp problems.

1007. 升降浮沉 [升降浮沉] *shēng jiàng fú chén*, **upbearing, downbearing, floating, and sinking** ['ʌpbɛrɪŋ, 'daʊnˌbɛrɪŋ, 'floʊtɪŋ ənd 'sɪŋkɪŋ]: Collectively referred to as "bearing." Upbearing means ascending to the upper body; downbearing means descending to the lower body. Floating means effusing and dissipating; sinking means draining and disinhibiting. Upbearing and floating medicinals (upfloaters) move upward and outward and have actions such as upbearing yáng, effusing the exterior, and dispersing cold. Downbearing and sinking medicinals (downsinkers) move downward and inward and have actions such as subduing yáng, downbearing counterflow, astriction, clearing heat, percolating dampness, and draining. Most yáng medicinals, which are warm or hot in nature and sweet and acrid in flavor, such as ephedra (*má huáng*), cinnamon twig (*guì zhī*), and astragalus (*huáng qí*), are upfloaters. Most yīn medicinals, which are cold in nature and bitter or sour in nature, such as rhubarb (*dà huáng*), mirabilite (*máng xiāo*), and phellodendron (*huáng bǎi*), are downsinkers. Generally, flowers and leaves and other light medicinals, such as asarum (*xì xīn*), mint (*bò hé*), and cimicifuga (*shēng má*), are upfloaters—inula flower (*xuán fù huā*) being an exception, whereas seeds, fruits, and heavy items, such as white perilla seed (*bái sū zǐ*), unripe bitter orange (*zhǐ shí*), and glauberite (*hán shuǐ shí*), are downsinkers—vitex (*màn jīng zǐ*) being an exception. Bearing can be imparted to other medicinals. Stir-frying with wine causes medicinals to bear upward; stir-frying with bran causes medicinals to downbear; stir-frying with ginger causes medicinals to dissipate; and stir-frying with vinegar causes medicinals to astringe.

8.2. 炮炙
Processing

1008. 炮炙 [炮炙] *páo zhì*, **processing of medicinals** [ˈprɑcɛsɪŋ əv mə-ˈdɪsɪnlz]: The processing of medicinal materials by washing, cutting, frying, etc.

1009. 饮片 [飲片] *yǐn piàn*, **decocting pieces** [dɪˈkɑktɪŋ–ˌpisɪz]: Medicinal materials cut to size and if necessary processed, as by stir-frying in preparation for decoction.

1010. 切 [切] *qiē*, **cutting** [ˈkʌtɪŋ]: Dividing (medicinal materials) with a knife into two or more pieces. Cutting is a commonly used basic method of medicinal processing. It facilitates drying and storage, increases weighing accuracy, and makes it easier for active constituents to be extracted during preparation processes such as decoction. Cutting is often facilitated by soaking or steeping. Kitchen knives, herb knives, guillotines, and nowadays, cutting machines are used to cut materials into lumps or slices of various sizes, usually known as decocting pieces. Herb cutters save labor time, but cut less cleanly than an experienced hand cutter using a sharp knife. Cutting includes cross-cutting (横切 *héng qiē*), oblique cutting (斜切 *xié qiē*), and lengthwise cutting (纵切 *zòng qiē*). The length or thickness and shape to which materials are cut depends on the material. Roots, rhizomes, stems, vines, and woody materials that are hard in substance are cut into thin slices, i.e., about 0.15 cm, whereas softer, less dense materials are cut into thick slices (about 0.3 cm) or in lengths of 1–1.5 cm. Materials that are long and thin, such as imperata (*bái máo gēn*), can be cut into lengths of 1–1.5 cm. Skins and barks that are hard and thick, such as phellodendron (*huáng bǎi*), can be cut into shreds of 0.6 cm. Thinner, less dense barks, such as eucommia (*dù zhòng*), are cut into broad strips of 1–1.5 cm. Brittle, fragile materials like lycium bark (*dì gǔ pí*) need not be cut. Leaves that are thick and flexible, such as pyrrosia (*shí wéi*), are cut into strips of 1–1.5 cm. Thick ones that are brittle after drying, such as mulberry leaf (*sāng yè*) and perilla leaf (*zǐ sū yè*), are either not cut or are simply rubbed between the hands. Whole plants with thin stems are cut into lengths of 1.5 cm; ones with thicker stems are cut into shorter lengths. Flowers and small fruits and seeds are generally not cut. Large fruits or ones that do not dry easily, such as crataegus (*shān zhā*), are cut into three or four slices. Some pericarps, such as trichosanthes rind (*guā lóu pí*), are roughly shredded.

1011. 切片 [切片] *qiē piàn*, **slicing** [ˈslaɪsɪŋ]: See preceding item.

1012. **捣碎** [搗碎] *dǎo suì,* **crushing** [ˈkrʌʃɪŋ]: To damage or destroy the structure of medicinal materials such as with a pestle and mortar. Some small fruits and seeds are crushed just before decocting with a pestle and mortar. Gardenia (*shān zhī zǐ*), amomum (*shā rén*), and Katsumada's galangal seed (*cǎo dòu kòu*) are crushed in small quantities before decoction to ensure that the active constituents are extracted. Medicinals should not be stored for long periods after crushing since they may lose their oil content and other constituents, thus becoming less effective.

1013. **为末** [爲末] *wéi mò,* **grinding to a powder** [ˈɡraɪndɪŋ tu ə ˈpaʊdɚ]: Reduction to powder with a pestle and mortar, or in an electric grinder.

1014. **为细末** [爲細末] *wéi xì mò,* **grinding to a fine powder** [ˈɡraɪndɪŋ tu ə faɪn ˈpaʊdɚ]: See grinding to a powder.

1015. **生** [生] *shēng,* **raw** [rɔ]: Not processed with heat (vegetable matter).

1016. **生** [生] *shēng,* **crude** [krud]: Not processed with heat (mineral matter).

1017. **熟** [熟] *shú,* **cooked** [kʊkt]: Having been subjected to processing with heat.

1018. **制霜** [製霜] *zhì shuāng,* **frosting** [ˈfrɔstɪŋ]: The production of a fine crisp powder by methods other than simple grinding is known as frosting. The following methods exist: (1) One method is the defatting and grinding of seeds. The seeds are first sun-dried or stir-fried, the husks are removed, and the kernels are pounded to an almost paste-like consistency. The materials are sandwiched between layers of paper and then sun-dried, baked, or pressed so that the paper absorbs the oil. The paper is repeatedly changed until the materials are light and loose and no longer stick together. Medicinals processed in this way include croton frost (*bā dòu shuāng*) and trichosanthes seed frost (*guā lóu rén shuāng*). (2) Another method, used to treat certain gourds, is efflorescence. For example, watermelon (*xī guā*) is frosted by gouging out a small lump to form a hole in which a small amount of mirabilite (*máng xiāo*) is placed. The lump is then replaced, and the watermelon is hung up to air. The mirabilite (*máng xiāo*) comes out and effloresces, so that a fine, white frost forms on the surface of the watermelon, which when brushed off is ready to use. (3) The production of persimmon frost (*shì shuāng*) represents a third method of frosting: dried persimmon (*shì bǐng*) is exposed to the sun in the day and to the dew at night and then is covered to allow the skin to saccharify and form a frost.

8.2.1. 水制 Water Processing

1019. 水制 [水製] *shuǐ zhì,* **water processing** ['wɔtɚ 'prɑcɛsɪŋ]: Any of various methods of treating medicinal materials with clean water to remove impurities, foreign bodies, unwanted elements (such as sand, earth, salt, unpleasant odors), to increase suppleness to facilitate cutting, to refine minerals, and to reduce toxicity. Methods must be carefully chosen to prevent loss of active constituents.

1020. 洗 [洗] *xǐ,* **washing** ['wɔʃɪŋ]: To remove earth or unwanted parts by dipping, rubbing, or scrubbing in water. With the exception of flowers, whose active constituents are easily lost in water, most materials are washed before use. The main aim of washing is to remove earth. Materials should not be left in water too long otherwise they lose their active constituents. Light, soft materials in particular should be washed as quickly as possible.

1021. 浸泡 [浸泡] *jìn pào,* **steeping** ['stipɪŋ]: Allow medicinal materials to stand in clear water or other fluid for a certain time. Steeping facilitates slicing, as in the case of areca (*bīng láng*) and lindera (*wū yào*). It can also reduce toxicity, as in the case of arisaema (*tiān nán xīng*) and pinellia (*bàn xià*).

1022. 漂 [漂] *piǎo,* **long-rinsing** ['lɔŋ rɪnsɪŋ]: Steeping materials in clean water that is continuously replaced to eliminate toxic constituents, salts, or malodor, or to remove foreign matter. Sargassum (*hǎi zǎo*), cistanche (*ròu cōng róng*), salted aconite (*xián fù zǐ*), and pinellia (*bàn xià*) are processed in this way.

1023. 闷润 [悶潤] *mèn rùn,* **covered moistening** ['kʌvɚd 'mɔɪsnɪŋ]: To allow materials that have been washed or steeped to stand in a receptacle covered with hemp sacking or a bag of moist straw and frequently sprinkle them with water so that they gradually become thoroughly moistened.

1024. 水飞 [水飛] *shuǐ fēi,* **water grinding** ['wɔtɚ–ˌɡrɑɪndɪŋ]: Fine grinding of medicinal materials in water. The materials are first roughly crushed. They are then placed in a porcelain mortar, covered with water, and ground until the grating sound of rough lumps ceases. At this point, more water is mixed in, and the water that contains suspended particles is poured off and reserved. More water and materials are added to the mortar, and the process is repeated. The reserved suspension is allowed to stand until the particles have settled, and the excess water is poured off. The remaining sludge is sun-dried, after which it is ready for use. This method is used for minerals and shells. Its advantage over dry grinding is that fine particles do not blow away or get lost, and that impurities dissolved in the water are (at least partly) removed. The much finer powder it produces makes for greater assimilation of orally taken medicinals and reduces irritation in topical applications. Cinnabar (*zhū shā*), talcum (*huá shí*), calamine (*lú gān shí*), and realgar (*xióng huáng*) are treated in this way for laryngeal insufflation, topical eye medication, or for coating pills.

8.2.2. 火制 Fire Processing

1025. 火制 [火製] *huǒ zhì*, **fire processing** [faɪr ˈprɑːsɛsɪŋ]: Processing medicinals by the application of heat. Fire processing methods involve either direct or indirect contact of the materials with a heat source, sometimes with adjuvants. Care is required in controlling time and temperature and in gauging the quantity of any additive used; excessively high temperatures can cause undesirable changes in a medicinal's characteristics. The most common forms of fire processing are the various forms of stir-frying and mix-frying. Less commonly used methods are roasting and stone-baking.

1026. 炒 [炒] *chǎo,* **stir-frying** [ˈstɝfraɪɪŋ]: Tossing (medicinal materials) in a heated wok. Stir-frying is the most commonly used method of heat processing. It is dry frying: oil should never be used unless specifically stated. The aims of stir-frying are threefold: (1) To eliminate unwanted constituents, change the nature of medicinals (such as reducing extreme cold or dryness), or minimize irritation or other side-effects. For example, the fierce draining precipitant action of rhubarb (*dà huáng*) in its raw form is moderated by stir-frying and even more markedly reduced by char-frying. (2) To increase the aromatic and spleen-fortifying qualities. For example, white atractylodes (*bái zhú*) and barley sprout (*mài yá*) are stir-fried until yellow, whereas crataegus (*shān zhā*) and medicated leaven (*shén qū*) are scorch-fried. (3) To facilitate crushing, storage, and extraction of active constituents through decoction. For example, some seeds crispen and crack open to facilitate decoction when lightly fried. Some materials become looser after stir-frying, so that they are not only more easily crushed, but also their active constituents are more easily extracted. Also, stir-frying reduces moisture content and destroys ferments, thus preventing the breakdown of active constituents during storage. Stir-frying includes plain stir-frying (light-stir-frying, scorch-frying, char-frying, etc.), and stir-frying with adjuvants such as bran, earth, oven earth (*fú lóng gān*), or rice. Stir-frying with liquid adjuvants, especially honey, is usually referred to as mix-frying.

1027. 清炒 [清炒] *qīng chǎo*, **plain stir-frying** [plen ˈstɝˈfɹaɪŋ]: Stir-frying without any adjuvants. It includes light stir-frying, scorch-frying, and blast-frying.

1028. 炒焦 [炒焦] *chǎo jiāo*, **scorch-frying** [ˈskɔrtʃfɹaɪŋ]: Stir-frying materials in a wok over a high flame until they become burnt on the outside and emit a burnt smell. Abductive dispersing medicinals such as medicated leaven (*shén qū*) and crataegus (*shān zhā*) are scorch-fried to strengthen their spleen-fortifying food-dispersing action.

1029. 微炒 [微炒] *wēi chǎo*, **light stir-frying** [laɪt ˈstɝˈfɹaɪŋ]: Stir-frying of short duration to remove the moisture content of medicinal materials so that they are left dry, at least on the outer surface, but without producing any change in form or medicinal characteristics.

1030. 炒黄 [炒黃] *chǎo huáng*, **stir-frying until yellow** [ˈstɝˈfɹaɪŋ ʌnˈtɪl ˈyɛlo]: Stir-frying medicinal materials until they turn slightly golden on the outside.

1031. 炮 [炮] *páo*, **blast-frying** [ˈbæst–fɹaɪŋ]: Stir-frying (medicinal materials) vigorously in an iron wok over a fierce fire until they give off smoke and their surface becomes scorched, swollen, and cracked. Dried ginger (*gān jiāng*), aconite (*fù zǐ*), and tianxiong aconite (*tiān xióng*) may be processed in this way to reduce their harshness.

1032. 炒炭 [炒炭] *chǎo tàn*, **char-fry** [ˈtʃɑrfɹaɪŋ]: A medicinal processing method similar to scorch-frying, but using an even higher flame. The aim of char-frying is to make the materials charred and black on the outside, brown on the inside, and brittle. Although a large proportion of the material is charred, the original properties are still present. This is what is known as "nature-preservative burning" (烧存性 *shāo cún xìng*). To ensure that the nature is partially preserved in this way, it is important that the material should not be completely carbonized. Because of the high temperature used in char-frying, materials easily catch fire. In this event, water should be sprinkled over the material until no sparks are seen. Some materials, such as typha pollen (*pú huáng*), require particularly vigorous stirring to clear the smoke they produce. Char-frying moderates the properties of a medicinal and increases its ability to promote contraction and check bleeding. Some modern experiments show that blood-stanching properties may in some cases be destroyed through this process.

1033. 烧存性 [燒存性] *shāo cún xìng*, **nature-preservative burning** [ˈnetʃɚ prɪˈzɝˈvətɪv ˈbɝnɪŋ]: See preceding item.

1034. 炙 [炙] *zhì*, **mix-fry** [ˈmɪksfɹaɪŋ]: The aim of mix-frying is to change medicinal characteristics, improve effectiveness, improve the flavor and smell, resolve toxicity, and prevent rotting. Usually, the adjuvant and materials are first blended, covered, and left to stand for a short time before frying so that the adjuvant soaks well into the materials. The most commonly used adjuvants are honey, vinegar, wine, and brine.

1035. 焙 [焙] *bèi*, **stone-baking** ['stonbekɪŋ]: Heating medicinal materials on a slab (or in a pan) without allowing them to change color.

1036. 煨 [煨] *wēi*, **roasting** [rostɪŋ]: A method of drawing out unwanted oils or irritants from medicinal materials and reducing their toxicity by exposure to heat. Materials are usually wrapped in wet paper or coated in flour and water paste, and then placed in hot embers until the wrapping becomes burnt and black. They may also be put at the side of the fire, in an oven, or tossed in a wok. Nutmeg (*ròu dòu kòu*) and kansui (*gān suì*) may be treated in this way.

1037. 煅 [煅] *duàn*, **calcine (v.); calcination (n.)** [kæl'sɑmɪŋ, ˌkælsɪ'ne-ʃən]: A medicinal processing method whereby medicinal materials are heated until red hot by charcoal, coal, or the like, in order to make them crisp, soft, and easily crushed, and to facilitate the extraction of their active constituents in decoction. Materials such as dragon bone (*lóng gǔ*), oyster shell (*mǔ lì*), gypsum (*shí gāo*), and chlorite/mica (*méng shí*) that come in large lumps and do not crumble easily under heat are calcined by being placed directly in the fire. Materials such as hematite (*dài zhě shí*) and pyrite (*zì rán tóng*) that easily crumble are calcined in crucibles called "*dūlǔ*" (嘟噜). Some materials such as borax (*péng shā*), calamine (*lú gān shí*), and alum (*bái fán*) may be simply heated in a wok. Soft materials such as juncus (*dēng xīn cǎo*) and old trachycarpus (*chén zōng pí*) are calcined in a mud-sealed wok to char. Especially hard materials such as hematite (*dài zhě shí*), white quartz (*bái shí yīng*), pyrite (*zì rán tóng*), tortoise shell (*guī bǎn*), and loadstone (*cí shí*) are dipped in vinegar after heating to make them softer; actinolite (*yáng qǐ shí*) can be dipped in wine.

8.2.3. 水火制 Fire and Water Processing

1038. 水火制 [水火製] *shuǐ huǒ zhì*, **fire and water processing** [fɑɪr ənd 'wɔtɚ'prɑcɛsɪŋ]: Processing that uses heat and water, such as boiling or steaming.

1039. 煮 [煮] *zhǔ*, **boiling** [bɔɪlɪŋ]: Cooking (foods or medicines) in boiling water or other liquid. Boiling, as a method of processing individual medicinals, has the aim of eliminating toxicity and irritants, preventing side-effects, increasing effectiveness, or facilitating storage. For example, boiling genkwa (*yuán huā*) in vinegar reduces its toxicity; boiling impure mirabilite (*pò xiāo*) with radish removes impurities, making it into refined mirabilite (*xuán míng fěn*). Boiling is also the method of making a formula into a decoction.

1040. 蒸 ［蒸］ *zhēng,* **steaming** [ˈstimɪŋ]: A method of processing medicinals whereby medicinal materials are placed in pots or baskets, with or without adjuvants, over boiling water. The aim is to change the nature of the medicinal, improve its effectiveness, and facilitate slicing and storage.

1041. 炖 ［燉］ *dùn,* **double-boiling** [ˈdʌbl̩–ˌbɔɪlɪŋ]: To boil in a container placed in boiling water rather than directly over a fire; to cook or heat in a double boiler.

1042. 煅淬 ［煆淬］ *duàn cuì,* **calcining and quenching** [kælˈsɑɪnɪŋ ənd kwɛntʃɪŋ]: To heat (medicinal materials) to a high temperature and then dip them in water or vinegar.

8.3. 剂型
Preparations

1043. 剂型 ［劑型］ *jì xíng,* **preparation** [ˌprɛpəˈreʃən]: The form in which medication is taken by a patient, e.g., docoction, pill, or paste.

1044. 汤 ［湯］ *tāng,* **decoction** [dɪˈkɑkʃən]: A medicinal preparation made by boiling the ingredients of a formula in water and then straining off the dregs. Because it was recognized that decoctions prepared in iron pots could have reduced effects, traditional literature stipulates the use of earthenware pots. Pyrex, ceramic, or enamel are now used. The decoction is the most common medicinal preparation. Decoctions are quickly absorbed by the body and so are particularly suitable for acute diseases of recent onset. In contrast to ready-prepared pills and powders, decoctions enable the formula to be tailored to the patient's individual needs. Materials can usually be boiled twice. The first time, add enough water to cover the materials and bring the pot to a boil. Boil 20–30 minutes, stirring occasionally. Then strain off the decoction and reserve the dregs. Any materials that swell on absorbing water will have done so during the first boiling, so that for the second boiling only enough water is added to cover the materials and a duration of 20 minutes only is required. The two boilings may be mixed together before the patient takes them, in order to ensure even doses. The water quantities, boiling times, and size of flame given above represent a general guide only. Ideally they are varied according to the medicinals used to ensure maximum benefit. Exterior-effusing and qì-rectifying medicinals are used for their qì rather than their flavor and are cooked over a fierce fire for a relatively short period to prevent loss of active constituents. Supplementing medicinals are used for their flavor and are therefore boiled for a longer period (about 10 minutes longer) over a low flame to ensure complete extraction of active constituents.

1045. 煎 [煎] *jiān,* **decoct** (v.); **brew** (v.) [dɪˈkɑkt]: To boil medicinal materials to make a decoction.

1046. 饮 [飲] *yǐn,* **beverage** [ˈbɛvərɪdʒ]: A decoction that is left to cool before being taken, e.g., Mosla Beverage (*xiāng rú yǐn*). Compare drink.

1047. 饮子 [飲子] *yǐn zi,* **drink** [drɪŋk]: A beverage (a decoction left to cool) that can be taken at any time.

1048. 丸 [丸] *wán,* **pill** [pɪl]: A medicinal preparation made by mixing finely ground medicinals with a binding medium (usually honey, water, or flour and water paste) and forming them into small round balls. The pill preparation has the advantage of being more convenient for the patient than the decoction, especially when medication has to be taken over a long period of time. The active constituents are absorbed into the body more slowly, but their effect is longer lasting. Pills are therefore most commonly used in the treatment of enduring diseases, especially concretions and accumulations. They are also used for certain acute patterns since they can be kept at hand ready for occasional use. Pills are taken by swallowing with, or dissolving in, water.

1049. 水丸 [水丸] *shuǐ wán,* **water pill** [ˈwɔtɚ-pɪl]: A preparation made by mixing the finely ground ingredients with cold water, yellow wine, vinegar or fresh herb juice, as the formula stipulates, before forming pills either by hand or by machine.

1050. 散 [散] *sǎn,* **powder** [ˈpɑudɚ]: A medicinal preparation made by finely grinding medicinal materials. Powders are suitable for both internal and external use. They are convenient for the patient. Orally taken powders are more easily absorbed than pills. Materials that cannot be heated, or do not easily dissolve in water are particularly suitable for preparation in powder form. The materials are first carefully dried, then blended and ground together. The coarser particles are sifted off and reground until everything has been ground to a uniformly fine powder. High oil content materials such as bitter apricot kernel (*kŭ xìng rén*) or spiny jujube (*suān zǎo rén*) that are not suited to baking are first set aside while the other medicinals are ground. They are then ground together with a part of the preground powder, which absorbs the oil and facilitates the grinding process. Soft sticky agents such as cooked rehmannia (*shú dì huáng*), cornus (*shān zhū yú*), and lycium berry (*gǒu qǐ zǐ*) may also be ground with part of the preground agents, then sun-dried or oven-dried, and finally ground to a fine powder. Agents such as bovine bezoar (*niú huáng*) and borneol (*bīng piàn*), which, being used in such small quantities, may be lost if ground together with the other medicinals, may be ground in a porcelain mortar and added to the other powdered agents. Finally, medicinals such as realgar (*xióng huáng*), sulfur (*shí liú huáng*), and niter (*xiāo shí*) should not be ground since they may catch fire or explode.

1051. 酒剂 [酒劑] *jiǔ jì,* **wine preparation** ['waɪn-ˌpreɛpə're ʃ ən]: Any preparation made by steeping medicinals in grain wine or liquor. There are two methods of making wine preparations, cold steeping and hot steeping. (1) Cold steeping: The medicinal materials are cut, crushed, or ground, and steeped in white liquor (liquor distilled usually from sorghum or maize) or yellow wine (wine made from rice or millet) in a sealed large stone jar. The preparation is stirred each day, either with a ladle or by shaking the jar. When ready to drink, which is after a minimum of 30 days, but ideally for most wines much longer, the clear wine near the surface may be removed and strained to be made ready for drinking. Grubs are almost inevitably brought out from the materials by the liquor. It suffices that these should be filtered out in the process of straining. Some formulas allow the materials to be reused. (2) Hot steeping: The materials and wine are placed in a receptacle and brought to a boil either in a steamer or double-boiler before they are placed in the jar to steep. In this method, the clear wine may be removed and strained for use after 15–20 days. Medicinal wines promote flow in the blood vessels and are used in wind-damp impediment patterns (rheumatism) and other chronic conditions.

1052. 膏 [膏] *gāo,* **paste** [pest]: Any semi-liquid or virtually solid pharmaceutical preparation. Distinction is made between rich pastes, which are taken orally, and medicinal pastes, which are applied topically. Rich pastes are made by reducing decoctions of agents to a thick consistency and then adding honey or rock candy. Medicinal pastes are made by adding powdered agents to heated mixtures of vegetable oil and wax. A plaster is a kind of topically applied medicinal paste that has to be softened by heating before being applied.

1053. **膏滋** [膏滋] *gāo zī,* **rich paste** ['rɪtʃ–pest]: A paste preparation to be taken orally. The ingredients are usually boiled 2–3 times, for 2–3 hours each time, until the smell is only faint. After each boiling, the decoction should be strained off, and fresh water added to the pot for the next boiling. Then, all the decoctions are slow-boiled together until they are reduced to a thick, viscous paste. The correct consistency is reached as soon as no water separates out from a globule of the paste when dropped on paper. If the paste becomes too thick, it is likely to stick to the pot and burn. If too thin, it is difficult to store. Then, a quantity of honey or sugar, equal to a specified proportion of the original materials (usually an equal proportion) is added before a final boiling. The paste is then put in earthenware or glass jars. Pastes keep for long periods and are usually used for chronic diseases.

1054. **药膏** [藥膏] *yào gāo,* **medicinal paste** [mə'dɪsɪnļ–pest]: A preparation made with vegetable oil and bee's wax and that is applied topically in the treatment of sores or burns. Medicinal pastes are made by first heating the oil, blending in the wax, and adding the ground medicinals while the mixture is still hot. The paste is ready for use when cool. Some formulas stipulate that certain medicinals be added in the form of decocting slices. These are first fried in the oil and the dregs removed before the wax and powdered medicinals are blended in. Aromatic medicinals such as borneol (*bīng piàn*) and camphor (*zhāng nǎo*) are added after the paste has cooled to ensure that they retain their full strength. Nowadays, finely ground materials are often combined with a petroleum jelly (Vaseline) and glycerin base to make "ointment" (软膏 *ruǎn gāo*).

1055. **膏药** [膏藥] *gāo yào,* **plaster** ['plæstɚ]: A topical paste that is mounted on cloth. It is made by slicing or pounding the ingredients and steeping them in sesame seed oil or tung-oil (*tóng yóu*) for 3–5 days. The mixture is then heated to fry the materials until they char. Flowers, leaves, and pericarps that cannot withstand heat should not be included. The materials are strained off, and the oil is returned to the fire, where it is continuously heated and stirred until the smoke given off turns from white to blue-green. When the temperature reaches 250-300°C (when the oil is dropped in water at this temperature it will stay together in a globule), the fire is turned down, and yellow up-borne elixir (*huáng shēng*) or processed galenite (*qiān fěn*) is slowly stirred in. The pot is removed from the fire when all the yellow up-borne elixir (*huáng shēng*) has dissolved. It is then sprinkled with water and stirred and then steeped in cold water to eliminate the fire toxin. Before use it is melted over a small flame or in water so that it can be spread on cloth or animal skin ready for topical application. Plasters are used for sores and wind-damp pain. They are available ready made and mounted on cloth and require only warming prior to application.

1056. 露 [露] *lù,* **distillate** [ˈdɪstɪlət]: The condensed vapor obtained when medicinals are boiled in water. Lonicera (*jīn yín huā*), agastache (*huò xiāng*), and mint (*bò hé*) can all be made into distillates. Distillates are bland in flavor and are taken as a beverage in the summer. They rapidly lose their effectiveness and so are best used as soon as possible.

1057. 露 [露] *lù,* **dew** [du]: See distillate.

1058. 锭 [錠] *dìng,* **lozenge** [ˈlɑzɪndʒ]: A solid preparation made by blending finely ground medicinals with flour paste and forming them into spindle shapes, cones, or oblongs. If taken orally, lozenges are crushed and swallowed with water. If to be applied topically, they are crushed and mixed with vinegar or sesame oil.

1059. 片 [片] *piàn,* **tablet** [ˈtæblɪt]: A medicinal preparation made by mixing a powder of ground medicinal materials with a formative medicinal and compressing them into a mold. Tablets are convenient to carry and use. Since they easily absorb dampness, they should be kept in a dry place. Tablets may be hand or machine made. To make tablets by hand, the constituents are ground to a fine powder, and blended with flour and water paste or viscous rice water, pressed in a mold, and either oven-dried or left to dry in the shade. Less commonly, some of the constituents are boiled, and, after the dregs are strained off, the decoction is reduced to a paste, which is then mixed with the dry medicinals.

1060. 热熨 [熱熨] *rè yùn,* **hot pack** [ˈhɑ–pæk]: A method of treatment in which a cloth bag containing medicinals that have been warmed, usually by stir-frying, is applied to the body to relieve pain. The hot pack method is used to treat wind-cold-damp impediment and cold pain in the stomach duct and abdomen. For example, stomach qì pain can be treated with a hot pack of stir-fried tangerine leaves. Salt, sand, or earth can also be used. Care should be taken not to burn the patient.

1061. 胶 [膠] *jiāo,* **glue** [glu]: The reduced extract of boiled skins, bone, shells, or horns. While glues are hard and even somewhat brittle at normal temperature, heating them brings out their gluey quality. Most glues are supplementing medicinals.

Examples of glues:

阿胶 *ē jiāo,* ass hide glue (Asini Corii Colla)
虎骨胶 *hǔ gǔ jiāo,* tiger bone glue (Tigris Ossis Gelatinum)

鳖甲胶 *biē jiǎ jiāo*, turtle shell glue (Trionycis Caparacis Gelatinum)

龟版胶 *guī bǎn jiāo*, tortoise shell glue (Testudinis Carapacis et Plastri Gelatinum)

鹿角胶 *lù jiǎo jiāo*, deerhorn glue (Cervi Cornus Gelatinum)

8.4. 药物用法
Methods of Use

1062. 服 [服] *fú*, **take** [tek]: To ingest (medicines).

1063. 冲服 [冲服] *chōng fú*, **take drenched** [tek drentʃ'd]: To swallow a medicine (powder, paste, or glue) mixed with several times its volume of cold, warm, or hot water or other fluid. Medicinals that should not or need not be decocted are taken drenched to facilitate swallowing. Some medicinals such as amber (*hǔ pò*), cinnabar (*zhū shā*), or notoginseng (*sān qī*) that are expensive or that should not be decocted are ground to a fine powder and mixed with warm water or an accompanying decoction and swallowed. Some gelatinous medicinals or mineral salts such as ass hide glue (*ē jiāo*), mirabilite (*máng xiāo*), or malt sugar (*yí táng*) can be dissolved in warm water or an accompanying decoction.

1064. 送服 [送服] *sòng fú*, **swallow with fluid** ['swɑlo wið 'fluɪd]: To ingest a solid medicine with water, a medicinal decoction, or other fluid.

1065. 频服 [頻服] *pín fú*, **take in frequent small doses** [tek ɪn 'frikwɛnt smɔl 'dosɪz]

1066. 顿服 [頓服] *dùn fú*, **quaff** [kwɔf]: Take in one go.

1067. 食远服 [食遠服] *shí yuǎn fú*, **take between meals** [tek bɪ'twin milz]

1068. 饭前服 [飯前服] *fàn qián fú*, **take before meals** [tek bɪ'fɔr milz]

1069. 临睡前服 [臨睡前服] *lín shuì qián fú*, **take before sleeping** [tek bɪ'fɔr 'slipɪŋ]

1070. 调敷 [調敷] *tiáo fú*, **apply mixed** [ə'plɑɪ mɪkst]: To topically apply a powder blended with fluid.

8.5. 方剂组成
Formula Composition

1071. 君〔君〕*jūn,* **sovereign** [ˈsɑvrɪn]: The sovereign performs the principal action of the formula, addressing the principal pattern. The sovereign may be one or more medicinals.

1072. 臣〔臣〕*chén,* **minister** [ˈmɪnɪstɚ]: The minister provides direct assistance to the sovereign.

1073. 佐〔佐〕*zuǒ,* **assistant** [əˈsɪstənt]: The assistant addresses secondary patterns or reduces the toxicity or harshness of the sovereign.

1074. 使〔使〕*shǐ,* **courier** [ˈkurɪɚ]: The courier makes other medicinals act on the desired part of the body or harmonizes the other medicinals.

习题
Questions

Answer the following questions in English:

811. What is a "plaster"? ....

812. What is a "drink"? ....

813. What do we call a reduced extract of boiled animal skins? ....

814. What is the term denoting a decoction left to cool before being taken? ....

815. What does "take drenched" mean? ....

816. What does "quaff" mean? ....

817. What do we call a paste preparation that is taken orally? ....

818. What is the name given to the ingredient of a formula that performs the principal action? ....

819. The condensed vapor obtained when medicinals are boiled is called what?

   ....

820. What preparation is most suited for the treatment of enduring illnesses? ....

Give the Pīnyīn and English for the following Chinese terms:

821. 散 ....

822. 使 ....

823. 蒸 ....

824. 酒剂 ....

825. 膏滋 ....

826. 热熨 ....

827. 烧存性 ....

828. 胶 ....

829. 片 ....

830. 临睡前服 ....

831. 顿服 ....

Supply the Chinese and English for the following:

832. *Tiáo fū.* ....

833. *Yào gāo.* ....

834. *Mèn rùn.* ....

835. *Piàn.* ....

836. *Sòng fú.* ....

837. *Zhì shuāng.* ....

838. *Zuǒ.* ....

839. *Tāng.* ....

840. *Chōng fú.* ....

841. *Chén.* ....

Give the Chinese and Pīnyīn for the following:

842. Preparation. ....

843. Double-boiling. ....

844. Water pill. ....

845. Calcining and quenching. ....

846. Char-frying. ....

847. Channel entry. ....

第九章　针灸
Acumoxatherapy

9.1. 针灸器材
Acumoxatherapy Materials

1075. **毫针** [毫針] *háo zhēn*, **filiform needle** [ˈfɪlɪfɔrm n ˈnidl̩]: One of the nine needles of ancient China that has been developed into a variety of fine needles of varying length most commonly used in performing acupuncture today. The filiform needle is now generally made from a stainless steel wire that is sharpened at one end and has a thin wire of copper, stainless steel, or silver wrapped around its opposite end as a handle. Stainless steel is chosen for the body of the needle because of its flexibility, strength, and resistance to oxidation. Though silver and gold also resist oxidation, they are expensive and are relatively soft metals. Thus, they are used only in specific systems of practice when their pliability does not impede treatment. Filiform needles range in size from 15 mm to 150 mm in length and 0.22 mm to 0.30 mm (30 to 34 gauge) in diameter.

1076. **火针** [火針] *huǒ zhēn*, **fire needle** [ˈfɑɪr–nidl̩]: A needle 8–10 cm long with a pointed tip and a handle made of horn, bamboo, or wood. Fire needle is used in fire needling.

1077. **电针** [電針] *diàn zhēn*, **electroacupuncture** [ɪˈlɛktro͵ækju͵pʌnk-tʃɚ]: A method of acupuncture in which an electrical current is applied to needles inserted in the body in order to produce a combined needle and electrical stimulus. Electroacupuncture was first reported in the PRC in the 1970s and over recent years has come to be widely used. Method: Select two suitable acupuncture points, insert needles, and obtain qi. Next, wire the needles to the electrical stimulator and apply a stimulus of appropriate intensity and duration. Then turn off the electrical stimulus and remove the needles. Electroacupuncture can be used in regular body acupuncture, ear acupuncture, head acupuncture, facial acupuncture, and acupuncture anesthesia. In patients suffering from heart disease, it is important not to allow the current to pass through the region of the heart.

1078. 三棱针 [三棱針] *sān léng zhēn,* **three-edged needle** [θri edʒd ˈnidl̩]: A thick needle with a sharp, three-edged tip used for letting blood. The use of presterilized, disposable lancets has replaced the three-edged needle for bloodletting in many acupuncture clinics.

1079. 皮肤针 [皮膚針] *pí fū zhēn,* **cutaneous needle** [kjuˈtenɪəs–ˌnidl̩]: An instrument traditionally made by binding five or seven sewing needles to a bamboo stick (traditionally called plum-blossom needle and seven-star needle, now made by mounting needles on a metal or plastic hammer) and used to tap the skin to move qì and quicken the blood in the affected area or on the pathway of an affected channel. The cutaneous needle is especially suitable for treating children and others where pain or fear of needle insertion may be a necessary consideration. The tapping can be light (no bleeding) or heavy (slight bleeding), depending on the patient's condition and the disease being treated. Nowadays in China, heavy tapping is employed to move stagnant blood in a local area. Cutaenous needling can be used to treat a number of internal medical diseases including digestive disorders, headache, menstrual pain, and certain skin diseases. Legal factors limit the applicability of this method in the West since cutaneous needles are difficult to sterilize. Method: The needle should be held about two inches above the skin and manipulated by a loose movement of the wrist. The needle must strike the skin perpendicularly and without excessive force to prevent bleeding. In general, tapping is performed from the top downward and from the medial toward the lateral aspect. Cutaneous tapping is contraindicated on ulcerations or external injuries. The two most common types of cutaneous needle now used are the plum blossom and the seven-star needle.

1080. 梅花针 [梅花針] *méi huā zhēn,* **plum-blossom needle** [ˈplʌmblɑsəm–ˌnidl̩]: See cutaneous needle.

1081. 七星针 [七星針] *qī xīng zhēn,* **seven-star needle** [ˈsɛvən stɑr ˈnidl̩]: See cutaneous needle.

1082. 揿针 [撳針] *qìn zhēn,* **thumbtack needle** [ˈθʌmtæk–ˌnɪdl̩]: A small needle about 2–3 mm long, continuous with and perpendicular to a circle of wire that forms the head. Thumbtack needles are mostly used in ear acupuncture or facial acupuncture; they are implanted into the skin using tweezers and then held in position with tape.

1083. 艾绒 [艾絨] *ài róng,* **moxa floss** ['mɑksə–flɔs]: Mugwort leaves rubbed to a woolly consistency.

1084. 艾条 [艾條] *ài tiáo,* **moxa pole** ['mɑksə–pol]: A roll of rubbed moxa leaves enclosed in paper that forms a cylinder about six inches in length and half an inch in diameter. The lighted moxa pole is held about one inch above the point to be warmed and is moved slowly in a circular motion to spread the heat over a small area. Alternately, the roll may be moved quickly up and down to increase thermal stimulation in what is called the pecking sparrow method. Moxa pole therapy can be combined with acupuncture by warming the area around the needle. Moxa pole is generally applied for 3–15 minutes or until the skin turns red. The proper distance must be maintained to avoid reddening the skin too quickly or burning the patient. Moxa pole treatment, or poling, is commonly employed to provide mild heat and move qì and blood in a local area; it thus treats wind-damp impediment pain and similar patterns.

1085. 艾炷 [艾炷] *ài zhù,* **moxa cone** ['mɑksə–kon]: A hand-rolled, conical lump of moxa. Large cones are about the size of a broad bean and are used only in indirect moxibustion; medium cones are the size of a soybean; and small cones are the size of a wheat grain. Moxa cones can be burnt on the skin (direct moxibustion) or separated from it by garlic, ginger, or salt (indirect moxibustion).

9.2. 针刺法
Acupuncture Needling

1086. 进针 [進針] *jìn zhēn,* **needle insertion** ['nidl̩–ɪn,sɝˈʃən]: To introduce a needle or needles into the body.

1087. 出针 [出針] *chū zhēn,* **needle removal** ['nidl̩ reɪˈmuvl̩]: The removal of an acupuncture needle from the body.

1088. 留针 [留針] *liú zhēn,* **needle retention** ['nidl̩–rɪˌtɛnʃən]: Leaving acupuncture needles inserted for a certain time. In modern practice, needles are often left in place for a period ranging from several minutes to two hours depending on the particular condition. This allows for application of other stimulation methods such as warming the needle, electrical stimulation, or intermittent manipulation. Often needles are retained with little or no additional manipulation. Needle retention in general can increase the ability of a point to relieve pain and quiet the spirit. Some specific treatments require needle retention to achieve satisfactory results. For example, treatment of intestinal welling-abscess (appendicitis) or panting generally involves the retention of needles for at least half an hour. The patient must be instructed not to move while the needles are in place. Pain that results from a change in posture can be relieved by withdrawing the needle to a level just beneath the skin and then reinserting it to the proper depth.

1089. 退针 [退針] *tuì zhēn,* **needle retraction** [ˈnidl̩–rɪˌtrækʃən]: The lifting of an inserted needle so that the point of the needle approaches but does not leave the skin.

1090. 捣针 [搗針] *dǎo zhēn,* **needle pounding** [ˈnidl̩–ˌpɑʊndɪŋ]: A needle manipulation technique whereby the needle, after insertion, is repeatedly raised and thrust between two levels of the flesh. Needle pounding differs from lifting and thrusting by absence of variation in speed between retraction and thrusting and by a shorter span of movement. It produces even supplementation and drainage, whereas lifting and thrusting is normally used to supplement or drain.

1091. 捻针 [捻針] *niǎn zhēn,* **needle twirling** [ˈnidl̩–twɝlɪŋ]: A method of needle manipulation whereby the practitioner grasps the handle of the needle between his thumb and forefinger and twists the needle first one way and then the other, in an arc between 180° and 360°. One should avoid turning the needle in a single direction in order to prevent the needle from adhering to fibrous tissue and causing unnecessary pain. Rotating the needle rapidly in a wide arc drains; a narrow arc with slow motion supplements; a medium arc with medium speed produces even supplementation and drainage. The rotation method can be combined with the lifting and thrusting method described above.

1092. 刮针 [刮針] *guā zhēn,* **needle scratching** [ˈnidl̩–ˌskrætʃɪŋ]: Scratching the handle of the needle upward or downward with the finger nail after insertion to encourage the obtaining of qì and intensify the needle sensation.

1093. 摇针 [搖針] *yáo zhēn,* **needle waggling** [ˈnidl̩–ˌwæglɪŋ]: A needle manipulation technique whereby, after insertion of the needle, the acupuncture point is held firmly with one hand, while the body of the needle is moved to and fro with the other hand.

1094. 得气 [得氣] *dé qì,* **obtaining qì** [əbˈtenɪŋ tʃi]: Causing the acupuncture needle to elicit needle sensation, i.e., any of the sensations associated with the presence of qì at or near the insertion site. These sensations include subjective sensations in the patient and an objective sensation felt by the practitioner's fingers. Depending on the acupunture point in question and the condition of the patient, the subjective sensation experienced by the patient can be described as twinging (酸 *suān*), distention, heaviness, tingling, or numbness. This should not be confused with the local sensation of pricking pain that may accompany needle insertion. Obtaining qì is a deeper sensation, duller in nature, and less localized than the sharp pain associated with the stimulation of subcutaneous nerves. The objective sensation felt by the practitioner can be described, to use the metaphor of *Song to Elucidate Mysteries (Biāo Yōu Fù)*, as a sudden deep tightening that resembles the feeling of a fish biting on a fishing line. As long as the needle moves easily, qì cannot be obtained. Since some patients report the slightest sensation in order to avoid further probing by the acupuncturist, it is better to rely on the subtle objective sensation. Channel-freeing manipulation and needle flicking are techniques designed to help obtain qì.

1095. 气至 [氣至] *qì zhì*, **arrival of qì** [əˈraɪvl̩ əv tʃi]: See obtaining qì.

1096. 针感 [針感] *zhēn gǎn*, **needle sensation** [nidl̩ sɛnˈseʃən]: The physical sensation felt in response to needling.

1097. 循摄法 [循攝法] *xún shè fǎ*, **channel-freeing manipulation** [ˈtʃæn-l̩–ˌfriɪŋ məˌnɪpjəˈleʃən]: An acupuncture technique used to help obtain qì that involves the application of light pressure along the course of the channel above and below the point being needled; this hastens the movement of qì and blood in the channel.

1098. 弹针 [彈針] *tán zhēn*, **needle flicking** [ˈnidl̩–ˌflɪkɪŋ]: A needle manipulation involving the flicking of the handle of an acupuncture needle as a method of obtaining qì.

1099. 呼吸补泻 [呼吸補瀉] *hū xī bǔ xiè*, **respiratory supplementation and drainage** [ˈrɛspɪrəˌtɔri ˌsʌpləmɛnˈteʃən ənd ˈdrenɪdʒ]: An acupuncture method whereby the patient breathes in or out on insertion or extraction of the acupuncture needle to produce a supplementing or a draining needle stimulus. Insertion on exhalation and extraction on inhalation supplement, whereas insertion on inhalation and extraction on exhalation drain.

1100. 迎随补泻 [迎隨補瀉] *yíng suí bǔ xiè*, **directional supplementation and drainage** [dəˈrɛkʃən̩l ˌsʌpləmɛnˈteʃən ənd ˈdrenɪdʒ]: An acupuncture technique whereby the needle is angled with or against the flow of qì in a channel to produce a supplementing or a draining needle stimulus. A needle pointing in the direction of the channel flow produces supplementation, whereas one pointing counter to the direction of the flow produces drainage.

1101. **疾徐补泻** [疾徐補瀉] *jí xú bǔ xiè*, **quick and slow supplementation and drainage** [kwɪk ənd slo ˌsʌpləmɛnˈteʃən ənd ˈdrenɪdʒ]: A method of achieving supplementation and drainage that involves varying the relative speed of insertion and extraction of the needle. A slow insertion followed by a quick extraction supplements, whereas a quick insertion followed by a slow extraction drains.

1102. **捻转补泻** [捻轉補瀉] *niǎn zhuǎn bǔ xiè*, **twirling supplementation and drainage** [ˈtwɝlɪŋˌsʌpləmɛnˈteʃən ənd ˈdrenɪdʒ]: A method of achieving supplementation or drainage by rotating the needle between the thumb and index finger. Forward movement of the thumb and backward movement of the index finger making the needle rotate clockwise produces supplementing stimulus. Forward movement of the index finger and backward movement of the thumb making the needle rotate counterclockwise produces a draining needle stimulus.

1103. **提插补泻** [提插補瀉] *tí chā bǔ xiè*, **lift-and-thrust supplementation and drainage** [lɪft ənd θrʌst ˌsʌpləmɛnˈteʃən ənd ˈdrenɪdʒ]: A method of achieving supplementation and drainage that involves varying the emphasis on lifting the needle (retracting without extracting) and re-thrusting the needle after insertion. Emphasis on thrusting supplements, whereas emphasis on lifting drains. In other words, vigorous thrusts followed by gentle lifts have a supplementing effect, whereas vigorous lifts followed by gentle thrusts have a draining effect.

1104. **开阖补泻** [開闔補瀉] *kāi hé bǔ xiè*, **open and closed supplementation and drainage** [ˈopən ənd klozd ˌsʌpləmɛnˈteʃən ənd ˈdrenɪdʒ]: A method of achieving supplementation and drainage that involves pressing or not pressing the finger (or an alcohol-soaked swab) on the point after needle extraction. Supplementation is achieved by lightly pressing and rubbing the point after needle extraction to close the hole and prevent channel qì from discharging. Draining is achieved by waggling the needle on extraction and not pressing the insertion site; this opens the hole and allows channel qì to discharge. Alternatively, slow needle extraction after which the point is quickly pressed with the finger supplements, whereas swift needle extraction with slow pressing of the point drains.

1105. **透天凉** [透天涼] *tòu tiān liáng*, **heaven-penetrating cooling method** [ˈhɛvn̩–ˌpɛnəˌtretɪŋ ˈkulɪŋ–mɛθəd]: A draining needle manipulation method that combines the lift-and-thrust, quick and slow, and open and closed techniques. The heaven-penetrating cooling method is used to treat heat pathoconditions such as heat impediment, welling-abscess swelling, and steaming bone. Method: (1) Determine the depth to which the needle will be inserted, and divide this depth into heaven, human, and earth levels. (2) Ask the patient to inhale deeply and slowly. (Steps 2 through 6 are performed during inhalation.) (3) Thrust slowly and lift quickly at the earth level six times. Insert the needle to the earth level six times. (4) Bring the needle up to the human level. Thrust slowly and lift quickly at the human level six times. (5) Bring the needle up to the heaven level. Thrust the needle slowly and lift the needle quickly at this level six times. (6) Repeat steps 3 through 5. (7) Ask the patient to exhale, and withdraw the needle quickly, leaving the point uncovered.

1106. 烧山火 [燒山火] *shāo shān huǒ,* **burning mountain fire method** ['bɜˑnɪŋ 'maʊntɪn faɪr 'mɛθəd]: A complex needle manipulation technique that combines a number of simple supplementing techniques such as lifting and thrusting and open and closed needle extraction to treat vacuity cold diseases such as the three yīn stages of cold damage disease, impotence, incontinence, yīn protrusion, and swelling and sagging of one testicle. Method: (1) Determine the depth to which the needle will be inserted. Divide this depth into three equal segments. Proceeding from the surface of the skin, these depths are labeled the level of heaven, the level of human, and the level of earth, respectively. (2) Ask the patient to inhale deeply. Steps 3 and 4 are performed during exhalation. Upon exhalation, thrust the needle quickly and lift slowly nine times to the level of heaven. (3) Thrust the needle quickly and lift slowly nine times in the level of human. (4) Thrust the needle quickly and lift slowly nine times in the level of earth. (5) Ask the patient to exhale, and slowly withdraw the needle. If the procedure is to be repeated, withdraw the needle to the level of heaven and repeat steps 2, 3, and 4; if not, withdraw the needle fully from the skin. (6) Press the site gently with a cotton swab after the needle has been withdrawn.

1107. 回阳九针 [回陽九針] *huí yáng jiǔ zhēn,* **nine needles for returning yáng** [nɑɪn 'nidḷz fər rɪ'tɜˑnɪŋ jæŋ/jɑŋ]: Nine points used in the treatment of yáng collapse. See the list below.

哑门 *yǎ mén,* GV-15 Mute's Gate
大陵 *dà líng,* PC-7 Great Mound
三阴交 *sān yīn jiāo,* SP-6 Three Yīn Intersection
涌泉 *yǒng quán,* KI-1 Gushing Spring
太溪 *tài xī,* KI-3 Great Ravine
中脘 *zhōng wǎn,* CV-12 Center Stomach Duct
环跳 *huán tiào,* GB-30 Jumping Round

足三里 *zú sān lǐ,* ST-36 Leg Three Li
合谷 *hé gǔ,* LI-4 Union Valley

1108. 火针 [火針] *huǒ zhēn,* **fire needling** ['faɪr–nidlɪŋ]: A method of acupuncture involving the swift pricking of the skin with a red hot needle. Fire needling is used in the treatment of welling-abscess, scrofula, stubborn lichen, and impediment.

9.3. 针刺意外
Acupuncture Accidents

1109. 晕针 [暈針] *yùn zhēn,* **needle sickness** ['nidl̩-ˌsɪknɪs]: Sickness induced by acupuncture treatment and characterized by dizziness, vomiting, oppression in the chest, somber white complexion, fixed eyes and torpid spirit, and, in severe cases, cold sweating and reversal cold in the limbs. Needle sickness is usually the result of excessively strong needle manipulation in persons who are unused to acupuncture treatment or who are nervous, tired, hungry, or in a weak state of health.

1110. 滞针 [滯針] *zhì zhēn,* **stuck needle** [stʌk 'nidl̩]: A needle inserted in the body that resists turning, lifting, thrusting, or performance of any other needle manipulation. Stuck needle occurs in spasm due to nervousness or to rotation in too wide an arc that causes tissue to catch on the needle.

1111. 折针 [折針] *zhé zhēn,* **needle breakage** ['nidl̩–ˌbrekɪdʒ]: Breaking of an acupuncture needle below the skin; usually occurs with eroded, chipped, or otherwise damaged needles in patients who move unduly after needle insertion.

9.4. 灸法
Moxibustion

1112. 艾灸 [艾灸] *ài jiǔ,* **moxibustion** ['mɑksəˌbʌstʃən]: A method of applying a heat stimulus to the body by burning the dried and sifted leaf particles from the herb mugwort (*ài yè*) on or close to the skin, with the aim of freeing qì and blood, coursing qì, dispersing cold, eliminating dampness, and warming yáng. Moxibustion is divided into two distinct methods: indirect moxibustion and direct moxibustion. Caution: (1) Moxibustion should not be performed on persons who are hungry, have just overeaten, or are intoxicated. (2) Most points for which moxibustion is contraindicated are near large blood vessels, on the face, on prominent skin creases, and at or near mucus membranes or sensory organs. Direct moxibustion is especially contraindicated at these sites. (3) Pregnant women should not receive moxibustion on their abdomen or lumbus. (4) If small blisters form as a result of moxibustion, they should be protected and allowed to heal without treatment. Large blisters, however, should be punctured and drained, and in case of infection appropriate dressing should be applied.

1113. 艾条灸 [艾條灸] *ài tiáo jiǔ,* **poling** [ˈpolɪŋ]: Warming the surface of the body with a moxa pole.

1114. 温针 [溫針] *wēn zhēn,* **warm needling** [ˈwɔrm–nidlɪŋ]: Burning moxa on the handle of an acupuncture needle that is inserted in the body. This method, whereby the needle conducts the heat into the flesh, is appropriate for vacuity cold diseases and wind-damp impediment patterns. Method: Warm needling is performed by first inserting the needle and placing a small piece of paper or aluminum foil around the needle. (Make a hole in the center of the piece of paper.) Moxa floss is then wrapped around the wire handle and lit. The paper will catch any ashes. The moxa is allowed to burn completely, and when no more heat radiates from the handle, the paper and moxa can be removed, and the needle withdrawn. One common practice is to snip a small cylindrical piece of moxa pole and press a pointed object such as a pencil into the center of the cylinder, thus forming a hole that allows the moxa to be placed on the handle of the needle. This latter method is safer and more convenient because the ash is firmer and less likely to fall from the handle.

1115. 直接灸 [直接灸] *zhí jiē jiǔ,* **direct moxibustion** [ˈdaɪrɛkt ˈmɑksə‚bʌstʃən]: The burning of hand-rolled moxa cones directly on the skin at selected points. This method includes scarring moxibustion and nonscarring moxibustion.

1116. 瘢痕灸 [瘢痕灸] *bān hén jiǔ,* **scarring moxibustion** [ˈskɑrɪŋˈmɑksə‚bʌstʃən]: The method of treatment whereby moxa is burned on the body and leaves a scar. Scarring moxibustion employs a small cone of moxa floss usually less than 1 cm in diameter that is placed directly on the skin and completely burned. The area is then wiped clean with a cloth and the process is repeated until the prescribed number of cones has been burned. When this has been done, the area should be carefully cleaned and dressed. Within three days, the patient will develop a blister that will eventually leave a small scar. The blister generally takes about a month to heal. During this time, the patient must keep the area clean and frequently change the dressing to prevent infection. The scarring method is the most drastic form of moxibustion. The formation of a blister was traditionally considered important in the healing process and thus it is said that if moxibustion does not form a blister, the disease will not be cured. This method is currently used in China to treat severe vacuity cold or cold-damp diseases. When performing scarring moxibustion, note the following: (1) Partially burning a cone or two not quite down to the skin is a way to gradually inure the patient to the burning pain. These pre-burned cones, however, should not be counted toward the prescribed number. (2) When the moxa is burning, the practitioner should scratch or tap the area around the point to reduce the burning pain. (3) The number of recommended cones should be adjusted to the patient's condition. Strong and young patients can withstand more burnings and larger cones than weak and elderly patients. (4) The patient should be given a full explanation about the procedure and be forewarned of the formation of a scar. (5) Garlic juice or some other liquid is usually placed on the point being treated in order to secure the moxa cone.

1117. 无瘢痕灸 [無瘢痕灸] *wú bān hén jiǔ*, **nonscarring moxibustion** ['nɔn–'skɑrɪŋ'mɑksə,bʌstʃən]: A method of direct moxibustion whereby the moxa cone is removed before it burns the skin. Cones are burned until the skin at the point turns red. Take care to avoid accidental scarring when using this technique. Nonscarring moxibustion is less drastic than scarring moxibustion and is used for mild vacuity cold patterns. Some sources state that extinguishing the cone by pressing it to the skin supplements and that removing it before extinguishing it drains.

1118. 艾炷灸 [艾炷灸] *ài zhù jiǔ*, **cone moxibustion** [kon 'mɑksə,bʌstʃən]: Moxibustion using moxa cones.

1119. 壮数 [壯數] *zhuàng shù*, **number of cones** ['nʌmbɚ əv konz]: The number of cones burned on a single site.

1120. 间接灸 [間接灸] *jiān jiē jiǔ*, **indirect moxibustion** [ɪndɑɪrɛkt 'mɑksə,bʌstʃən]: Moxibustion performed on an insulating material such as crushed garlic or a slice of ginger that spreads the heat and reduces its intensity, as well as protecting skin from burning.

1121. 隔附子灸 [隔附子灸] *gé fù zǐ jiǔ*, **moxibustion on aconite** ['mɑksə,bʌstʃən ɔn 'ækənɑɪt]: The application of moxibustion using cakes of aconite (*fù zǐ*) as an insulating medium. The cakes are made by grinding the aconite to a powder, mixing it with yellow wine (rice or millet wine), and forming it into a dry, crustlike substance about 2 mm thick. The cake crust is perforated and placed on the point, and moxa is burnt on top of it. Because aconite is acrid and hot, this method can treat yáng vacuity diseases. It is most commonly administered on enduring sores (and boils) to stop suppuration and permit healing.

1122. **隔姜灸** [隔薑灸] *gé jiāng jiǔ,* **moxibustion on ginger** [ˈmɑksə,-bʌstʃən ɔn ˈdʒɪndʒɚ]: Burning of moxa cones on ginger as an insulating medium. A slice of ginger about 4 mm thick (slightly thicker than a quarter dollar) is perforated with a sewing needle and placed on the point. Large cones of moxa are burnt on the slice (which is lifted from the skin momentarily when the heat exceeds the patient's tolerance) until the skin at the point is moist and red. This method is ideal for center burner vacuity, abdominal fullness, stomach pain, mounting pain, diarrhea, vomiting, wind-cold impediment pain, wind-cold exterior patterns, and yáng vacuity diseases in general.

1123. **隔蒜灸** [隔蒜灸] *gé suàn jiǔ,* **moxibustion on garlic** [ˈmɑksə,-bʌstʃən ɔn ˈgɑrlɪk]: The application of moxibustion on a thick slice of garlic as an insulating medium. Method: A slice of garlic about 4 mm thick that has been perforated with several holes is placed on the site. The moxa is placed on the garlic and ignited with incense, the garlic being changed after four to five cones have been burnt. In general, five to seven burnings constitute one treatment. This method is used to treat vacuity taxation (tuberculosis), toxicity from sores, scrofula, and abdominal accumulation masses. The patient should be informed that this method sometimes causes blisters.

1124. **隔盐灸** [隔鹽灸] *gé yán jiǔ,* **moxibustion on salt** [ˈmɑksə,bʌstʃən ɔn sɔlt]: Burning of moxa cones on salt as an insulating medium. Moxibustion on salt is usually performed on the umbilicus. The umbilicus is filled with table salt, and a large cone of moxa is burned on top of the salt. This method is effective for treatment of cold damage yīn patterns, cholera, and wind stroke desertion patterns. It can return yáng, stem counterflow, and stem desertion.

9.5. 拔火罐
Cupping

1125. **拔火罐** [拔火罐] *bá huǒ guàn,* **fire cupping** [ˈfɑɪr–ˌkʌpɪŋ]: A method of treatment involving the application of suction to skin to draw out blood and sometimes pus. Cupping is also called "fire cupping" because the suction is produced when, for example, a lighted alcohol swab placed inside the cup burns the oxygen to create a vacuum after the cup has been placed on the skin. Fire cups used to be made of animal horn, bamboo, or earthenware, but globe-shaped glass ones are now preferred because they enable the practitioner to see the flame and so prevent it from burning the patient. The recent development of cups with suction pumps (suction cups) makes cupping safer and more convenient than before. Cupping is used to treat wind-damp impediment pain, colds, phlegm-rheum, cough and panting; for stomach pain, abdominal pain, back and lumbar pain, leg qì pain; and for initial-stage welling-abscesses and flat-abscesses. Individual forms of cupping include stationary cupping, push-cupping, flash-cupping, and pricking and cupping. Contraindications: Cupping should not be applied where there is generalized heat [effusion] with headache, clouded vision and heavy head, convulsions, arched-back rigidity, or clenched jaw. It should not be used on parts of the body affected by skin disease or areas where the flesh is thin or bones show through, or on major blood vessels. It should not be applied to the abdomen in pregnancy or to areas affected by water swelling.

1126. **坐罐法** [坐罐法] *zuò guàn fǎ,* **stationary cupping** [ˈsteʃənɛrɪ ˈkʌpɪŋ]: A method of cupping whereby the cups are left in place for about ten minutes after they have been applied.

1127. **推罐** [推罐] *tuī guàn,* **push-cupping** [ˈpuʃ–ˌkʌpɪŋ]: A method of cupping whereby the cup is pushed back and forth over a wide area that has been lubricated with sesame oil, and now often petroleum jelly (Vaseline). This method is applied to large flat fleshy areas such as the back, lumbus, or thighs. It is used for impediment or other patterns of pain or numbness. Method: First, smear the area to be cupped with petroleum jelly or other lubricant, and then apply the cup in the same manner as for regular stationary cupping. Once the cup is firmly attached, hold it firmly in two hands and move it around over the affected area. Remove the cup once the skin is evenly reddened to the desired degree.

1128. 闪罐 [閃罐] *shǎn guàn,* **flash cupping** [ˈflæʃ-ˌkʌpɪŋ]: A method of cupping whereby the cup is swiftly removed after application and repeatedly reapplied until the required degree of reddening or static blood appears. This method is used for local pain or numbness or for impaired functions.

1129. 刺络拔罐 [刺絡拔罐] *cì luò bá guàn,* **pricking and cupping** [ˈprɪkɪŋ ənd ˈkʌpɪŋ]: A method of cupping whereby a cup is applied to an area of skin that has been pricked with a cutaneous needle (e.g., a plum blossom needle). This method, which can draw large amounts of blood if the area has been heavily pricked, is used for cinnabar toxin, sprain, or mammary welling-abscess.

习题
Questions

Answer the following questions in English:

852. What is the name of the cupping method whereby the cups are swiftly moved after being applied? ....

853. What do we call a hand-rolled conical lump of moxa? ....

854. What is the name of the technique of burning moxa that is mounted on the handle of an acupuncture needle? ....

855. What are the two kinds of direct moxibustion? ....

856. What is the needle traditionally used for bloodletting? ....

857. What do we call the method of cupping whereby the cups are left in place after they have been applied? ....

858. What do we call the application of a red-hot needle to the skin? ....

859. Which is the most commonly used needle in acupuncture today? ....

860. What needle is 2–3 mm long and continuous with and perpendicular to a circle of wire that forms the head? ....

861. What do we call the method of cupping whereby a cup is applied to an area of skin that has been pricked with a cutaneous needle?

Give the Pīnyīn and English for the following Chinese terms:

862. 无瘢痕灸 ....

863. 留针 ....

864. 间接灸 ....

865. 艾条灸 ....

866. 烧山火 ....

867. 开阖补泻 ....

868. 得气 ....

869. 捣针 ....

870. 退针 ....

871. 隔蒜灸 ....

872. 直接灸 ....

Supply the Chinese and English for the following:

873. *Jìn zhēn.* ....

874. *Yíng suí bǔ xiè.* ....

875. *Tòu tiān liáng.* ....

876. *Niǎn zhuǎn bǔ xiè.* ....

877. *Zhēn cì.* ....

878. *Chū zhēn.* ....

879. *Kāi hé bǔ xiè.* ....

880. *Huí yáng jiǔ zhēn.* ....

881. *Dé qì.* ....

882. *Aì róng.* ....

Give the Chinese and Pīnyīn for the following:

883. Respiratory supplmentation and drainage. ....

884. Moxibustion. ....

885. Warm needling. ....

886. Lift-and-thrust supplementation and drainage. ....

附录一：汉语拼音与发音
Appendix I: Pīnyīn and Pronunciation

China has many different dialects, but Mandarin Chinese, or 普通话 Pǔtōnghuà ("common language") as it is now called in the People's Republic of China, is the lingua franca of the Chinese world. It is the dialect most commonly learned by Westerners, and the one most useful for students of Chinese medicine to learn.

Pīnyīn is the system now most commonly used to represent the sound of Mandarin words in the Roman alphabet. This system has largely replaced Wade-Giles and other systems of transcription.

Chinese is often loosely described as being a "monosyllabic language." This means that the smallest unit of meaning is represented in sound by a single syllable (and in writing by a single Chinese character). Chinese syllables are vowel sounds (e.g., *a, ou, e*), which may or may not be preceded by a consonant (e.g., *da, dou, de*) and/or followed by consonants (e.g., *ang, dang, eng, deng*).

Chinese is a tonal language. This means that each syllable, in addition to having a sound, which in Pīnyīn is represented in letters of the alphabet, also has a tone. Mandarin has four basic tones, which are represented by accents placed over the letters. In this appendix, discussion of the tones is contained in a special section after that dealing with sounds.

Sounds

Accurate pronunciation in any language can only be learned from native speakers of that language. When learning Chinese, you should seek out a good native speaker of Mandarin. The best Mandarin is spoken in Běijīng, and someone from Běijīng will provide you with the best model for pronunciation. If no courses in Mandarin are being offered in your locality, and you cannot find a good Mandarin speaker to help you with your pronunciation, you can purchase teach-yourself Chinese texbooks with tapes or CDs that teach the pronunciation. These are usually available in the larger bookstores and can be easily ordered anywhere.

Most of the sounds of Mandarin are quite easy for English speakers to reproduce. Only a few are difficult. Never be afraid to ask Chinese people to help you how to pronounce words. They always give oodles of encouragement to anyone learning their language, and always tell you how good your pronunciation is!

In what follows, the sounds of Mandarin are explained in rough English equivalents. Sounds in other European languages are given where they are closer to the Chinese sounds. In some cases, phonetic symbols have been added in brackets, e.g., [æ], [ɑ], to clarify the value of certain sounds.

b : Like the English *b*, but unaspirated, so that it actually sounds more like the *p* in *spay*. The Chinese 八 *bā*, meaning 'eight', resembles the *ba* in "Ba, ba, black sheep"; 痹 *bì*, 'impediment', sounds like the English *bee*.

p : Like the English *p*, but well aspirated such as when uttering the word *pig* as an invective (as in "You pig!"). The Chinese 脾 *pí*, 'spleen', resembles the *p* in *pea*. Note that in English *b* and *p* are distinguished in normal speech by the presence and absence of voicing, while in Chinese they are distinguished by the absence and presence of aspiration. A similar difference exists between *d* and *t* and between *g* and *k*.[2]

m : As the English *m*. The Chinese 母 *mǔ*, 'mother', is pronounced like *moo*, the sound made by a cow.

f : Exactly as the English *f*. Thus 非 *fēi*, 'not', sounds like the name *Fay*.

d : Roughly as the *d* of the English *dog*, but unaspirated, so that it actually sounds more like the *t* in *stow*. The Chinese 斗 *dǒu*, 'to shake', is pronounced like the English *doe* (a female deer).

t : Roughly as the *t* of the English *ten*, but more strongly aspirated. (It is never pronounced as the *t* in the American English *better*.) Thus the Chinese 头 *tóu*, 'head', resembles the *t* in *tow*; 土 *tǔ*, 'earth' or 'soil', resembles the English *two*; 体 *tǐ*, 'body', resembles the English *tea*.

l : Initial *l*-, as in 累 *lèi*, 'tired', which sounds like the English *lay*.

n : As the English *n*. The Chinese 内 *nèi*, 'inside', is pronounced like the archaic English *nay*; 脑 *nǎo*, 'brain', sounds like the English *now*; 逆 *nì*, 'counterflow', sounds like the English *knee*.

g : As the English *g* in *get* (not as the *g* of *genial*). Thus the Chinese 根 *gēn*, 'root', resembles the English *gun*. The Chinese *g* sound is unaspirated and sounds more like the *k* in *skin*.

---

[2] Wade-Giles transcription represented the unaspirated sounds as *p*, *t*, *k* and the aspirated sounds as *p'*, *t'*, *k'*. This difference in transcription system explains why *Dao* and *Daoism* used to be written as *Tao* and *Taoism*, and why *dāng guī* was borrowed into English in the form *tangkuei*.

k : As the English *k*, though more strongly aspirated. The Chinese 哭 *kū*, 'to weep', sounds similar to the English in *coo*; 开 *kāi* sounds like the *ki* of *kite*.

h : Approximately as the English *h*, so that 黑 *hēi*, 'black', resembles *hay*. A characteristic of good Mandarin, however, is a tendency toward a slight rasping sound like the *ch* in the Scottish pronunciation of *loch*, the German *Bach*, or the Spanish *jamón*.

j : Approximately as the *j* in *judge* or the *g* in *gemini*. Thus 悸 *jì*, 'palpitations', is pronounced like *gee*. If one listens carefully to native Mandarin speakers, one finds that the sound is not voiced like the English sound. The *j* in Pīnyin is always followed by an *i* or *u* pronounced as [ü]. Examples include: 降 *jiàng*, 'downbear', 结 *jié*, 'bind', 疖 *jié*, 'boil', 紧 *jǐn*, 'tight', 灸 *jiǔ*, 'moxibustion', 疽 *jū*, 'flat-abscess', 卷 *juǎn*, 'curled', and 君 *jūn*, 'sovereign'.

q : As the *ch* in *cheese*. The Chinese 气 *qì*, 'qì', 'air', is pronounced like the *chee* in *cheek*. Like *j*, *q* is followed by *i* or *u* pronounced as [ü]. Examples include 掐 *qiā*, 'fingernail pressing', 欠 *qiàn*, 'lack', 秋 *qiū*, 'autumn', 清 *qīng*, 'clear', 曲 *qū*, 'fermented leaven', 去 *qù*, 'remove', and 全 *quán*, 'complete'.

x : Similar to the English *sh*, so that 细 *xì*, 'thin, fine', resembles the English *she*. However, if you listen to Chinese speakers, you will discover that the sound is wispier than the English *sh*, so that *xì* sounds nearly as much like the English *see* as the English *she*. The *x* in Pīnyīn is always followed by an *i* or a *u* pronounced as [ü]. Examples: 下 *xià*, 'down', 泄 *xiè*, 'discharge', 涎 *xián*, 'drool', 胸 *xiōng*, 'chest', 羞 *xiū*, 'be shy of', 'aversion to', 心 *xīn*, 'heart', 虚 *xū*, 'vacuity', 循 *xún*, 'feel (one's way)', and 宣 *xuān*, 'diffuse'.

zh : As the *j* in the English *jowl*, but curling the tongue backward to make an *r* sound. Unlike the English *j* sound, the Chinese *zh* is not voiced. One example is 针 *zhēn*, 'needle', pronounced something like the last syllable of the English *dungeon*.

ch : As the *ch* in cheese, but curling the tongue backward to make an *r* sound. Unlike the English *ch* sound, the Chinese *ch* is not voiced. This sound occurs in 尺 *chǐ*, 'cubit', 肠 *cháng*, 'intestine', 潮 *cháo*, 'tidal', 冲 *chōng*, 'thoroughfare', and 喘 *chuǎn*, 'panting'.

sh : Produced like the *sh* in ship, but curling the tongue backward to make an *r* sound. This sound occurs in 疝 *shàn*, 'mounting', 伤 *shāng*, 'damage', 少 *shào*, 'lesser', 肾 *shèn*, 'kidney', 湿 *shī*, 'dampness', 手 *shǒu*, 'hand', and 水 *shuǐ*, 'water'.

r : As the *r* in *road*, but in some circumstances tending toward the sound of *g* in *beige*. The Chinese 肉 *ròu*, 'flesh', sounds like the English *roe*; 乳 *rǔ*, 'breast', sounds like the English *rue*. Other examples include 软 *ruǎn*, 'soft', 弱 *ruò*, 'weak', and 人 *rén*, 'human'.

z : As the *ds* in *heads*. The Chinese 杂 *zá*, 'miscellaneous', sounds like the *za* in *mozzarella* when pronounced by an Italian. This sound also occurs in 足 *zú*, 'foot', and 滋 *zī*, 'enrich'.

c : As the *ts* in *Whitsun*. This is also like the German *z*, as in *Zeitgeist*. This sound occurs in 刺 *cì*, 'to needle'.

s : As the *s* in *see*, never as the *s* in *easy*. Occurs in 三 *sān*, 'three', 四 *sì*, 'four', and 色 *sè*, 'color'.

-i, y : The final *-i* is pronounced in three different ways. 1) After *z-*, *c-*, and *s-*, it is a weakly buzzing, syllabic *z*. Examples include 子 *zǐ*, 'child,' 'son', 刺 *cì*, 'to needle', and 思 *sī*, 'thought'. 2) After *zh-*, *ch-*, and *sh-*, and *r-*, it is a syllabic American *r*. Examples include 肢 *zhī*, 'limb', 迟 *chí*, 'slow', 食 *shí*, 'food', and 日 *rì*, 'sun'. 3) After other consonants, it sounds like the *ee* in the English *see*. Thus as in 淋 *lín*, 'strangury', it sounds like the English *lean*, though shorter. Other examples include 病 *bìng*, 'disease', 津 *jīn*, 'liquid', 情 *qíng*, 'affect'. The sound *yi*, which occurs in the initial position only, is pronounced as the archaic English pronoun *ye*. Before *ao*, *an*, *ang*, *u*, and *e* it is pronounced as the English *y*, e.g., 表 *biǎo*, 'exterior', 跷 *qiāo*, 'springing (vessel)', 钱 *qián*, 'money', 'qián (weight)', 点 *diǎn*, 'speckle', 绛 *jiàng*, 'crimson', 久 *jiǔ*, 'for a long time or 'enduring', 跌 *dié*, 'fall', and 液 *yè*, 'humor'.

-u, w : The final *u* is pronounced as the *oo* in *food* or as the *o* in *do*. More precisely it is like the *u* in the German *nu* or Spanish *su* since the rounding of the lips is kept the same throughout the syllable. Examples include 母 *mǔ*, 'mother', 毒 *dú*, 'poison', 补 *bǔ*, 'supplement', 浮 *fú*, 'floating', 腑 *fǔ*, 'bowel', 腹 *fù*, 'abdomen', 颅 *lù*, 'skull', 骨 *gǔ*, 'bone', 谷 *gǔ*, 'grain', 固 *gù*, 'secure', 主 *zhǔ*, 'govern', 搐 *chù*, 'convulsions', 暑 *shǔ*, 'summerheat', and 促 *cù*, 'skipping'. When *-u* is not the last sound in the syllable, it is pronounced as the English *w*, e.g., 酸 *suān*, 'sour', 窜 *cuàn*, 'scurry', 乱 *luàn*, 'chaotic', 短 *duǎn*, 'short,' 光 *guáng*, 'light', 滑 *huá*, 'slippery', 化 *huà*, 'transform', and 黄 *huáng*, 'yellow'. When this sound occurs as an initial, it is written as *w*, e.g., 五 *wǔ*, 'five', 脘 *wǎn*, 'stomach duct'. Finally, the combination *ui* is pronounced as the English *way* (not as the English *we*).[3] Examples include 回 *huí*, 'return', 归 *guī*, 'return', 水 *shuǐ*, 'water', and 睡 *shuì*, 'sleep'.

-ü, -u, yu : Final *-ü*, as *qù*, 'to go', or *lǜ*, 'green', pronounced like a French *u* or a German *ü*, that is often represented as [ü] in phonetic scripts. No equivalent of this sound exists in English except in the Scottish pronunciation of the vowel sound appearing in *choose* or *lute*. This sound is spelled as *ü* (with an umlaut on the *u*) after *l* or *n*, e.g., 女 *nǚ*, 'female', or 绿 *lǜ*, 'green', to distinguish the sound from the *u* representing the English *oo* [u]. The umlaut is not used when the sound of the initial is *j*, *q*, *x* or *y*; in this position it is always pronounced as [ü], never as [u]. Examples include: 菊 *jú*, 'chrysanthemum', 曲 *qū*, 'fermented leaven', 倦 *juàn*, 'fatigued', 蜷 *quán*, 'curled-up', 血 *xuè*, 'blood', 元 *yuán*, 'origin', 晕 *yūn*, 'dizziness', and 运 *yùn*, 'move'.

a : As the *a* in French, Spanish, or Italian (or in the Northern English pronunciation of *grass*). It is often represented in phonetic notation as [ɑ]. It is like the *a* in *father*, but shorter and more open. It is not pronounced like the *a* in *bad*. Examples include 八 *bā*, 'eight', 发 *fā*, 'effuse', 法 *fǎ*, 'method', and 大 *dà*, 'great'.

-o, -uo, wo : The final *-o* sounds like *awe* in the British rather than the American pronunciation. This sound can directly follow *b*, *p*, *m*, and *f*, e.g., 剥 *bō*, 'peeling' (tongue fur), 薄 *bó*, 'thin', 破 *pò*, 'break', 磨 *mó*, 'grind', and 佛 *fó*, 'Buddha'. After all other initials (*d*, *t*, *n*, *l*, *h*, *zh*, *ch*, *sh*, *r*, *z*, *c*, and *s*) *o* does not occur alone, but is preceded by *u* and sounds like the *wa* of *war* in the British pronunciation. Examples include 多 *duō*, 'much,' 脱 *tuō*, 'shed', 'dessertion,' 络 *luò*, 'network vessel', 火 *huǒ*, 'fire', 浊 *zhuó*, 'turbid', 说 *shuō*, 'a dictum', 弱 *ruò*, 'weak', 左 *zuǒ*, 'left', 错

---

[3] The convention of using *ui* to represent a sound similar to the English *way* is apparently explicable in terms of economy of letters. Older transcriptions represented the sound, somewhat more clearly, as *uei*, as in English loanward *tangkuei*.

cuò, 'cross', and 所 *suǒ*, 'place'. The same sound occurring in the initial position is written as *wo*, as in 我 *wǒ*, 'I', 'me'.

e : The Pīnyīn *e* is used to represent two distinct sounds. Final -*e*, after *i* or *u*, like the *e* in *bed* [ε]. In all other positions, it is like vowel in *bird* without any *r* sound, or like *œ* in the French *hors d'œuvre*, a sound which is often represented in phonetic notation as [œ]. Examples: 阿 *ē* of 阿胶 *ē jiāo*, 'ass-hide glue', 蛾 *é*, 'moth', 恶 *è*, 'malign', 得 *dé*, 'obtain', 膈 *gé*, 'diaphragm', 和 *hé*, 'harmonize', 克 *kè*, 'restrain'.

ai : As the English *eye* (actually more closely to the German *ei* of *Heim*). It occurs in 艾 *ài*, 'moxa', 'mugwort', 脉 *mài*, 'vessel' 'pulse', 苔 *tāi*, 'tongue fur', and 开 *kāi*, 'open'.

ei : As the *ei* in the English *feint*. The Chinese 胃 *wèi*, 'stomach', is pronounced as the English *weigh* or *way*, while 累 *lèi*, 'tired', sounds like the English *lay*. Other examples include 黑 *hēi*, 'black', 肥 *féi*, 'obese', and 肺 *fèi*, 'lung'.

ao : As the *ow* of *how*. Thus, 脑 *nǎo*, 'brain', is pronounced more or less like the English *now*. In actual fact, the sound is closer to the *au* of the German *Haus* or the Spanish *jaula*. Another examples is 膏 *gāo*, 'unctuous' (as in 膏淋 *gāo lín*, 'unctuous strangury').

ou : As the English *oh!*, especially in the American pronunciation rather than the standard British pronunciation. This sound can occur in the initial position, as in 呕 *ǒu*, 'retching', which sounds like *oh!* It more often occurs as a final, as in 抽 *chōu* 'tug', 稠 *chóu*, 'thick', 'viscous', 腠 *còu*, 'interstice', 漏 *lòu* 'to leak', 'spotting', 痘 *dòu*, 'pox', 喉 *hóu*, 'larynx', 厚 *hòu* 'thick', 后 *hòu*, 'after', and 垢 *gòu*, 'grimy'.

an : As the *an* in the Spanish for bread, *pan*. The *n* sound tend to be rather nasal and indistinct. It occurs in 安 *ān*, 'to quiet' 寒 *hán*, 'cold', 烦 *fán*, 'vexation', 反 *fǎn*, 're(flux)' (as in 反 胃 *fǎn wèi*, 'stomach reflux'), 肝 *gān*, 'liver', 甘 *gān*, 'sweet' 满 *mǎn*, 'fullness', and 缓 *huǎn*, 'moderate'. After *yi* or *i*, it is pronounced, depending on the speaker, either like the English pronunciation of *Anne* (with [æ] as the vowel sound) or as *en* in the English *yen*. Examples include 前 *qián*, 'before', 先 *xiān* 'advanced', 'earlier', 弦 *xián*, 'stringlike', 宣 *xuān*, 'diffuse' and 蜷 *quán*, 'curled-up'.

en : As the *un* of the English *undo*, with the mouth less widely opened. Thus 本 *běn*, 'root', resembles the English *bun* (never as the English name *Ben*). Similarly, 分 *fēn*, 'fēn' (a weight), is pronounced like the English *fun*. The *n* sound tends to be rather nasal and indistinct. This sound also occurs in 奔 *bēn*, 'running' (as in running piglet), and 身 *shēn*, 'body'.

ang : As the *ang* in *sang*, but with the *a* pronounced like the *a* in *father* (though not so long). This sound occurs in 脏 *zàng*, 'viscus', 胀 *zhàng*, 'distention', 胖 *pàng*, 'obese', 养 *yǎng*, 'nourish', and 肠 *cháng*, 'intestine'.

-eng : The final *-eng* is similar to the *ung* in the English *sung*. (Beware, it is not pronounced like the *eng* in the English *length*). Thus, 崩 *beng*, 'flooding' (metrorrhagia), is pronounced like the English *bung*, though with the mouth less widely opened. This sound also occurs in 蒸 *zhēng*, 'steam', 风 *fēng*, 'wind', 癥 *zhēng*, 'concretion', and 证 *zhèng*, 'pattern'.

er : The final *-er* is pronounced as the *er* in the American English *her*. Examples include 儿 *ér*, 'child', and 耳 *ěr*, 'ear'.

-r : The final *-r* is a characteristic of Běijīng speech which in most cases is considered optional in Mandarin. In Chinese characters, it is represented by the character 儿 *ér*, which is a noun suffix. In speech, however, it is not pronounced as a distinct syllable, but as a rhotacization of the syllable it follows. Examples include 小孩儿 *xiǎo háir*, 'child', 开方儿 *kāi fāngr*, 'write a prescription'. Noun forms ending in 儿 *-r* regularly heard in conversation, but seen in literature only in novels in which the author wishes highlight speech idiosyncrasy of a character. In Chinese medical literature, such forms rarely seen, and other forms are used instead (e.g., 小儿 *xiǎo ér*, 'child'; 开处方 *kāi chǔ fāng*, 'write a prescription').

Tones

The notion of tonality is by no means an alien concept in English. We pronounce words with different intonation to express slight nuances in meaning such as inquiry, doubt, affirmation, etc. English question sentences, for example, are often characterized by a rising intonation at the end (In "Is he coming?" the word *coming* is usually pronounced with a rising intonation.) Chinese tones differ in that each syllable has a fixed tone that is an integral part of the pronunciation rather than expressing nuances. Westerners usually find the tones are relatively easy to reproduce. The difficulty lies only in abandoning our native habit of varying intonation in running speech and in giving each word the correct tone.

1st Tone (第一声 *dì yī shēng***)** : A syllable in the first tone has a high level sound.

2nd Tone (第二声 *dì èr shēng***)** : A syllable in the second tone has a high rising tone. As in the English "Yes?" or "Oh?"

3rd Tone (第三声 *dì sān shēng***)** : A syllable in the third tone has a low dipping tone.

4th Tone (第四声 *dì sì shēng***)** : A syllable in the fourth tone falls from a high level to a low level. As in the English "No!"

These tones are fixed in all cases except the third tone, which changes to a second tone when it precedes a syllable in third tone. Thus, 解表 *jiě biǎo* is read as *jié biǎo* (even though it is not written like that).

In modern Mandarin, there is also what is called a neutral tone, which occurs in compounds that are largely confined to colloquial expression. The neutral tone, which is marked in Pīnyīn by the absence of any tone mark, in fact not one, but two distinct tones. After a syllable in first, second, and fourth tones, a neutral tone is a low falling tone, like the first half of a full third tone, e.g., 狮子 *shī zi*, 'lion'; 孩子 *hái zi*, 'child'; 杏子 *xìng zi*, 'apricot'. After a third tone, it is like a first tone but slightly lower, e.g., 饺子 *jiǎo zi*. The noun suffix 子 *zi* accounts for most occurrences of the neutral tone. But the final element in certain compounds is also conventionally pronounced (especially in Běijīng) in the neutral tone. Examples include 太太 *tài tai*, 'Mr.'; 先生 *xiān sheng*, 'Mr.'; 老鸹 *lǎo gua*, 'crow'; and 老顽固 *lǎo wán gu*, 'old stick-the-mud'.

Homophony

A feature of Chinese is that many of its monosyllabic words are homophonic, i.e., share the same sound. This feature stemmed from a reduction of the number of sounds in the ancient language and has resulted in two words often having to be used instead of one. (This is why, for example, 耳 *ěr* has been replaced by *ěr duo* in the modern spoken language.) Vast numbers of words are distinguished by tone alone, but many words have exactly the same sound and tone. The homophony of Chinese poses considerable difficulties to the foreign student learning language.

Examples of Chinese Medical Words Distinguished by Tone Alone

ban 斑 *bān*, 'macules'; 半 *bàn*, 'half'

bei 悲 *bēi*, 'sorrow'; 背 *bèi*, 'back'

ben 奔 *bēn*, 'running'; 本 *běn*, 'root'

bi 鼻 *bí*, 'nose'; 闭 *bì*, 'block', 'close'

biao 标 *biāo*, 'tip'; 表 *biǎo*, 'exterior'

bo 剥 *bō*, 'peeling'; 薄 *bó*, 'thin'

cang 苍 *cāng*, 'somber-white'; 藏 *cáng*, 'store'

chi 迟 *chí*, 'slow'; 齿 *chǐ*, 'tooth'; 赤 *chì*, 'red'

chou 抽 *chōu*, 'tugging'; 稠 *chóu*, 'thick'

dai 呆 *dai*, 'torpor'; 带 *dài*, 'girdle'

dan 丹 *dān*, 'cinnabar'; 胆 *dǎn*, 'gallbladder'; 淡 *dàn*, 'pale'

dao 导 *dǎo*, 'abduct'; 道 *dào*, 'way'

dian 癫 *diān*, 'epilepsy'; 点 *diǎn*, 'speckle'

e 蛾 *é*, 'moth'; 恶 *ě*, 'nausea'; 恶 *è*, 'malign'; 呃 *è*, 'hiccup'

er 儿 *ér*, 'child'; 耳 *ěr*, 'ear'; 二 *èr*, 'two'

fa 发 *fā*, 'effuse'; 法 *fǎ*, 'method'

fan 烦 *fán*, 'vexation'; 反 *fǎn*, 'reflux'; 犯 *fàn*, 'invade'

fei 肥 *féi*, 'obese'; 肺 *fèi*, 'lung'

fu 浮 *fú*, 'floating'; 腑 *fǔ*, 'bowel'; 腹 *fù*, 'abdomen'

gan 肝 *gān*, 'liver'; 感 *gǎn*, 'contract'

gu 骨 *gǔ*, 'bone'; 固 *gù*, 'secure'

han 寒 *hán*, 'cold'; 汗 *hàn*, 'sweat'

he 呵 *hē*, 'yawn'; 和 *hé*, 'harmonize'

hou 喉 *hóu*, 'larynx'; 厚 *hòu*, 'thick'

hua 滑 *huá*, 'slippery'; 化 *huà*, 'transform'

huang 黄 *huáng*, 'yellow'; 晄 *huǎng*, 'bright white'

huo 火 *huǒ*, 'fire'; 霍 *huò*, 'sudden'

ji 积 *jī*, 'accumulate'; 急 *jí*, 'urgent'; 悸 *jì*, 'palpitations'

jie 结 *jié*, 'bind'; 解 *jiě*, 'resolve'

ke 咳 *ké*, 'cough'; 渴 *kě*, 'thirst'

kou 芤 *kōu*, 'scallion'; 口 *kǒu*, 'mouth'

ku 哭 *kū*, 'weep'; 苦 *kǔ*, 'bitter'

li 里 *lǐ*, 'interior'; 利 *lì*, 'disinhibit'

liu 留 *liú*, 'settle'; 六 *liù*, 'six'

luo 瘰 *luǒ*, 'scrofula' 络 *luò*, 'network vessel'

mei 梅 *méi*, 'plum'; 寐 *mèi*, 'sleep'

men 门 *mén*, 'gate'; 闷 *mèn*, 'oppression'

mian 眠 *mián*, 'sleep'; 面 *miàn*, 'face'

pi 皮 *pí*, 'skin'; 痞 *pǐ*, 'glomus'

qi 七 *qī*, 'seven'; 脐 *qí*, 'umbilicus'; 气 *qì*, 'qi'

qian 前 *qián*, 'before'; 欠 *qiàn*, 'lack'

qiao 跷 *qiāo*, 'springing'; 窍 *qiào*, 'orifice'

qing 清 *qīng*, 'clear'; 情 *qíng*, 'affect'

ru 濡 *rú*, 'soggy'; 乳 *rǔ*, 'breast'

san 三 *sān*, 'three'; 散 *sàn*, 'dissipate'

shao 少 *shǎo*, 'scant'; 少 *shào*, 'lesser'

shen 身 *shēn*, 'body'; 神 *shén*, 'spirit'; 肾 *shèn*, 'kidney'

sheng 生 *shēng*, 'engender'; 胜 *shèng*, 'prevail'

shi 湿 *shī*, 'dampness'; 食 *shí*, 'food'; 使 *shǐ*, 'courier' 视 *shì*, 'look', 'stare'

shou 手 *shǒu*, 'hand'; 受 *shòu*, 'contract'

shui 水 *shuǐ*, 'water'; 睡 *shuì*, 'sleep'

tai 胎 *tāi*, 'fetus'; 太 *tài*, 'greater'

tang 汤 *tāng*, 'decoction'; 溏 *táng*, 'sloppy'

tong 统 *tǒng*, 'manage', 'control'; 痛 *tòng*, 'pain'

tou 头 *tóu*, 'head'; 透 *tòu*, 'outthrust'

tu 土 *tǔ*, 'earth', 'soil'; 吐 *tù*, 'vomit'

tuo 脱 *tuō*, 'shed', 'desert'; 唾 *tuò*, 'spittle'

wai 喎 *wāi*, 'deviated'; 外 *wào*, 'out'

wan 丸 *wán*, 'pill'; 脘 *wǎn*, 'stomach duct'; 腕 *wàn*, 'wrist'

wang 亡 *wáng*, 'collapse'; 妄 *wàng*, 'frenetic'

wei 微 *wēi*, 'slight'; 维 *wéi*, 'link'; 痿 *wěi*, 'wilting'; 卫 *wèi*, 'defense'

wu 五 *wǔ*, 'five'; 恶 *wù*, 'aversion to'; 侮 *wǔ*, 'rebel'

x 熄 *xī*, 'extinguish'; 喜 *xǐ*, 'joy'; 细 *xì*, 'fine'

xian 先 *xiān*, 'earlier'; 弦 *xián*, 'stringlike' (of pulse); 癣 *xiǎn*, 'lichen'; 陷 *xiàn*, 'fall'

xiang 相 *xiāng*, 'each other'; 相 *xiàng*, 'minister'

xiao 消 *xiāo*, 'disperse'; 小 *xiǎo*, 'small'

xie 邪 *xié*, 'evil'; 泄 *xiè*, 'discharge'

xin 心 *xīn*, 'heart'; 囟 *xìn*, 'fontanel'

xuan 宣 *xuān*, 'diffuse'; 眩 *xuàn*, 'dizziness'

xue 穴 *xué*, 'acupuncture point'; 血 *xuè*, 'blood'

yan 咽 *yān*, 'pharynx'; 言 *yán*, 'speak'; 眼 *yǎn*, 'eye'; 厌 *yàn*, 'aversion to'

yang 阳 *yáng*, 'yáng'; 养 *yǎng*, 'nourish'

ye 噎 *yē*, 'dysphagia'; 液 *yè*, 'humor'

yin 阴 *yīn*, 'yīn'; 淫 *yín*, 'excess'; 饮 *yǐn*, 'drink', 'rheum'

ying 营 *yíng*, 'construction'; 瘿 *yǐng*, 'goiter'

yu 瘀 *yū*, 'stasis'; 于 *yú*, 'at'; 语 *yǔ*, 'speech'; 郁 *yù*, 'depression'

yun 晕 *yūn*, 'dizziness'; 孕 *yùn*, 'pregnancy'

zao 糟 *zāo*, 'waste'; 早 *zǎo*, 'early', 'premature'; 燥 *zào*, 'dryness'

zhen 疹 *zhěn*, 'papule'; 镇 *zhèn*, 'settle'

zheng 癥 *zhēng*, 'concretion'; 证 *zhèng*, 'pattern'

zhi 肢 *zhī*, 'limb'; 止 *zhǐ*, 'stop'; 滞 *zhì*, 'stagnation'

zhong 中 *zhōng*, 'center'; 中 *zhòng*, 'strike'

zhu 逐 *zhú*, 'expel'; 注 *zhù*, 'pour'
zi 紫 *zǐ*, 'purple'; 自 *zì*, 'spontaneous'

zu 足 *zú*, 'foot'; 阻 *zǔ*, 'obstruct'

Examples of Complete Homophones
in Chinese Medical Terminology

bì 闭 'block,' 'close'; 痹 'impedi-ment'; 辟 'repel'

cháng 肠 'intestine'; 长 'long'

chǐ 齿 'tooth'; 尺 'cubit'

chōng 冲 'thoroughfare'; 充 'full-ness'

dài 带 'girdle'; 怠 'fatigued'

dǎn 胆 'gallbladder'; 疸 'jaun-dice'

dào 道 'way'; 盗 'thief'

dòng 动 'stir'; 冻 'freeze'

dú 独 'alone'; 毒 'toxin'

è 恶 'malign'; 呃 'hiccup'; 饿 'hunger'

fàn 犯 'invade'; 泛 'flood'

fú 浮 'floating'; 伏 'hidden'

gān 干 'dry'; 甘 'sweet'; 肝 'liver'

gé 革 'drumskin' (pulse); 膈 'di-aphragm'

gǔ 骨 'bone'; 谷 'grain'; 鼓 'drum'

hé 和 'harmonize'; 核 'node'; 阖 'close'

hóng 红 'red'; 洪 'surging' (of pulse)

hòu 后 'after'; 厚 'thick'

huá 滑 'slippery'; 华 'bloom'

jī 积 'accumulate'; 肌 'flesh'

jí 疾 'disease'; 急 'urgent'; 极 'ex-treme'

jiān 肩 'shoulder'; 间 'period', 'interval'; 煎 'brew'; 坚 'hard'

jiàng 降 'downbear'; 强 'stiff'; 绛 'crimson'

jié 结 *jié*, 'bind'; 节 'joint'; 疖 'boil'

jīn 金 'metal'; 筋 'sinew'; 紧 'tight'

jiǔ 九 'nine', 久 'for a long time', 'enduring'; 灸 'moxibustion'; 酒 'liquor'

láo 劳 'taxation'; 牢 'firm' (pulse)

lǐ 里 'interior'; 理 'rectify'

lì 疬 'pestilence'; 力 'strength'; 利 'disinhibit'; 痢 'dysentery'; 疬 'scrofula'

liú 流 'flow'; 留 'settle'

mù 木 'wood'; 目 'eye'

nì 逆 'counterflow'; 腻 'slimy'

qì 气 'qì'; 瘛 'pulling' (a type of spasm)

qīng 清 'clear'; 青 'blue-green'

sè 色 'color', 'complexion'; 涩 'rough' (of pulse); 塞 'conges-tion'

shēng 生 'engender'; 声 'voice'; 升 'upbear'

shī 失 'lose'; 湿 'dampness'

shí 时 'time'; 十 'shí'; 实 'reple-tion'; 食 'food'

tāi 胎 'fetus'; 苔 'tongue fur'

tì 涕 'snivel'; 嚏 'sneeze'

wèi 卫 'defense'; 胃 'stomach'

xī 膝 'knee'; 息 'breath'; 稀 'thin' (of fluids)

xián 弦 'stringlike'; 涎 'drool'; 咸 'salty'

xiàng 相 'ministerial'; 象 'sign'; 项 'nape'

xiāo 消 'disperse'; 哮 'wheezing'

xié 胁 'rib-side'; 斜 'deviated'

xīn 心 'heart'; 辛 'acrid'

xíng 行 'move', 'phase'; 形 'form', 'body'

yán 言 'speech'; 炎 'to flame'

yīn 因 'cause'; 阴 'yīn'

yín 淫 'excess'; 龈 'gum'

yù 郁 'depression'; 育 'foster'

yuán 原 'source'; 元 'origin'

yùn 运 'move'; 孕 'pregnancy'

zào 燥 'dryness'; 躁 'agitation'

zhèng 正 'straight'; 证 'pattern'

zhì 治 'treat'; 滞 'stagnation'

zhù 助 'assist'; 注 'pour'

zǐ 子 'child'; 紫 'purple'

Non-Standard Pronunciation

Although China is a land of many different dialects, many of which are not mutually intelligible, Mandarin is not only taught in all elementary schools but it also provides the medium of all education throughout China and Táiwān. Whatever dialect Chinese people may learn from their parents or from their local community, most people now have a command of Mandarin that facilitates communication with anyone in the Chinese world. Nevertheless, the speech of many Chinese does not conform to standard Mandarin pronunciation and contains elements from local dialects. In particular, the retroflex sound *zh*, *ch*, and *sh*, which are unique to Mandarin, are difficult for native speakers of other dialects to produce and tend to be replaced with the non-retroflex equivalents *z*, *c*, and *s*. This tendency is common to people as far apart as Sìchuān, Shànghǎi, Guǎngzhōu, and Táiwān.

Some southern Chinese (notably Fujianese and Taiwanese) who are not native speakers of Mandarin have difficulty making the sound *f*, and tend to pronounce it is *hw*. In addition, they often fail to distinguish *l* from *n*, pronouncing both as *n*.

附錄二：國語注音符號與漢語拼音對照表

Appendix II: Pīnyīn Conversion Table for Mandarin Phonetic Symbols

ㄅ b	玻 *bo*	ㄘ ci, c	雌 *ci*; 粗 *cu*; 錯 *cuo*
ㄆ p	坡 *po*	ㄙ si, s	思 *si*; 蘇 *su*; 撒 *sa*
ㄇ m	摸 *mo*	ㄧ yi, y, i	一 *yi*; 陰 *yin*; 先 *xian*
ㄈ f	發 *fa*	ㄨ w, u, o	屋 *wu*; 書 *shu*; 中 *zhong* 完 *wan*
ㄉ d	搭 *da*	ㄩ yu, u, yo, io	瘀 *yu*; 拘 *ju*; 用 *yong*; 女 *nü*; 綠 *lü*
ㄊ t	他 *ta*	ㄚ a	阿 *a*;
ㄋ n	糯 *nuo*	ㄛ o	我 *wo*;
ㄌ l	落 *luo*	ㄜ e	餓 *e*; 科 *ke*
ㄍ g	歌 *ge*	ㄝ e	學 *xue*; 坐 *xie*
ㄎ k	科 *ke*	ㄞ ai	唉 *ai*;
ㄏ h	喝 *he*	ㄟ ei, i	黑 *hei*; 追 *zhui*
ㄐ j	雞 *ji*	ㄠ ao	凹 *ao*;
ㄑ q	七 *qi*	ㄡ ou	歐 *ou*;
ㄒ x	西 *xi*	ㄢ an	安 *an*;
ㄓ zhi, zh	之 *zhi*; 朱 *zhu*; 渣 *zha*	ㄣ en, n	恩 *en*; 奔 *ben*; 檳 *bin*;
ㄔ chi, ch	吃 *chi*; 出 *chu*; 差 *cha*	ㄤ ang	骯 *ang*; 陽 *yang*; 床 *chuang*
ㄕ shi, sh	失 *shi*; 書 *shu*; 殺 *sha*	ㄥ eng, ng	風 *feng*; 清 *qing*;
ㄖ n, r	日 *n*; 入 *ru*; 熱 *re*	ㄦ er, r	兒 *er*; 會兒 *huir*
ㄗ zi, z	滋 *zi*; 租 *zu*; 臧 *zei*		

- ㄓ、ㄔ、ㄕ、ㄖ、ㄗ、ㄘ、ㄙ 如果爲單音(首音無尾)，漢語拼音拼爲 *zhi*，*chi*，*shi* 等；若其後有尾音，則 *i* 不寫(如ㄓㄤ *zhang*，ㄓㄨㄤ *zhuang*)。

- ㄧ若爲單音，拼爲*yi*；ㄧ如果是首音，而其後之尾音爲ㄣ或ㄥ時，以 *yi* 拼之，(如ㄧㄣ *yin*)，至於以其他注音符號爲尾音時，則一律拼爲 *y*，(如ㄧㄤ *yang*)；若ㄧ位於首尾兩個注音符號之間則拼寫爲*i* (如ㄒㄧㄢ *xian*、ㄅㄧㄠ *biao*)。

- ㄨ爲單音時，拼爲*wu*；若其後有尾音，則以*w* 拼之 (如ㄨㄢ *wan*、ㄨㄥ *weng*)；而當ㄨ夾處於前後的首音與尾音之中，除了以ㄥ爲尾音時 (如 ㄓㄨㄥ *zhong*)，將ㄨ 以*o* 拼出之外[4]，一律將ㄨ拼爲*u*。

- ㄩ爲單音或首音，則拼爲*yu* (如ㄩ *yu*，ㄩㄣ *yun*)；非爲單音或首音時，單以*u* 拼之，(如ㄐㄩ *ju*、ㄐㄩㄢ *juan*)；而當ㄩ之後的尾音爲ㄥ時，出現以下之例外情形：當ㄩ爲首音而尾音爲ㄥ時，以*yo*來拼出ㄩ (如ㄩㄥ *yong*)；ㄩ之前有其他首音而ㄥ爲尾音時，則將ㄩ拼爲*io*，(如ㄒㄩㄥ *xiong*)。[5] 另一個例外情形

---

[4] *zhong* 用*o* 來代表ㄨ，是因爲其發音非如撲字ㄆㄨ的ㄨ。

[5] ㄩㄥ (-ㄩㄥ) 寫爲 *yong* (*-iong*) 將其音解釋爲 "ㄧㄨㄥ"，其實是比較接近確實的念法！

乃ㄩ為尾音，而首音為ㄋ或ㄌ時，則將ㄩ拼為 *ü*（如ㄋㄩ *nü*、ㄌㄩ *lü*）。

- ㄣ與ㄥ為單音或尾音時，通常各別被拼為 *en*、*eng*，但若ㄣ、ㄥ為尾音，其前以一、ㄩ為首音或以一、ㄩ為中間音，而領首以其他符號時，則將ㄣ、ㄥ分別拼為 *n*、*ng*，（如一ㄣ *yin*、一ㄥ *ying*；ㄑ一ㄣ *qin*、ㄑ一ㄥ *qing*；ㄩㄣ *yun*、ㄩㄥ *yong*；ㄒㄩㄣ *xun*、ㄒㄩㄥ *xiong*)。而當ㄣ、ㄥ為尾音，其前以ㄨ為首音時，ㄣ、ㄥ仍分別拼為 *en*、*eng*，（如ㄨㄣ *wen*、ㄨㄥ *weng*)，但若以ㄨ為中間音，而領首以其他符號時則則將ㄣ、ㄥ分別拼為 *n*、*ng*，（如ㄓㄨㄣ *zhun*、ㄓㄨㄥ *zhong*)。

- ㄟ為單音或尾音時，拼為 *ei*，但例外之情況出現在其前以ㄨ為中間音，並以其他符號為首時，ㄟ被拼為 *i*，（如ㄓㄨㄟ *zhui*)。

- 四聲符號之一、二、三、四聲分別為 *ā*、*á*、*ǎ*、*à*，標示於母音之上，若出現母音有兩個的情形，則標示於重音之上，如 *āo*、*āi*、*ēi*、*ēi*、*ōu*、*uō*、*uā*、*uē*、*üē*；輕聲則不標示任何符號。此與國語注音之差別僅在於第一聲與輕聲之標示。

※注意: 中華人民共和國的標準"普通話"與中華民國"國語"不同
發音字主要是如下：

萆ㄅㄧˋ (bì)
柏ㄅㄞˇ (bǎi)
髮ㄈㄚˋ (fà)
斂ㄌㄧㄢˇ (liǎn)
期ㄑㄧ(qī)
息ㄒㄧ(xī)
熄ㄒㄧ(xī)

血ㄒㄩㄝˋ (xuè)
穴ㄒㄩㄝˊ (xué)
熟ㄕㄨˊ (shú)
脘ㄨㄢˇ (wǎn)
喎ㄨㄞ(wāi)
殼ㄎㄜˊ (qiào)

※注意: 下列文字，請注意其讀法：

痹ㄅㄧˋ (bì)
婢ㄅㄧˋ (bì)
瀕ㄅㄧㄣ(bīn)
朴ㄆㄛˋ (pò)
腓ㄈㄟˊ (féi)
膻ㄕㄢ(shān)
衄ㄋㄩˋ (nù)
瘰ㄌㄨㄛˇ (luǒ)
訶ㄏㄜ(hē)
穢ㄏㄨㄟˋ (huì)
紺ㄍㄢˋ (gàn)
扣ㄎㄡ(kōu)
灸ㄐㄧㄡˇ (jiǔ)
疽ㄐㄩ(jū)
鐲ㄐㄩㄢ(juān)
怯ㄑㄧㄝˋ (qiè)
觩ㄑㄧㄡˊ (qiú)
癇ㄒㄧㄢˊ (xián)

弦ㄒㄧㄢˊ (xián)
痃ㄒㄧㄢˊ (xián)
癬ㄒㄧㄢˇ (xiǎn)
薤ㄒㄧㄝˋ (xiè)
薢ㄒㄧㄝˋ (xiè)
芎ㄒㄩㄥ(xiōng)
妊ㄖㄣˋ (rèn)
娠ㄕㄣ(shēn)
痤ㄘˋ (cì)
噯ㄞˋ (ài)
藁ㄍㄠˇ (gǎo)
蠹ㄋㄧˋ (ni)
郗; ㄒㄧ(xī)
嗅ㄒㄧㄡˋ (xiù)
腘 ㄐㄩㄣˋ (jùn)、ㄐㄩㄥˇ (jiǒng)
恍ㄏㄨㄤˇ (huǎng)
痦ㄆㄟˊ (péi)

注音符號漢語拼音對照

ㄅ

ㄅㄚ	ba
ㄅㄛ	bo
ㄅㄞ	bai
ㄅㄟ	bei
ㄅㄠ	bao
ㄅㄢ	ban
ㄅㄣ	ben
ㄅㄤ	bang
ㄅㄥ	beng
ㄅㄧ	bi
ㄅㄧㄝ	bie
ㄅㄧㄠ	biao
ㄅㄧㄢ	bian
ㄅㄧㄣ	bin
ㄅㄧㄥ	bing
ㄅㄨ	bu

ㄆ

ㄆㄚ	pa
ㄆㄛ	po
ㄆㄞ	pai
ㄆㄟ	pei
ㄆㄠ	pao
ㄆㄢ	pan
ㄆㄣ	pen
ㄆㄤ	pang
ㄆㄥ	peng
ㄆㄧ	pi
ㄆㄧㄝ	pie
ㄆㄧㄠ	piao
ㄆㄧㄢ	pian
ㄆㄧㄣ	pin
ㄆㄧㄥ	ping
ㄆㄨ	pu

ㄇ

ㄇㄚ	ma
ㄇㄛ	mo
ㄇㄜ	me
ㄇㄞ	mai
ㄇㄟ	mei
ㄇㄠ	mao
ㄇㄡ	mou
ㄇㄢ	man
ㄇㄣ	men
ㄇㄤ	mang
ㄇㄥ	meng
ㄇㄧ	mi
ㄇㄧㄝ	mie
ㄇㄧㄠ	miao
ㄇㄧㄡ	miu
ㄇㄧㄢ	mian
ㄇㄧㄣ	min
ㄇㄧㄥ	ming
ㄇㄨ	mu

ㄈ

ㄈㄚ	fa
ㄈㄛ	fo
ㄈㄟ	fei
ㄈㄡ	fou
ㄈㄢ	fan
ㄈㄣ	fen
ㄈㄤ	fang
ㄈㄥ	feng
ㄈㄨ	fu

ㄉ

ㄉㄚ	da
ㄉㄜ	de
ㄉㄞ	dai
ㄉㄠ	dao
ㄉㄡ	dou
ㄉㄢ	dan
ㄉㄤ	dang
ㄉㄥ	deng
ㄉㄧ	di
ㄉㄧㄝ	die
ㄉㄧㄠ	diao
ㄉㄧㄡ	diu
ㄉㄧㄢ	dian
ㄉㄧㄥ	ding
ㄉㄨ	du

ㄉ (ㄉㄨ column)

ㄉㄨㄛ	duo
ㄉㄨㄟ	dui
ㄉㄨㄢ	duan
ㄉㄨㄣ	dun
ㄉㄨㄥ	dong

ㄊ

ㄊㄚ	ta
ㄊㄜ	te
ㄊㄞ	tai
ㄊㄠ	tao
ㄊㄡ	tou
ㄊㄢ	tan
ㄊㄤ	tang
ㄊㄥ	teng
ㄊㄧ	ti
ㄊㄧㄝ	tie
ㄊㄧㄠ	tiao
ㄊㄧㄢ	tian
ㄊㄧㄥ	ting
ㄊㄨ	tu
ㄊㄨㄛ	tuo
ㄊㄨㄟ	tui
ㄊㄨㄢ	tuan
ㄊㄨㄣ	tun
ㄊㄨㄥ	tong

ㄋ

ㄋㄚ	na
ㄋㄜ	ne
ㄋㄞ	nai
ㄋㄟ	nei
ㄋㄠ	nao
ㄋㄢ	nan
ㄋㄣ	nen
ㄋㄤ	nang
ㄋㄥ	neng
ㄋㄧ	ni
ㄋㄧㄝ	nie
ㄋㄧㄠ	niao
ㄋㄧㄡ	niu
ㄋㄧㄢ	nian
ㄋㄧㄤ	niang
ㄋㄧㄥ	ning
ㄋㄨ	nu
ㄋㄨㄛ	nuo
ㄋㄨㄢ	nuan
ㄋㄨㄥ	nong
ㄋㄩ	nü
ㄋㄩㄝ	nüe

ㄌ

ㄌㄚ	la
ㄌㄜ	le
ㄌㄞ	lai
ㄌㄟ	lei
ㄌㄠ	lao
ㄌㄡ	lou
ㄌㄢ	lan
ㄌㄤ	lang
ㄌㄥ	leng
ㄌㄧ	li
ㄌㄧㄚ	lia
ㄌㄧㄝ	lie
ㄌㄧㄠ	liao
ㄌㄧㄡ	liu
ㄌㄧㄢ	lian
ㄌㄧㄣ	lin
ㄌㄧㄤ	liang
ㄌㄧㄥ	ling
ㄌㄨ	lu
ㄌㄨㄛ	luo
ㄌㄨㄢ	luan
ㄌㄨㄣ	lun
ㄌㄨㄥ	long
ㄌㄩ	lü
ㄌㄩㄝ	lüe

ㄍ

ㄍㄚ	ga
ㄍㄜ	ge
ㄍㄞ	gai
ㄍㄠ	gao
ㄍㄟ	gei

《ㄡ gou
《ㄢ gan
《ㄣ gen
《ㄤ gang
《ㄥ geng
《ㄨ gu
《ㄨㄚ gua
《ㄨㄛ guo
《ㄨㄞ guai
《ㄨㄟ gui
《ㄨㄢ guan
《ㄨㄣ gun
《ㄨㄤ guang
《ㄨㄥ gong

ㄎ

ㄎㄚ ka
ㄎㄜ ke
ㄎㄞ kai
ㄎㄠ kao
ㄎㄡ kou
ㄎㄢ kan
ㄎㄣ ken
ㄎㄤ kang
ㄎㄥ keng
ㄎㄨ ku
ㄎㄨㄚ kua
ㄎㄨㄛ kuo
ㄎㄨㄞ kuai
ㄎㄨㄟ kui
ㄎㄨㄢ kuan
ㄎㄨㄣ kun
ㄎㄨㄤ kuang
ㄎㄨㄥ kong

ㄏ

ㄏㄚ ha
ㄏㄜ he
ㄏㄞ hai
ㄏㄟ hei
ㄏㄠ hao
ㄏㄡ hou
ㄏㄢ han
ㄏㄣ hen

ㄏㄤ hang
ㄏㄥ heng
ㄏㄨ hu
ㄏㄨㄚ hua
ㄏㄨㄛ huo
ㄏㄨㄞ huai
ㄏㄨㄟ hui
ㄏㄨㄢ huan
ㄏㄨㄣ hun
ㄏㄨㄤ huang
ㄏㄨㄥ hong

ㄐ

ㄐㄧ ji
ㄐㄧㄚ jia
ㄐㄧㄝ jie
ㄐㄧㄠ jiao
ㄐㄧㄡ jiu
ㄐㄧㄢ jian
ㄐㄧㄣ jin
ㄐㄧㄤ jiang
ㄐㄧㄥ jing
ㄐㄨ ju
ㄐㄨㄣ jun
ㄐㄨ juan
ㄐㄨㄝ jue
ㄐㄨㄥ jiong

ㄑ

ㄑㄧ qi
ㄑㄧㄚ qia
ㄑㄧㄝ qie
ㄑㄧㄠ qiao
ㄑㄧㄡ qiu
ㄑㄧㄢ qian
ㄑㄧㄣ qin
ㄑㄧㄤ qiang
ㄑㄧㄥ qing
ㄑㄨ qu
ㄑㄨㄣ qun
ㄑㄨ quan
ㄑㄨㄝ que
ㄑㄨㄥ qiong

ㄒ

ㄒㄧ xi
ㄒㄧㄚ xia
ㄒㄧㄝ xie
ㄒㄧㄠ xiao
ㄒㄧㄡ xiu
ㄒㄧㄢ xian
ㄒㄧㄣ xin
ㄒㄧㄤ xiang
ㄒㄧㄥ xing
ㄒㄨ xu
ㄒㄨㄢ xuan
ㄒㄨㄣ xun
ㄒㄨㄝ xue
ㄒㄨㄥ xiong

ㄓ

ㄓ zhi
ㄓㄚ zha
ㄓㄜ zhe
ㄓㄞ zhai
ㄓㄟ zhei
ㄓㄠ zhao
ㄓㄡ zhou
ㄓㄢ zhan
ㄓㄣ zhen
ㄓㄤ zhang
ㄓㄥ zheng
ㄓㄨ zhu
ㄓㄨㄚ zhua
ㄓㄨㄛ zhuo
ㄓㄨㄞ zhuai
ㄓㄨㄟ zhui
ㄓㄨㄢ zhuan
ㄓㄨㄣ zhun
ㄓㄨㄤ zhuang
ㄓㄨㄥ zhong

ㄔ

ㄔ chi
ㄔㄚ cha
ㄔㄜ che
ㄔㄞ chai
ㄔㄠ chao

ㄔㄡ chou
ㄔㄢ chan
ㄔㄣ chen
ㄔㄤ chang
ㄔㄥ cheng
ㄔㄨ chu
ㄔㄨㄞ chuai
ㄔㄨㄟ chui
ㄔㄨㄢ chuan
ㄔㄨㄣ chun
ㄔㄨㄤ chuang
ㄔㄨㄥ chong

ㄕ

ㄕ shi
ㄕㄚ sha
ㄕㄜ she
ㄕㄞ shai
ㄕㄟ shei
ㄕㄠ shao
ㄕㄡ shou
ㄕㄢ shan
ㄕㄣ shen
ㄕㄤ shang
ㄕㄥ sheng
ㄕㄨ shu
ㄕㄨㄚ shua
ㄕㄨㄛ shuo
ㄕㄨㄞ shuai
ㄕㄨㄟ shui
ㄕㄨㄢ shuan
ㄕㄨㄣ shun
ㄕㄨㄤ shuang

ㄖ

ㄖ ri
ㄖㄜ re
ㄖㄠ rao
ㄖㄡ rou
ㄖㄢ ran
ㄖㄣ ren
ㄖㄤ rang
ㄖㄥ reng
ㄖㄨ ru

ㄖㄨㄛ ruo
ㄖㄨㄟ rui
ㄖㄨㄢ ruan
ㄖㄨㄣ run
ㄖㄨㄥ rong

ㄗ

ㄗ zi
ㄗㄚ za
ㄗㄜ ze
ㄗㄞ zai
ㄗㄟ zei
ㄗㄠ zao
ㄗㄡ zou
ㄗㄢ zan
ㄗㄣ zen
ㄗㄤ zang
ㄗㄥ zeng
ㄗㄨ zu
ㄗㄨㄛ zuo
ㄗㄨㄟ zui
ㄗㄨㄢ zuan
ㄗㄨㄣ zun
ㄗㄨㄥ zong

ㄘ

ㄘ ci
ㄘㄚ ca
ㄘㄜ ce
ㄘㄞ cai
ㄘㄠ cao
ㄘㄡ cou
ㄘㄢ can
ㄘㄤ cang
ㄘㄥ ceng
ㄘㄨ cu
ㄘㄨㄛ cuo
ㄘㄨㄟ cui
ㄘㄨㄢ cuan
ㄘㄨㄣ cun
ㄘㄨㄥ cong

ㄙ

ㄙ si
ㄙㄚ sa
ㄙㄜ se
ㄙㄞ sai
ㄙㄠ sao
ㄙㄡ sou
ㄙㄢ san

ㄙㄣ sen
ㄙㄤ sang
ㄙㄥ seng
ㄙㄨ su
ㄙㄨㄛ suo
ㄙㄨㄟ sui
ㄙㄨㄢ suan
ㄙㄨㄣ sun
ㄙㄨㄥ song

一

一 yi
一ㄚ ya
一ㄝ ye
一ㄠ yao
一ㄡ you
一ㄢ yan
一ㄣ yin
一ㄤ yang
一ㄥ ying

ㄨ

ㄨ wu
ㄨㄚ wa
ㄨㄚ wa

ㄨㄛ wo
ㄨㄞ wai
ㄨㄟ wei
ㄨㄢ wan
ㄨㄣ wen
ㄨㄤ wang
ㄨㄥ weng

ㄩ

ㄩ yu
ㄩㄝ yue
ㄩㄢ yuan
ㄩㄣ yun
ㄩㄥ yong

ㄚ 一 ㄢ

ㄚ a
ㄜ e
ㄞ ai
ㄠ ao
ㄡ ou
ㄢ an
ㄣ en
ㄤ ang
ㄦ er

汉语拼音注音符号对照

a ㄚ
ai ㄞ
an ㄢ
ang ㄤ
ao ㄠ
ba ㄅㄚ
bai ㄅㄞ
ban ㄅㄢ
bang ㄅㄤ
bao ㄅㄠ
bei ㄅㄟ
ben ㄅㄣ
beng ㄅㄥ
bi ㄅ一
bian ㄅ一ㄢ

biao ㄅ一ㄠ
bie ㄅ一ㄝ
bin ㄅ一ㄣ
bing ㄅ一ㄥ
bo ㄅㄛ
bu ㄅㄨ
ca ㄘㄚ
cai ㄘㄞ
can ㄘㄢ
cang ㄘㄤ
cao ㄘㄠ
ce ㄘㄜ
cen ㄘㄣ
ceng ㄘㄥ
cha ㄔㄚ

chai ㄔㄞ
chan ㄔㄢ
chang ㄔㄤ
chao ㄔㄠ
che ㄔㄜ
chen ㄔㄣ
cheng ㄔㄥ
chi ㄔ
chong ㄔㄨㄥ
chou ㄔㄡ
chu ㄔㄨ
chua ㄔㄨㄚ
chuai ㄔㄨㄞ
chuan ㄔㄨㄢ
chuang ㄔㄨㄤ

chui ㄔㄨㄟ
chun ㄔㄨㄣ
chuo ㄔㄨㄛ
ci ㄘ
cong ㄘㄨㄥ
cou ㄘㄡ
cu ㄘㄨ
cuan ㄘㄨㄢ
cui ㄘㄨㄟ
cun ㄘㄨㄣ
cuo ㄘㄨㄛ
da ㄉㄚ
dai ㄉㄞ
dan ㄉㄢ
dang ㄉㄤ

dao ㄉㄠ	gua ㄍㄨㄚ	kao ㄎㄠ	me ㄇㄜ
de ㄉㄜ	guai ㄍㄨㄞ	ke ㄎㄜ	mei ㄇㄟ
dei ㄉㄟ	guan ㄍㄨㄢ	ken ㄎㄣ	men ㄇㄣ
den ㄉㄣ	guang ㄍㄨㄤ	keng ㄎㄥ	meng ㄇㄥ
deng ㄉㄥ	gui ㄍㄨㄟ	kong ㄎㄨㄥ	mi ㄇㄧ
di ㄉㄧ	gun ㄍㄨㄣ	kou ㄎㄡ	mian ㄇㄧㄢ
dian ㄉㄧㄢ	guo ㄍㄨㄛ	ku ㄎㄨ	miao ㄇㄧㄠ
diao ㄉㄧㄠ	ha ㄏㄚ	kua ㄎㄨㄚ	mie ㄇㄧㄝ
die ㄉㄧㄝ	hai ㄏㄞ	kuai ㄎㄨㄞ	min ㄇㄧㄣ
ding ㄉㄧㄥ	han ㄏㄢ	kuan ㄎㄨㄢ	ming ㄇㄧㄥ
diu ㄉㄧㄡ	hang ㄏㄤ	kuang ㄎㄨㄤ	miu ㄇㄧㄡ
dong ㄉㄨㄥ	hao ㄏㄠ	kui ㄎㄨㄟ	mo ㄇㄛ
dou ㄉㄡ	he ㄏㄜ	kun ㄎㄨㄣ	mou ㄇㄡ
du ㄉㄨ	hei ㄏㄟ	kuo ㄎㄨㄛ	mu ㄇㄨ
duan ㄉㄨㄢ	hen ㄏㄣ	la ㄌㄚ	na ㄋㄚ
dui ㄉㄨㄟ	heng ㄏㄥ	lai ㄌㄞ	nai ㄋㄞ
dun ㄉㄨㄣ	hong ㄏㄨㄥ	lan ㄌㄢ	nan ㄋㄢ
duo ㄉㄨㄛ	hou ㄏㄡ	lang ㄌㄤ	nang ㄋㄤ
e ㄜ	hu ㄏㄨ	lao ㄌㄠ	nao ㄋㄠ
ei ㄟ	hua ㄏㄨㄚ	le ㄌㄜ	ne ㄋㄜ
en ㄣ	huai ㄏㄨㄞ	lei ㄌㄟ	nei ㄋㄟ
eng ㄥ	huan ㄏㄨㄢ	leng ㄌㄥ	nen ㄋㄣ
er ㄦ	huang ㄏㄨㄤ	li ㄌㄧ	neng ㄋㄥ
fa ㄈㄚ	hui ㄏㄨㄟ	lia ㄌㄧㄚ	ni ㄋㄧ
fan ㄈㄢ	hun ㄏㄨㄣ	lian ㄌㄧㄢ	nian ㄋㄧㄢ
fang ㄈㄤ	huo ㄏㄨㄛ	liang ㄌㄧㄤ	niang ㄋㄧㄤ
fei ㄈㄟ	ji ㄐㄧ	liao ㄌㄧㄠ	niao ㄋㄧㄠ
fen ㄈㄣ	jia ㄐㄧㄚ	lie ㄌㄧㄝ	nie ㄋㄧㄝ
feng ㄈㄥ	jian ㄐㄧㄢ	lin ㄌㄧㄣ	nin ㄋㄧㄣ
fo ㄈㄛ	jiang ㄐㄧㄤ	ling ㄌㄧㄥ	ning ㄋㄧㄥ
fou ㄈㄡ	jiao ㄐㄧㄠ	liu ㄌㄧㄡ	niu ㄋㄧㄡ
fu ㄈㄨ	jie ㄐㄧㄝ	long ㄌㄨㄥ	nong ㄋㄨㄥ
ga ㄍㄚ	jin ㄐㄧㄣ	lou ㄌㄡ	nu ㄋㄨ
gai ㄍㄞ	jing ㄐㄧㄥ	lu ㄌㄨ	nou ㄋㄡ
gan ㄍㄢ	jiong ㄐㄩㄥ	lü ㄌㄩ	nu ㄋㄨ
gang ㄍㄤ	jiu ㄐㄧㄡ	luan ㄌㄨㄢ	nü ㄋㄩ
gao ㄍㄠ	ju ㄐㄩ	lüe ㄌㄩㄝ	nuan ㄋㄨㄢ
ge ㄍㄜ	juan ㄐㄩㄢ	lun ㄌㄨㄣ	nüe ㄋㄩㄝ
gei ㄍㄟ	jue ㄐㄩㄝ	luo ㄌㄨㄛ	nuo ㄋㄨㄛ
gen ㄍㄣ	jun ㄐㄩㄣ	ma ㄇㄚ	o ㄛ
geng ㄍㄥ	ka ㄎㄚ	mai ㄇㄞ	ou ㄡ
gong ㄍㄨㄥ	kai ㄎㄞ	man ㄇㄢ	pa ㄆㄚ
gou ㄍㄡ	kan ㄎㄢ	mang ㄇㄤ	pai ㄆㄞ
gu ㄍㄨ	kang ㄎㄤ	mao ㄇㄠ	

pan ㄆㄢ	sai ㄙㄞ	tie ㄊㄧㄝ	yu ㄩ
pang ㄆㄤ	san ㄙㄢ	ting ㄊㄧㄥ	yuan ㄩㄢ
pao ㄆㄠ	sang ㄙㄤ	tong ㄊㄨㄥ	yue ㄩㄝ
pei ㄆㄟ	sao ㄙㄠ	tou ㄊㄡ	yun ㄩㄣ
pen ㄆㄣ	se ㄙㄜ	tu ㄊㄨ	za ㄗㄚ
peng ㄆㄥ	sen ㄙㄣ	tuan ㄊㄨㄢ	zai ㄗㄞ
pi ㄆㄧ	seng ㄙㄥ	tui ㄊㄨㄟ	zan ㄗㄢ
pian ㄆㄧㄢ	sha ㄕㄚ	tun ㄊㄨㄣ	zang ㄗㄤ
piao ㄆㄧㄠ	shai ㄕㄞ	tuo ㄊㄨㄛ	zao ㄗㄠ
pie ㄆㄧㄝ	shan ㄕㄢ	wa ㄨㄚ	ze ㄗㄜ
pin ㄆㄧㄣ	shang ㄕㄤ	wa ㄨㄚ	zei ㄗㄟ
ping ㄆㄧㄥ	shao ㄕㄠ	wai ㄨㄞ	zen ㄗㄣ
po ㄆㄛ	she ㄕㄜ	wan ㄨㄢ	zeng ㄗㄥ
pou ㄆㄡ	shei ㄕㄟ	wang ㄨㄤ	zha ㄓㄚ
pu ㄆㄨ	shen ㄕㄣ	wei ㄨㄟ	zhai ㄓㄞ
qi ㄑㄧ	sheng ㄕㄥ	wen ㄨㄣ	zhan ㄓㄢ
qia ㄑㄧㄚ	shi ㄕ	weng ㄨㄥ	zhang ㄓㄤ
qian ㄑㄧㄢ	shou ㄕㄡ	wo ㄨㄛ	zhao ㄓㄠ
qiang ㄑㄧㄤ	shu ㄕㄨ	wu ㄨ	zhe ㄓㄜ
qiao ㄑㄧㄠ	shua ㄕㄨㄚ	xi ㄒㄧ	zhei ㄓㄟ
qie ㄑㄧㄝ	shuai ㄕㄨㄞ	xia ㄒㄧㄚ	zhen ㄓㄣ
qin ㄑㄧㄣ	shuan ㄕㄨㄢ	xian ㄒㄧㄢ	zheng ㄓㄥ
qing ㄑㄧㄥ	shuang ㄕㄨㄤ	xiang ㄒㄧㄤ	zhi ㄓ
qiong ㄑㄩㄥ	shui ㄕㄨㄟ	xiao ㄒㄧㄠ	zhong ㄓㄨㄥ
qiu ㄑㄧㄡ	shun ㄕㄨㄣ	xie ㄒㄧㄝ	zhou ㄓㄡ
qu ㄑㄩ	shuo ㄕㄨㄛ	xin ㄒㄧㄣ	zhu ㄓㄨ
quan ㄑㄩ	si ㄙ	xing ㄒㄧㄥ	zhua ㄓㄨㄚ
que ㄑㄩㄝ	song ㄙㄨㄥ	xiong ㄒㄩㄥ	zhuai ㄓㄨㄞ
qun ㄑㄩㄣ	sou ㄙㄡ	xiu ㄒㄧㄡ	zhuan ㄓㄨㄢ
ran ㄖㄢ	su ㄙㄨ	xu ㄒㄩ	zhuang ㄓㄨㄤ
rang ㄖㄤ	suan ㄙㄨㄢ	xuan ㄒㄩㄢ	zhui ㄓㄨㄟ
rao ㄖㄠ	sui ㄙㄨㄟ	xue ㄒㄩㄝ	zhun ㄓㄨㄣ
re ㄖㄜ	sun ㄙㄨㄣ	xun ㄒㄩㄣ	zhuo ㄓㄨㄛ
ren ㄖㄣ	suo ㄙㄨㄛ	ya ㄧㄚ	zi ㄗ
reng ㄖㄥ	ta ㄊㄚ	yan ㄧㄢ	zong ㄗㄨㄥ
ri ㄖ	tai ㄊㄞ	yang ㄧㄤ	zou ㄗㄡ
rong ㄖㄨㄥ	tan ㄊㄢ	yao ㄧㄠ	zu ㄗㄨ
rou ㄖㄡ	tang ㄊㄤ	ye ㄧㄝ	zuan ㄗㄨㄢ
ru ㄖㄨ	tao ㄊㄠ	yi ㄧ	zui ㄗㄨㄟ
ruan ㄖㄨㄢ	te ㄊㄜ	yin ㄧㄣ	zun ㄗㄨㄣ
rui ㄖㄨㄟ	teng ㄊㄥ	ying ㄧㄥ	zuo ㄗㄨㄛ
run ㄖㄨㄣ	ti ㄊㄧ	yo ㄧㄛ	
ruo ㄖㄨㄛ	tian ㄊㄧㄢ	yong ㄩㄥ	
sa ㄙㄚ	tiao ㄊㄧㄠ	you ㄧㄡ	

附录三：单字
Appendix III: Single Characters

This appendix presents basic characters used in the terminology of Chinese medicine in Pīnyīn order, with their English equivalents and examples of terms in which they each appear. Note that in some of the terms given as examples the single character has no equivalent in English (e.g., 舌苔白如积粉 *shé tāi bái rú jī fěn* is translated as "mealy white tongue fur," in which 积 *jī*, accumulate, does not appear).

This appendix is mainly intended for English-speaking students learning the Chinese terminology, and for this reason, the characters are presented in large print (the complex forms in parentheses). It is also helpful to anyone learning the terminological correspondences at the level of individual words.

嗳〔噯〕ài [1]
belch, belching

嗳气酸腐〔噯氣酸腐〕*ài qì suān fǔ*, belching of sour putrid qì (gas)

安〔安〕ān [2]
quiet, quieting

重镇安神〔重鎮安神〕*zhòng zhèn ān shén*, quieting the spirit with heavy settlers

按〔按〕àn [3]
press, pressure

脘腹痛喜按〔脘腹痛喜按〕*wǎn fù tòng xǐ àn*, pain in the stomach duct and abdomen that likes pressure

八〔八〕bā [4]
eight

八法〔八法〕*bā fǎ*, eight methods

拔〔拔〕bá [5]
pluck

拔火罐〔拔火罐〕*bá huǒ guàn*, fire cupping

把〔把〕bǎ [6]
take

把脉〔把脈〕*bǎ mài*, take the pulse

白〔白〕bái [7]
white

面色白〔面色白〕*miàn sè bái*, white facial complexion

面色淡白〔面色淡白〕*miàn sè dàn bái*, pale white facial complexion

舌苔白如积粉〔舌苔白如積粉〕*shé tāi bái rú jī fěn*, mealy white tongue fur

斑〔斑〕bān [8]
macules

斑疹〔斑疹〕*bān zhěn*, maculopapular eruption

半〔半〕bàn [9]
half, hemi-

半表半里证〔半表半裡證〕*bàn biǎo bàn lǐ zhèng*, midstage pattern; half-interior half-exterior pattern

半身不遂〔半身不遂〕*bàn shēn bù suì*, hemiplegia

胞〔胞〕bāo 10
bladder, uterus

转胞〔轉胞〕*zhuǎn bāo*, shifted bladder

女子胞〔女子胞〕*nǚ zǐ bāo*, uterus

暴〔暴〕bāo 11
fulminant

阴液暴脱〔陰液暴脱〕*yīn yè bào tuō*, fulminant desertion of yīn humor

悲〔悲〕bēi 12
sorrow

背〔背〕bèi 13
back

背俞〔背俞〕*bèi shū*, back transport [point]

焙〔焙〕bèi 14
stone-baking

奔〔奔〕bēn 15
running

奔豚〔奔豚〕*bēn tún*, running piglet

本〔本〕běn 16
root

治本〔治本〕*zhì běn*, treating the root

崩〔崩〕bēng 17
flooding

崩漏〔崩漏〕*bēng lòu*, flooding and spotting

鼻〔鼻〕bí 18
nose

肺开窍于鼻〔肺開竅於鼻〕*fèi kāi qiào yú bí*, lung opens at the nose

鼻翼煽动〔鼻翼煽動〕*bí yì shān dòng*, flaring nostrils

闭〔閉〕bì 19
block, close

气闭〔氣閉〕*qì bì*, qì block

闭经〔閉經〕*bì jīng*, menstrual block; amenorrhea

囟门迟闭〔囟門遲閉〕*xìn mén chí bì*, retarded closure of the fontanel gate

秘〔秘〕bì 20
constipation

便秘〔便秘〕*biàn bì*, constipation

痹〔痹〕bì 21
impediment

寒痹〔寒痹〕*hán bì*, cold impediment

心痹〔心痹〕*xīn bì*, heart impediment

辟〔辟〕bì 22
repel, repelling

辟秽开窍〔辟穢開竅〕*bì huì kāi qiào*, repelling foulness and opening the orifices

标〔標〕biāo ▢23
tip

治标〔治標〕*zhì biāo,* treating the tip

表〔表〕biǎo ▢24
exterior

肺与大肠相表里〔肺與大腸相表裡〕*fèi yǔ dà cháng xiāng biǎo lǐ,* lung and large intestine stand in interior-exterior relationship

表证〔表證〕*biǎo zhèng,* exterior pattern

病〔病〕bìng ▢25
disease

太阳病〔太陽病〕*tài yáng bìng,* greater yáng disease

阳明病〔陽明病〕*yáng míng bìng,* yáng brightness disease

剥〔剝〕bō ▢26
peeling

苔剥〔苔剝〕*tāi bō,* peeling fur

薄〔薄〕bó ▢27
thin (tongue fur, stool)

苔薄〔苔薄〕*tāi bó,* thin fur

补〔補〕bǔ ▢28
supplement

补气〔補氣〕*bǔ qì,* supplementing qì

补血〔補血〕*bǔ xuè,* supplementing the blood

苍〔蒼〕cāng ▢29
somber

面色苍白〔面色蒼白〕*miàn sè cāng bái,* somber white facial complexion

藏〔藏〕cáng ▢30
store

心藏神〔心藏神〕*xīn cáng shén,* heart stores the spirit

肠〔腸〕cháng ▢31
intestine

小肠〔小腸〕*xiǎo cháng,* small intestine

大肠〔大腸〕*dà cháng,* large intestine

长〔長〕cháng ▢32
long

小便清长〔小便清長〕*xiǎo biàn qīng cháng,* long voidings of clear urine

长脉〔長脈〕*cháng mài,* long pulse

潮〔潮〕cháo ▢33
tidal

潮热〔潮熱〕*cháo rè,* tidal heat [effusion]; tidal fever

沉〔沉〕chén ▢34
sunken (pulse), deep (pulse)

沉脉〔沉脈〕*chén mài,* sunken pulse; deep pulse

臣〔臣〕chén ▢35
minister

乘〔乘〕chéng ▢36
overwhelm, overwhelming

相乘〔相乘〕*xiāng chéng*, overwhelming

迟〔遲〕chí ⟦37⟧
slow, retarded

迟脉〔遲脈〕*chí mài*, slow pulse

尺〔尺〕chǐ ⟦38⟧
cubit

齿〔齒〕chǐ ⟦39⟧
tooth; dental

牙齿〔牙齒〕*yá chǐ*, tooth (*n.*); dental (*adj.*)

齿龈〔齒齦〕*chǐ yín*, gum

舌边齿痕〔舌邊齒痕〕*shé biān chǐ hén*, dental impressions on the margins of the tongue

赤〔赤〕chì ⟦40⟧
red, reddish (urine)

面赤〔面赤〕*miàn chì*, red face

目赤〔目赤〕*mù chì*, red eyes

小便短赤〔小便短赤〕*xiǎo biàn duǎn chì*, short voidings of reddish urine

冲〔衝〕chōng ⟦41⟧
thoroughfare

冲脉〔衝脈〕*chōng mài*, thoroughfare vessel

冲〔沖〕chōng ⟦42⟧
drench

冲服〔沖服〕*chōng fú*, take drenched

充〔充〕chōng ⟦43⟧
fullness

肾，其充在骨〔腎，其充在骨〕*shèn, qí chōng zài gǔ*, kidney... its fullness is in the bone

抽〔抽〕chōu ⟦44⟧
tugging

抽风〔抽風〕*chōu fēng*, tugging wind

四肢抽搐〔四肢抽搐〕*sì zhī chōu chù*, convulsion of the limbs

稠〔稠〕chóu ⟦45⟧
thick (phlegm)

咳痰黄稠〔咳痰黃稠〕*ké tán huáng chóu*, cough with thick yellow phlegm

搐〔搐〕chù ⟦46⟧
convulsion

四肢抽搐〔四肢抽搐〕*sì zhī chōu chù*, convulsion of the limbs

喘〔喘〕chuǎn ⟦47⟧
panting

哮喘〔哮喘〕*xiāo chuǎn*, wheezing and panting

疮〔瘡〕chuāng ⟦48⟧
sore

疔疮〔疔瘡〕*dīng chuāng*, clove sore

口（中生）疮〔口（中生）瘡〕*kǒu (zhōng shēng) chuāng*, mouth sore

疮疡〔瘡瘍〕*chuāng yáng*, sore

唇〔唇〕chún ⟦49⟧
lips

脾，其华在唇四白〔脾，其華在唇四白〕*pí, qí huá zài chún sì bái*, spleen... its bloom is in the four whites of the lips

口唇淡白 〔口唇淡白〕 *kǒu chún dàn bái,* pale lips

刺 〔刺〕cì 　50
needle (*v.*)

刺络拔罐 〔刺絡拔罐〕 *cì luò bá guàn,* pricking and cupping

针刺 〔針刺〕 *zhēn cì,* acupuncture

腠 〔腠〕còu 　51
interstices

腠理 〔腠理〕 *còu lǐ,* interstices

粗 〔粗〕cū 　52
rough

气粗 〔氣粗〕 *qì cū,* rough breathing

促 〔促〕cù 　53
skipping; hasty

气促 〔氣促〕 *qì cù,* hasty breathing

促脉 〔促脈〕 *cù mài,* skipping pulse

窜 〔竄〕cuàn 　54
scurrying

脐周窜痛 〔臍周竄痛〕 *qí zhōu cuàn tòng,* scurrying pain around the umbilicus

淬 〔淬〕cuì 　55
quench

寸 〔寸〕cùn 　56
inch

同身寸 〔同身寸〕 *tóng shēn cùn,* body inch

寸口 〔寸口〕 *cùn kǒu,* wrist pulse; inch opening

打 〔打〕dǎ 　57
knock

跌打 〔跌打〕 *dié dǎ,* knocks and falls

大 〔大〕dà 　58
large (pulse, intestine), greater (abdomen)

大肠 〔大腸〕 *dà cháng,* large intestine

大腹 〔大腹〕 *dà fù,* greater abdomen

呆 〔呆〕dāi 　59
torpid, torpor

纳呆 〔納呆〕 *nà dāi,* torpid intake

带 〔帶〕dài 　60
girdling; vaginal discharge

带脉 〔帶脈〕 *dài mài,* girdling vessel

止带 〔止脈〕 *zhǐ dài,* checking vaginal discharge

怠 〔怠〕dài 　61
fatigue, fatigued

倦怠乏力 〔倦怠乏力〕 *juàn dài fá lì,* fatigue and lack of strength

代 〔代〕dài 　62
intermittent

代脉 〔代脈〕 *dài mài,* intermittent pulse

单 〔單〕dān 　63
single

单蛾〔單蛾〕*dān é*, single moth

丹〔丹〕dān [64]
cinnabar

丹毒〔丹毒〕*dān dú*, erysipelas; cinnabar toxin [sore]

丹田〔丹田〕*dān tián*, cinnabar field

胆〔膽〕dǎn [65]
gallbladder

肝与胆相表里〔肝與膽相表裡〕*gān yǔ dǎn xiāng biǎo lǐ*, liver and gallbladder stand in interior-exterior relationship

肝胆湿热〔肝膽濕熱〕*gān dǎn shī rè*, liver-gallbladder damp-heat

疸〔疸〕dǎn [66]
jaundice

黄疸〔黃疸〕*huáng dǎn*, jaundice

淡〔淡〕dàn [67]
pale

面色淡白〔面色淡白〕*miàn sè dàn bái*, pale white facial complexion

舌淡〔舌淡〕*shé dàn*, pale tongue

导〔導〕dǎo [68]
abduct, abducting, abduction

消导〔消導〕*xiāo dǎo*, abductive dispersion

捣〔搗〕dǎo [69]
crush, pound

道〔道〕dào [70]
way

肺主通调水道〔肺主通調水道〕*fèi zhǔ tōng tiáo shuǐ dào*, lung governs regulation of the waterways

穴道〔穴道〕*xué dào*, acupuncture point

盗〔盜〕dào [71]
thief

盗汗〔盜汗〕*dào hàn*, night sweating; thief sweating

癫〔癲〕diān [72]
withdrawal

癫狂〔癲狂〕*diān kuáng*, mania and withdrawal

点〔點〕diǎn [73]
speckles

瘀点〔瘀點〕*yū diǎn*, stasis speckles

跌〔跌〕dié [74]
fall

跌打〔跌打〕*dié dǎ*, knocks and falls

疔〔疔〕dīng [75]
clove sore

疔疮〔疔瘡〕*dīng chuāng*, clove sore

动〔動〕dòng [76]
stir, stirring, stirred

胎动不安〔胎動不安〕*tāi dòng bù ān*, stirring fetus

动脉〔動脈〕*dòng mài*, stirred pulse

肝风内动〔肝風內動〕*gān fēng nèi dòng,* liver wind stirring internally

冻〔凍〕**dòng** 77
frost

冻疮〔凍瘡〕*dòng chuāng,* frostbite

痘〔痘〕**dòu** 78
pox

督〔督〕**dū** 79
governing

督脉〔督脈〕*dū mài,* governing vessel

毒〔毒〕**dú** 80
toxin

丹毒〔丹毒〕*dān dú,* erysipelas; cinnabar toxin [sore]

独〔獨〕**dú** 81
alone

独语〔獨語〕*dú yǔ,* soliloquy; talking alone

短〔短〕**duǎn** 82
short

短气〔短氣〕*duǎn qì,* shortness of breath

小便短赤〔小便短赤〕*xiǎo biàn duǎn chì,* short voidings of reddish urine

小便短少〔小便短少〕*xiǎo biàn duǎn shǎo,* short voidings of scant urine

短脉〔短脈〕*duǎn mài,* short pulse

煅〔煅〕**duàn** 83
calcine; calcination

炖〔燉〕**dùn** 84
double-boiling

多〔多〕**duō** 85
copious, profuse

痰多清稀〔痰多清稀〕*tán duō qīng xī,* copious clear thin phlegm

夜间多尿〔夜間多尿〕*yè jiān duō niào,* profuse urination at night; nocturia

多梦〔多夢〕*duō mèng,* profuse dreaming

蛾〔蛾〕**é** 86
moth

乳蛾〔乳蛾〕*rǔ é,* nipple moth; baby moth

恶〔惡〕**ě** 87
nausea

恶心〔惡心〕*ě xīn,* nausea

呃〔呃〕**è** 88
hiccup

呃逆〔呃逆〕*è nì,* hiccup

恶〔惡〕**è** 89
malign

遏阻〔遏阻〕*è zǔ,* malign obstruction; morning sickness

儿〔兒〕**ér** 90
child

小儿惊风〔小兒驚風〕*xiǎo ér jīng fēng,* child fright wind

耳〔耳〕**ěr** 91
ear

肾开窍于耳〔腎開竅於耳〕*shèn kāi qiào yú ěr*, kidney opens at the ears

二〔二〕èr   92

two

肾开窍于二阴〔腎開竅於二陰〕*shèn kāi qiào yú èr yīn*, kidney opens at the two yīn

十二经〔十二經〕*shí èr jīng*, twelve channels

发〔發〕fā   93

effuse, effusion

发热〔發熱〕*fā rè*, heat effusion; fever

法〔法〕fǎ   94

method

治法〔治法〕*zhì fǎ*, method of treatment

发〔髮〕fà   95

hair (of the head)

肾，其华在发〔腎，其華在髮〕*shèn, qí huá zài fà*, kidney... its bloom is in the hair (of the head)

烦〔煩〕fán   96

vex, vexing, vexation

心烦〔心煩〕*xīn fán*, heart vexation

五心烦热〔五心煩熱〕*wǔ xīn fán rè*, vexing heat in the five hearts

反〔反〕fǎn   97

paradoxical (treatment), reflux (stomach)

反治〔反治〕*fǎn zhì*, paradoxical treatment

反胃〔反胃〕*fǎn wèi*, stomach reflux

犯〔犯〕fàn   98

invade

肝气犯脾〔肝氣犯脾〕*gān qì fàn pí*, liver qì invading the spleen

肝气犯胃〔肝氣犯胃〕*gān qì fàn wèi*, liver qì invading the stomach

泛〔泛〕fàn   99

flood, flooding; upflow

阳虚水泛〔陽虛水泛〕*yáng xū shuǐ fàn*, yáng vacuity water flood

泛酸〔泛酸〕*fàn suān*, acid upflow

肥〔肥〕féi   100

obese, fat

形体肥胖〔形體肥胖〕*xíng tǐ féi pàng*, obesity

过食肥甘〔過食肥甘〕*guò shí féi gān*, excessive consumption of sweet and fatty foods

肺〔肺〕fèi   101

lung, pulmonary

肺气不宣〔肺氣不宣〕*fèi qì bù xuān*, nondiffusion of lung qì

肺肾阴虚〔肺腎陰虛〕*fèi shèn yīn xū*, lung-kidney yīn vacuity

肺痈〔肺癰〕*fèi yōng*, pulmonary welling-abscess

粉〔粉〕fěn   102

meal(y)

舌苔白如积粉 〔舌苔白如積粉〕 *shé tāi bái rú jī fěn*, mealy white tongue fur

风 〔風〕fēng 　103
wind

抽风 〔抽風〕 *chōu fēng*, tugging wind

恶风 〔惡風〕 *wù fēng*, aversion to wind

肝风内动 〔肝風內動〕 *gān fēng nèi dòng*, liver wind stirring internally

肝阳化风 〔肝陽化風〕 *gān yáng huà fēng*, liver yáng transforming into wind

外感风邪 〔外感風邪〕 *wài gǎn fēng xié*, external contraction of wind evil

浮 〔浮〕fú 　104
floating (of pulse), superficial (network vessel), puffy (swelling)

浮络 〔浮絡〕 *fú luò*, superficial network vessel

浮脉 〔浮脈〕 *fú mài*, floating pulse

浮肿 〔浮腫〕 *fú zhǒng*, puffy swelling

伏 〔伏〕fú 　105
hidden (pulse)

伏脉 〔伏脈〕 *fú mài*, hidden pulse

服 〔服〕fú 　106
take (medicine)

冲服 〔沖服〕 *chōng fú*, take drenched

腑 〔腑〕fǔ 　107
bowel

脏腑之气 〔臟腑之氣〕 *zàng fǔ zhī qì*, bowel and visceral qì

腹 〔腹〕fù 　108
abdomen; abdominal

大腹 〔大腹〕 *dà fù*, greater abdomen

甘 〔甘〕gān 　109
sweet, sweetness

过食肥甘 〔過食肥甘〕 *guò shí féi gān*, excessive consumption of sweet and fatty foods

肝 〔肝〕gān 　110
liver

肝属木 〔肝屬木〕 *gān shǔ mù*, liver belongs to wood

肝藏血 〔肝藏血〕 *gān cáng xuè*, liver stores blood

肝火上炎 〔肝火上炎〕 *gān huǒ shàng yán*, liver fire flaming upward

干 〔乾〕gān 　111
dry, dryness

舌苔干燥 〔舌苔乾燥〕 *shé tāi gān zào*, dry tongue fur

感 〔感〕gǎn 　112
contract, contraction

外感风邪 〔外感風邪〕 *wài gǎn fēng xié*, external contraction of wind evil

肛 〔肛〕gāng 　113
anus

脱肛〔脱肛〕*tuō gāng*, prolapse of the rectum

膏〔膏〕gāo 　114

unctuous (stranguty); gāo (as in gāo-huāng); paste

膏肓〔膏肓〕*gāo huāng*, gāo-huāng

膏淋〔膏淋〕*gāo lín*, unctuous strangury

膏滋〔膏滋〕*gāo zī*, rich paste

膈〔膈〕gé 　115

diaphragm, diaphragmatic; occlusion

噎膈〔噎膈〕*yē gé*, dysphagia-occlusion

革〔革〕gé 　116

drumskin

革脉〔革脈〕*gé mài*, drumskin pulse

攻〔攻〕gōng 　117

attack

攻痰〔攻痰〕*gōng tán*, attacking phlegm

垢〔垢〕gòu 　118

grimy

苔垢〔苔垢〕*tāi gòu*, grimy fur

骨〔骨〕gǔ 　119

bone

肾生骨髓〔腎生骨髓〕*shèn shēng gǔ suí*, kidney engenders the bone and marrow

肾，其充在骨〔腎，其充在骨〕*shèn, qí chōng zài gǔ*, kidney... its fullness is in the bone

牙齿干燥如枯骨〔牙齒乾燥如枯骨〕*yá chǐ gān zào rú kū gǔ*, teeth dry as desiccated bones

谷〔穀〕gǔ 　120

grain, food

下利清谷〔下利清穀〕*xià lì qīng gǔ*, clear-grain diarrhea; clear-food diarrhea

纳谷不香〔納穀不香〕*nà gǔ bù xiāng*, no pleasure in eating

鼓〔鼓〕gǔ 　121

drum

鼓胀〔鼓脹〕*gǔ zhàng*, drum distention

固〔固〕gù 　122

secure, securing; stem, stemming

肾气不固〔腎氣不固〕*shèn qì bù gù*, insecurity of kidney qi

涩肠固脱〔澀腸固脫〕*sè cháng gù tuō*, astringing the intestines and stemming desertion

关〔關〕guān 　123

bar (pulse); pass (throat); gate (essence); joint

寸关尺〔寸關尺〕*cùn guān chǐ*, inch, bar, cubit

喉关〔喉關〕*hóu guān*, throat pass

关节疼痛〔關節疼痛〕*guān jié téng tòng*, joint pain

精关〔精關〕*jīng guān*, essence gate

罐〔罐〕guàn 　124

cup, container

拔火罐〔拔火罐〕*bá huǒ guàn,* fire cupping

光〔光〕guāng | 125 |
light, smooth, bare

恶光羞明〔惡光羞明〕*wù guāng xiū míng,* aversion to light

舌光红〔舌光紅〕*shé guāng hóng,* smooth bare red tongue

眼无光彩〔眼無光彩〕*yǎn wú guāng cǎi,* dull eyes

海〔海〕hǎi | 126 |
sea

气海〔氣海〕*qì hǎi,* sea of qi

寒〔寒〕hán | 127 |
cold

恶寒〔惡寒〕*wù hán,* aversion to cold

憎寒〔憎寒〕*zēng hán,* abhorrence of cold

表寒〔表寒〕*biǎo hán,* exterior cold

血寒〔血寒〕*xuè hán,* blood cold

汗〔汗〕hàn | 128 |
sweat, sweating

敛汗〔斂汗〕*liǎn hàn,* constraining sweat

自汗〔自汗〕*zì hàn,* spontaneous sweating

盗汗〔盜汗〕*dào hàn,* night sweating; thief sweating

呵〔呵〕hē | 129 |
yawn, yawning

呵欠〔呵欠〕*hē qiàn,* yawning

核〔核〕hé | 130 |
node (as in 'phlegm node'), pit (as in 'plum-pit')

喉核〔喉核〕*hóu hé,* throat node

梅核气〔梅核氣〕*méi hé qì,* plum-pit qi

痰核〔痰核〕*tán hé,* phlegm node

阖〔闔〕hé | 131 |
close, closing

肾主开阖〔腎主開闔〕*shèn zhǔ kāi hé,* kidney governs opening and closing

和〔和〕hé | 132 |
harmonize, harmonizing, harmonization, harmony

口中和〔口中和〕*kǒu zhōng hé,* harmony of mouth

和解半表半里〔和解半表半裡〕*hé jiě bàn biǎo bàn lǐ,* harmonizing (and resolving) midstage patterns; harmonizing (and resolving) half-exterior half-interior patterns

黑〔黑〕hēi | 133 |
black

面色黑〔面色黑〕*miàn sè hēi,* black facial complexion

痕〔痕〕hén | 134 |
impression

舌边齿痕〔舌邊齒痕〕*shé biān chǐ hén,* dental impressions on the margins of the tongue

红〔紅〕hóng | 135 |
red

面色红〔面色紅〕*miàn sè hóng,* red facial complexion

舌红〔舌紅〕*shé hóng,* red tongue

洪〔洪〕hóng [136]
surging

洪脉〔洪脈〕*hóng mài,* surging pulse

喉〔喉〕hóu [137]
larynx, laryngeal; throat

喉核〔喉核〕*hóu hé,* throat node

喉关〔喉關〕*hóu guān,* throat pass

结喉〔結喉〕*jié hóu,* laryngeal prominence

喉中有痰声〔喉中有痰聲〕*hóu zhōng yǒu tán shēng,* sound of phlegm in the throat

白喉〔白喉〕*bái hóu,* diphtheria

厚〔厚〕hòu [138]
thick (tongue fur); rich (food)

苔厚〔苔厚〕*tāi hòu,* thick fur

偏嗜油腻厚味〔偏嗜油膩厚味〕*piān shì yóu nì hòu wèi,* predilection for greasy and rich foods

后〔後〕hòu [139]
after, delayed, later, post

食后困顿〔食後困頓〕*shí hòu kùn dùn,* drowsiness after eating

午后潮热〔午後潮熱〕*wǔ hòu cháo rè,* postmeridian tidal heat [effusion]; postmeridian tidal fever

里急后重〔裡急後重〕*lǐ jí hòu zhòng,* tenesmus; abdominal urgency and rectal heaviness

花〔花〕huā [140]
flower

目花〔目花〕*mù huā,* flowery vision

梅花针〔梅花針〕*méi huā zhēn,* plum-blossom needle

华〔華〕huá [141]
bloom, luster

脾，其华在唇四白〔脾，其華在唇四白〕*pí, qí huá zài chún sì bái,* spleen. . . its bloom is in the four whites of the lips

面色无华〔面色無華〕*miàn sè wú huá,* lusterless facial complexion

滑〔滑〕huá [142]
slippery (pulse), efflux (stool, semen)

滑脉〔滑脈〕*huá mài,* slippery pulse

滑精〔滑精〕*huá jīng,* seminal efflux

化〔化〕huà [143]
transform, transforming, transformation

气化〔氣化〕*qì huà,* qì transformation

脾主运化〔脾主運化〕*pí zhǔ yùn huà,* spleen governs movement and transformation

活〔活〕huó [144]
quicken, quickening

活血化瘀 〔活血化瘀〕 *huó xuè huà yū*, quickening the blood and transforming stasis

踝 〔踝〕huái ⎡145⎤
ankle

缓 〔緩〕huǎn ⎡146⎤
moderate

缓脉 〔緩脈〕 *huǎn mài*, moderate pulse

肓 〔肓〕huāng ⎡147⎤
huāng (as in 'gāo-huāng')

膏肓 〔膏肓〕 *gāo huāng*, gāo-huāng

黄 〔黃〕huáng ⎡148⎤
yellow

面色黄 〔面色黃〕 *miàn sè huáng*, yellow facial complexion

黄苔 〔黃苔〕 *huáng tāi*, yellow fur

目黄 〔目黃〕 *mù huáng*, yellow eyes

皖 〔皖〕huǎng ⎡149⎤
bright

面色皖白 〔面色皖白〕 *miàn sè huǎng bái*, bright white facial complexion

回 〔回〕huí ⎡150⎤
return, returning

回阳救逆 〔回陽救逆〕 *huí yáng jiù nì*, returning yáng and stemming counterflow

昏 〔昏〕hūn ⎡151⎤
clouding, clouded

神昏 〔神昏〕 *shén hūn*, clouded spirit

昏睡 〔昏睡〕 *hūn shuì*, clouding sleep

昏倒 〔昏倒〕 *hūn dǎo*, clouding collapse

火 〔火〕huǒ ⎡152⎤
fire

君火 〔君火〕 *jūn huǒ*, sovereign fire

霍 〔霍〕huò ⎡153⎤
sudden

霍乱 〔霍亂〕 *huò luàn*, cholera; sudden turmoil

豁 〔豁〕huò ⎡154⎤
sweep

豁痰开窍 〔豁痰開竅〕 *huò tán kāi qiào*, sweeping phlegm and opening the orifices

肌 〔肌〕jī ⎡155⎤
flesh

肌肉 〔肌肉〕 *jī ròu*, flesh

肌肉瘦削 〔肌肉瘦削〕 *jī ròu shòu xuè*, emaciation

积 〔積〕jī ⎡156⎤
accumulate

肠胃积滞 〔腸胃積滯〕 *cháng wèi jī zhì*, gastrointestinal accumulation

癥瘕积聚 〔癥瘕積聚〕 *zhēng jiǎ jī jù*, concretions, conglomerations, accumulations, and gatherings

舌苔白如积粉〔舌苔白如積粉〕 *shé tāi bái rú jī fěn*, mealy white tongue fur

疾〔疾〕jí 157
disease; racing

疾脉〔疾脈〕 *jí mài*, racing pulse

疾病〔疾病〕 *jí bìng*, disease

急〔急〕jí 158
urgent, urgency; rapid; tension

里急后重〔裡急後重〕 *lǐ jí hòu zhòng*, tenesmus; abdominal urgency and rectal heaviness

气急〔氣急〕 *qì jí*, rapid breathing

筋脉拘急〔筋脈拘急〕 *jīn mài jū jí*, tension of the sinews

极〔極〕jí 159
extreme

热极生风〔熱極生風〕 *rè jí shēng fēng*, extreme heat engendering wind

悸〔悸〕jì 160
palpitations

心悸〔心悸〕 *xīn jì*, heart palpitations

剂〔劑〕jì 161
preparation

剂型〔劑型〕 *jì xíng*, preparation

济〔濟〕jì 162
help

水火相济〔水火相濟〕 *shuǐ huǒ xiāng jì*, fire and water help each other

假〔假〕jiǎ 163
false

假神〔假神〕 *jiǎ shén*, false spiritedness

瘕〔瘕〕jiǎ 164
conglomeration

癥瘕积聚〔癥瘕積聚〕 *zhēng jiǎ jī jù*, concretions, conglomerations, accumulations, and gatherings

肩〔肩〕jiān 165
shoulder

肩息〔肩息〕 *jiān xī*, raised-shoulder breathing

坚〔堅〕jiān 166
hard

软坚〔軟堅〕 *ruǎn jiān*, softening hardness

煎〔煎〕jiān 167
decoct; brew

健〔健〕jiàn 168
fortify, constant

健脾利水〔健脾利水〕 *jiàn pí lì shuǐ*, fortifying the spleen and disinhibiting water

健忘〔健忘〕 *jiàn wàng*, forgetfulness

降〔降〕jiàng 169
bear downward, downbear

肺主肃降〔肺主肅降〕 *fèi zhǔ sù jiàng*, lung governs depurative downbearing

绛〔絳〕jiàng 170
crimson

舌绛〔舌絳〕*shé jiàng*, crimson tongue

强〔強〕jiàng 〔171〕
stiff

颈项强直〔頸項強直〕*jǐng xiàng jiàng zhí*, rigidity of the neck

焦〔焦〕jiāo 〔172〕
burn, burnt (yellow tongue fur), burner; parched (lips)

三焦〔三焦〕*sān jiāo*, triple burner

口唇干焦〔口唇乾焦〕*kǒu chún gān jiāo*, parched lips

交〔交〕jiāo 〔173〕
interact, intersect

心肾不交〔心腎不交〕*xīn shèn bù jiāo*, noninteraction of the heart and kidney

交会穴〔交會穴〕*jiāo huì xué*, intersection point

胶〔膠〕jiāo 〔174〕
glue

节〔節〕jié 〔175〕
joint, temperance

关节疼痛〔關節疼痛〕*guān jié téng tòng*, joint pain

饮食不节〔飲食不節〕*yǐn shí bù jié*, dietary irregularities

房室不节〔房室不節〕*fáng shì bù jié*, sexual intemperance

结〔結〕jié 〔176〕
bind, binding, bound

大便干结〔大便乾結〕*dà biàn gān jié*, dry bound stool

肝气郁结〔肝氣鬱結〕*gān qì yù jié*, binding depression of liver qì

结脉〔結脈〕*jié mài*, bound pulse

齿龈结瓣〔齒齦結瓣〕*chǐ yín jié bàn*, petaled gums

结喉〔結喉〕*jié hóu*, laryngeal prominence

疖〔癤〕jié 〔177〕
boil

解〔解〕jiě 〔178〕
resolve, resolution (therapeutic action); ununited

解表〔解表〕*jiě biǎo*, resolving the exterior

解颅〔解顱〕*jiě lú*, ununited skull

金〔金〕jīn 〔179〕
metal

肺属金〔肺屬金〕*fèi shǔ jīn*, lung belongs to metal

津〔津〕jīn 〔180〕
liquid

津液〔津液〕*jīn yè*, liquid and humor (fluids)

筋〔筋〕jīn 〔181〕
sinew

肝主筋〔肝主筋〕*gān zhǔ jīn*, liver governs the sinews

筋惕肉眴〔筋惕肉瞤〕*jīn tì ròu shùn*, jerking sinews and twitching flesh

紧〔緊〕jǐn 〔182〕
tight

紧脉〔緊脈〕*jǐn mài,* tight pulse

噤〔噤〕jìn　183

clenched

口噤〔口噤〕*kǒu jìn,* clenched jaw

浸〔浸〕jìn　184

steep, steeping

经〔經〕jīng　185

channel; menses, menstruation, menstrual

经络〔經絡〕*jīng luò,* channels and network vessels

月经过少〔月經過少〕*yuè jīng guò shǎo,* scant menstruation

惊〔驚〕jīng　186

fright

惊悸〔驚悸〕*jīng jì,* fright palpitations

精〔精〕jīng　187

essence

肾藏精〔腎藏精〕*shèn cáng jīng,* kidney stores essence

颈〔頸〕jǐng　188

neck

颈项强直〔頸項強直〕*jǐng xiàng jiàng zhí,* rigidity of the neck

镜〔鏡〕jìng　189

mirror

镜面舌〔鏡面舌〕*jìng miàn shé,* mirror tongue

净〔淨〕jìng　190

clean

舌净〔舌淨〕*shé jìng,* clean tongue

痉〔痙〕jìng　191

tetany, tetanic

痉病〔痙病〕*jìng bìng,* tetany

痉厥〔痙厥〕*jìng jué,* tetanic reversal

九〔九〕jiǔ　192

nine

九窍〔九竅〕*jiǔ qiào,* nine orifices

酒〔酒〕jiǔ　193

wine; liquor

久〔久〕jiǔ　194

enduring

久泄〔久泄〕*jiǔ xiè,* enduring diarrhea

灸〔灸〕jiǔ　195

moxibustion

针灸〔針灸〕*zhēn jiǔ,* acupuncture and moxibustion

救〔救〕jiù　196

stem, stemming

回阳救逆〔回陽救逆〕*huí yáng jiù nì,* returning yáng and stemming counterflow

疽〔疽〕jū　197

flat-abscess

拒〔拒〕jù　198

refuse

腹痛拒按 〔腹痛拒按〕 *fù tòng jù àn*, abdominal pain that refuses pressure

聚 〔聚〕jù 199
gather, gathering

癥瘕积聚 〔癥瘕積聚〕 *zhēng jiǎ jī jù*, concretions, conglomerations, accumulations, and gatherings

卷 〔卷〕juǎn 200
curled

舌卷 〔舌卷〕 *shé juǎn*, curled tongue

倦 〔倦〕juàn 201
fatigue, fatigued

劳倦 〔勞倦〕 *láo juàn*, taxation fatigue

四肢困倦 〔四肢困倦〕 *sì zhī kùn juàn*, fatigued cumbersome limbs

厥 〔厥〕jué 202
reverse

痉厥 〔痙厥〕 *jìng jué*, tetanic reversal

君 〔君〕jūn 203
sovereign

君火 〔君火〕 *jūn huǒ*, sovereign fire

咯 〔咯〕kǎ 204
expectorate, hack

痰少不易咯 〔痰少不易咯〕 *tán shǎo bú yì kǎ*, scant phlegm expectorated with difficulty

开 〔開〕kāi 205
open, opening

心开窍于舌 〔心開竅於舌〕 *xīn kāi qiào yú shé*, heart opens at the tongue

肾主开阖 〔腎主開闔〕 *shèn zhǔ kāi hé*, kidney governs opening and closing

清心开窍 〔清心開竅〕 *qīng xīn kāi qiào*, clearing the heart and opening the orifices

亢 〔亢〕kàng 206
hyperactive

肝阳上亢 〔肝陽上亢〕 *gān yáng shàng kàng*, ascendant hyperactivity of liver yáng; ascendant liver yáng

窠 〔窠〕kē 207
nest

目窠上微肿 〔目窠上微腫〕 *mù kē shàng wēi zhǒng*, slight swelling of the eye nest

咳 〔咳〕ké 208
cough

咳痰黄稠 〔咳痰黃稠〕 *ké tán huáng chóu*, cough with thick yellow phlegm

渴 〔渴〕kě 209
thirst

口渴 〔口渴〕 *kǒu kě*, thirst

渴不欲饮 〔渴不欲飲〕 *kě bù yù yǐn*, thirst with no desire to drink

克 〔剋〕kè 210
restrain, restraining

恐 〔恐〕kǒng 211

fear

苃〔苃〕kōu 〔212〕
scallion-stalk

苃脉〔苃脈〕*kōu mài*, scallion-stalk pulse

口〔口〕kǒu 〔213〕
mouth; oral; opening

脾开窍于口〔脾開竅於口〕*pí kāi qiào yú kǒu*, spleen opens at the mouth

口眼喎斜〔口眼喎斜〕*kǒu yǎn wāi xié*, deviated eyes and mouth

寸口〔寸口〕*cùn kǒu*, wrist pulse; inch opening

枯〔枯〕kū 〔214〕
dry, desiccated

发枯〔髮枯〕*fà kū*, dry hair

牙齿干燥如枯骨〔牙齒乾燥如枯骨〕*yá chǐ gān zào rú kū gǔ*, teeth dry as desiccated bones

肾阴枯涸〔腎陰枯涸〕*shèn yīn kū hé*, desiccation of kidney yīn

苦〔苦〕kǔ 〔215〕
bitter, bitterness

口苦〔口苦〕*kǒu kǔ*, bitter taste in the mouth

胸胁苦满〔胸脅苦滿〕*xiōng xié kǔ mǎn*, chest and rib-side fullness

块〔塊〕kuài 〔216〕
lump

痞块〔痞塊〕*pǐ kuài*, glomus lump

狂〔狂〕kuáng 〔217〕
mania

狂躁〔狂躁〕*kuáng zào*, mania and agitation

亏〔虧〕kuī 〔218〕
depletion

肝肾阴亏〔肝腎陰虧〕*gān shèn yīn kuī*, liver-kidney yīn depletion

困〔困〕kùn 〔219〕
encumbrance

食后困顿〔食後困頓〕*shí hòu kùn dùn*, drowsiness after eating

脾虚湿困〔脾虛濕困〕*pí xū shī kùn*, spleen vacuity damp encumbrance

懒〔懶〕lǎn 〔220〕
lazy, laziness

懒言〔懶言〕*lǎn yán*, laziness to speak

劳〔勞〕láo 〔221〕
taxation

劳淋〔勞淋〕*láo lín*, taxation strangury

牢〔牢〕láo 〔222〕
firm

牢脉〔牢脈〕*láo mài*, firm pulse; confined pulse

老〔老〕lǎo 〔223〕
old

老黄〔老黃〕*lǎo huáng*, old yellow

泪〔淚〕lèi 〔224〕
tears

冷〔冷〕lěng 〔225〕
cold

四肢逆冷 〔四肢逆冷〕 *sì zhī nì lěng*, counterflow cold of the limbs

理〔理〕lǐ 226
rectify, rectifying

理气和营 〔理氣和營〕 *lǐ qì hé yíng*, rectifying qi and harmonizing construction

撮空理线 〔撮空理線〕 *cuō kōng lǐ xiàn*, groping in the air and pulling [invisible] strings

腠理 〔腠理〕 *còu lǐ*, interstices

里〔裡〕lǐ 227
interior

肝与胆相表里 〔肝與膽相表裡〕 *gān yǔ dǎn xiāng biǎo lǐ*, liver and gallbladder stand in interior-exterior relationship

里证 〔裡證〕 *lǐ zhèng*, interior pattern

疠〔癘〕lì 228
pestilence

疠气 〔癘氣〕 *lì qì*, pestilential qi

力〔力〕lì 229
force, strength

有力 〔有力〕 *yǒu lì*, forceful

倦怠乏力 〔倦怠乏力〕 *juàn dài fá lì*, fatigue and lack of strength

沥〔瀝〕lì 230
dribble

尿有余沥 〔尿有餘瀝〕 *niào yǒu yú lì*, dribble after voiding

利〔利〕lì 231
disinhibit, disinhibiting

清利湿热 〔清利濕熱〕 *qīng lì shī rè*, clearing heat and disinhibiting dampness

肺气不利 〔肺氣不利〕 *fèi qì bù lì*, inhibition of lung qi

小便不利 〔小便不利〕 *xiǎo biàn bù lì*, inhibited urination

下利清谷 〔下利清穀〕 *xià lì qīng gǔ*, clear-grain diarrhea; clear-food diarrhea

痢〔痢〕lì 232
dysentery

痢疾 〔痢疾〕 *lì jí*, dysentery

疬〔癧〕lì 233
scrofula

瘰疬 〔瘰癧〕 *luǒ lì*, scrofula

敛〔斂〕liǎn 234
constrain, constraining

敛汗 〔斂汗〕 *liǎn hàn*, constraining sweat

敛肺 〔斂肺〕 *liǎn fèi*, constraining the lung

凉〔涼〕liáng 235
cool, coolness, cooling

渴喜凉饮 〔渴喜涼飲〕 *kě xǐ liáng yǐn*, thirst with a liking for cool drinks

凉血 〔涼血〕 *liáng xuè*, cooling the blood

辛凉解表 〔辛涼解表〕 *xīn liáng jiě biǎo*, resolving the exterior with coolness and acridity

裂〔裂〕liè 236
fissured

舌裂 〔舌裂〕 *shé liè*, fissured tongue

淋 〔淋〕lín 237

strangury

淋证 〔淋證〕 *lín zhèng*, strangury pattern

流 〔流〕liú 238

run

鼻流清涕 〔鼻流清涕〕 *bí liú qīng tì*, runny nose with clear snivel (nasal mucus)

口角流涎 〔口角流涎〕 *kǒu jiǎo liú xián*, drooling from the corners of the mouth

流注 〔流注〕 *liú zhù*, streaming sore

留 〔留〕liú 239

lodge; retain

痰留经络 〔痰留經絡〕 *tán liú jīng luò*, phlegm lodged in the channels

留针 〔留針〕 *liú zhēn*, needle retention

六 〔六〕liù 240

six

六淫 〔六淫〕 *liù yín*, six excesses

颅 〔顱〕lú 241

skull

解颅 〔解顱〕 *jiě lú*, ununited skull

露 〔露〕lù 242

distillate; dew

癃 〔癃〕lóng 243

dribbling urination

癃闭 〔癃閉〕 *lóng bì*, dribbling urinary block

漏 〔漏〕lòu 244

spotting

崩漏 〔崩漏〕 *bēng lòu*, flooding and spotting

乱 〔亂〕luàn 245

chaotic, turmoil (sudden turmoil)

乱经 〔亂經〕 *luàn jīng*, chaotic menstruation

霍乱 〔霍亂〕 *huò luàn*, cholera; sudden turmoil

瘰 〔瘰〕luǒ 246

scrofula

瘰疬 〔瘰癧〕 *luǒ lì*, scrofula

络 〔絡〕luò 247

net, network [vessel]

络脉 〔絡脈〕 *luò mài*, network vessel

痰留经络 〔痰留經絡〕 *tán liú jīng luò*, phlegm lodged in the channels

麻 〔麻〕má 248

tingle, tingling; numb, numbness; measles

四肢麻木 〔四肢麻木〕 *sì zhī má mù*, numbness (and tingling) of the limbs

麻疹 〔麻疹〕 *má zhěn*, measles

脉 〔脈〕mài 249

vessel, pulse

络脉 〔絡脈〕 *luò mài*, network vessel

任脉〔任脈〕*rèn mài*, controlling vessel

满〔滿〕mǎn [250]
fullness

胸满〔胸滿〕*xiōng mǎn*, fullness in the chest

胸胁苦满〔胸脅苦滿〕*xiōng xié kǔ mǎn*, chest and rib-side fullness

腹满〔腹滿〕*fù mǎn*, abdominal fullness

芒〔芒〕máng [251]
prickle

舌起芒刺〔舌起芒刺〕*shé qǐ máng cì*, prickly tongue

梅〔梅〕méi [252]
plum

梅核气〔梅核氣〕*méi hé qì*, plum-pit qì

寐〔寐〕mèi [253]
sleep

不寐〔不寐〕*bù mèi*, sleeplessness

门〔門〕mén [254]
gate

囟门〔囟門〕*xìn mén*, fontanel gate, anterior fontanel

命门〔命門〕*mìng mén*, life gate

闷〔悶〕mèn [255]
oppression

胸闷〔胸悶〕*xiōng mèn*, oppression in the chest

梦〔夢〕mèng [256]
dream

多梦〔多夢〕*duō mèng*, profuse dreaming

梦遗〔夢遺〕*mèng yí*, dream emission

迷〔迷〕mí [257]
confound

痰迷心窍〔痰迷心竅〕*tán mí xīn qiào*, phlegm confounding the orifices of the heart

眠〔眠〕mián [258]
sleep

失眠〔失眠〕*shī mián*, insomnia

面〔面〕miàn [259]
face, facial

面色苍白〔面色蒼白〕*miàn sè cāng bái*, somber white facial complexion

面色黄〔面色黃〕*miàn sè huáng*, yellow facial complexion

鸣〔鳴〕míng [260]
rumbling; ringing; tinnitus

肠鸣〔腸鳴〕*cháng míng*, rumbling intestines

耳鸣〔耳鳴〕*ěr míng*, tinnitus; ringing in the ears

膜〔膜〕mó [261]
membrane

膜原〔膜原〕*mó yuán*, membrane source

末〔末〕mò [262]
powder

为末〔爲末〕*wéi mò*, grinding to a powder

木〔木〕**mù**   [263]
wood; numb, numbness

肝属木〔肝屬木〕*gān shǔ mù*, liver belongs to wood

四肢麻木〔四肢麻木〕*sì zhī má mù*, numbness (and tingling) of the limbs

目〔目〕**mù**   [264]
eye

肝开窍于目〔肝開竅於目〕*gān kāi qiào yú mù*, liver opens at the eyes

纳〔納〕**nà**   [265]
intake

胃主受纳〔胃主受納〕*wèi zhǔ shòu nà*, stomach governs intake

难〔難〕**nán**   [266]
difficult

便难〔便難〕*biàn nán*, difficult defecation

脑〔腦〕**nǎo**   [267]
brain

内〔內〕**nèi**   [268]
internal

内因〔內因〕*nèi yīn*, internal cause

肝风内动〔肝風內動〕*gān fēng nèi dòng*, liver wind stirring internally

嫩〔嫩〕**nèn**   [269]
tender-soft

舌淡胖嫩〔舌淡胖嫩〕*shé dàn pàng nèn*, pale tender-soft enlarged tongue

腻〔膩〕**nì**   [270]
slimy

苔腻〔苔膩〕*tāi nì*, slimy fur

逆〔逆〕**nì**   [271]
counterflow

四肢逆冷〔四肢逆冷〕*sì zhī nì lěng*, counterflow cold of the limbs

呃逆〔呃逆〕*è nì*, hiccup

捻〔捻〕**niǎn**   [272]
twirl

捻针〔捻針〕*niǎn zhēn*, needle twirling

捻转补泻〔捻轉補瀉〕*niǎn zhuǎn bǔ xiè*, twirling supplementation and drainage

尿〔尿〕**niào**   [273]
urine, urinary; urination

夜间多尿〔夜間多尿〕*yè jiān duō niào*, profuse urination at night; nocturia

缩尿〔縮尿〕*suō niào*, reducing urine

遗尿〔遺尿〕*yí niào*, enuresis

弄〔弄〕**nòng**   [274]
worry (in the sense of to move repeatedly)

吐弄舌〔吐弄舌〕*tù nòng shé*, protrusion and worrying of the tongue

怒〔怒〕**nù**   [275]
anger

易怒〔易怒〕*yì nù*, irascibility

衄〔衄〕nǜ 276
spontaneous external bleeding

衄〔衄〕*nǜ*, spontaneous external bleeding

疟〔瘧〕nüè 277
malaria

疟疾〔瘧疾〕*nüè jí*, malaria

呕〔嘔〕ǒu 278
retching, vomiting

呕吐痰饮〔嘔吐痰飲〕*ǒu tù tán yǐn*, vomiting of phlegm-rheum

胖〔胖〕pàng 279
obese, obesity

形体肥胖〔形體肥胖〕*xíng tǐ féi pàng*, obesity

舌胖大〔舌胖大〕*shé pàng dà*, enlarged tongue

炮〔炮〕páo 280
blast-fry

泡〔泡〕pào 281
steep, steeping

皮〔皮〕pí 282
skin

皮毛〔皮毛〕*pí máo*, skin and [body] hair

脾〔脾〕pí 283
spleen

脾主运化〔脾主運化〕*pí zhǔ yùn huà*, spleen governs movement and transformation

脾主肌肉、四肢〔脾主肌肉、四肢〕*pí zhǔ jī ròu, sì zhī*, spleen governs the flesh and limbs

肝气犯脾〔肝氣犯脾〕*gān qì fàn pí*, liver qì invading the spleen

痞〔痞〕pǐ 284
glomus

胸痞〔胸痞〕*xiōng pǐ*, glomus in the chest

偏〔偏〕piān 285
hemilateral (headache)

偏头痛〔偏頭痛〕*piān tóu tòng*, hemilateral headache

片〔片〕piàn 286
tablet

切片〔切片〕*qiē piàn*, slice

漂〔漂〕piǎo 287
long-rinsing

频〔頻〕pín 288
frequent

小便频数〔小便頻數〕*xiǎo biàn pín shuò*, frequent urination

平〔平〕píng 289
calm

平肝息风〔平肝息風〕*píng gān xī fēng*, calming the liver and extinguishing wind

破〔破〕pò 290
break, breaking

破血〔破血〕*pò xuè*, breaking blood

破气〔破氣〕*pò qì*, breaking qì

七〔七〕qī 291

seven

七情〔七情〕*qī qíng*, seven affects

脐〔臍〕qí 292

umbilicus

脐周窜痛〔臍周竄痛〕*qí zhōu cuàn tòng*, scurrying pain around the umbilicus

气〔氣〕qì 293

qì; breath, breathing

正气〔正氣〕*zhèng qì*, right qì

卫气〔衞氣〕*wèi qì*, defense qì

原气〔原氣〕*yuán qì*, source qì

邪气〔邪氣〕*xié qì*, evil qì

嗳气酸腐〔噯氣酸腐〕*ài qì suān fǔ*, belching of sour putrid qì (gas)

短气〔短氣〕*duǎn qì*, shortness of breath

气粗〔氣粗〕*qì cū*, rough breathing

瘛〔瘛〕qì 294

pulling

瘛瘲〔瘛瘲〕*qì zòng*, tugging and slackening

前〔前〕qián 295

before

饭前服〔飯前服〕*fàn qián fú*, take before meals

欠〔欠〕qiàn 296

lack

四肢欠温〔四肢欠溫〕*sì zhī qiàn wēn*, lack of warmth in the limbs

跷〔蹺〕qiāo 297

springing

阴跷（蹻）脉〔陰蹺（蹻）脈〕*yīn qiāo mài*, yīn springing vessel

蹻〔蹻〕qiāo 298

see previous entry

窍〔竅〕qiào 299

orifice

心开窍于舌〔心開竅於舌〕*xīn kāi qiào yú shé*, heart opens at the tongue

切〔切〕qiē 300

cut

切〔切〕qiè 301

take, feel

切脉〔切脈〕*qiè mài*, take the pulse

清〔清〕qīng 302

clear, clearing

脾主升清〔脾主升清〕*pí zhǔ shēng qīng*, spleen governs up-bearing of the clear

小肠主分别清浊〔小腸主分別清濁〕*xiǎo cháng zhǔ fēn bié qīng zhuó*, small intestine governs separation of the clear and turbid

痰多清稀〔痰多清稀〕*tán duō qīng xī*, copious clear thin phlegm

小便清长〔小便清長〕*xiǎo biàn qīng cháng*, long voidings of clear urine

清热解毒〔清熱解毒〕 *qīng rè jiě dú*, clearing heat and resolving toxin

青〔青〕qīng 303
green-blue

面色青紫〔面色青紫〕 *miàn sè qīng zǐ*, green-blue or purple facial complexion

轻〔輕〕qīng 304
light

轻宣润燥〔輕宣潤燥〕 *qīng xuān rùn zào*, moistening dryness by light diffusion

情〔情〕qíng 305
affects

七情〔七情〕 *qī qíng*, seven affects

内伤七情〔內傷七情〕 *nèi shāng qī qíng*, internal damage by the seven affects; affect damage

祛〔祛〕qū 306
dispel, dispelling

祛湿〔祛濕〕 *qū shī*, dispelling dampness

祛风化痰〔祛風化痰〕 *qū fēng huà tán*, dispelling wind and transforming phlegm

蜷〔踡〕quán 307
curled-up

向里蜷卧〔向裡踡臥〕 *xiàng lǐ quán wò*, lying in curled-up posture

扰〔擾〕rǎo 308
harass

痰浊上扰〔痰濁上擾〕 *tán zhuó shàng rǎo*, phlegm turbidity harassing the upper body

热〔熱〕rè 309
heat, fever

发热〔發熱〕 *fā rè*, heat effusion; fever

壮热〔壯熱〕 *zhuàng rè*, vigorous heat [effusion]; vigorous fever

表热〔表熱〕 *biǎo rè*, exterior heat

肝胆湿热〔肝膽濕熱〕 *gān dǎn shī rè*, liver-gallbladder damp-heat

任〔任〕rén 310
controlling

任脉〔任脈〕 *rèn mài*, controlling vessel

肉〔肉〕ròu 311
flesh

脱肉破䐃〔脫肉破䐃〕 *tuō ròu pò jiǒng (jùn)*, shedding of flesh and loss of bulk

濡〔濡〕rú 312
soggy

濡脉〔濡脈〕 *rú mài*, soggy pulse

乳〔乳〕rǔ 313
breast, nipple

乳头〔乳頭〕 *rǔ tóu*, nipple

乳蛾〔乳蛾〕 *rǔ é*, nipple moth; baby moth

入〔入〕rù 314
enter, entry

风邪入经〔風邪入經〕*fēng xié rù jīng*, wind evil entering the channels

热入心包〔熱入心包〕*rè rù xīn bāo*, heat entering the pericardium

软〔軟〕ruǎn 315

soften, softening; limp

软坚〔軟堅〕*ruǎn jiān*, softening hardness

腰膝软弱〔腰膝軟弱〕*yāo xī ruǎn ruò*, limp lumbus and knees

润〔潤〕rùn 316

moist

润下〔潤下〕*rùn xià*, moist precipitation

弱〔弱〕ruò 317

weak; limp

腰膝软弱〔腰膝軟弱〕*yāo xī ruǎn ruò*, limp lumbus and knees

弱脉〔弱脈〕*ruò mài*, weak pulse

三〔三〕sān 318

three, triple

三因〔三因〕*sān yīn*, three causes (of disease)

三焦〔三焦〕*sān jiāo*, triple burner

散〔散〕sǎn 319

powder

散〔散〕sàn 320

dissipate, dissipating, dissipated

散脉〔散脈〕*sàn mài*, dissipated pulse

色〔色〕sè 321

color; complexion

五色〔五色〕*wǔ sè*, five colors

塞〔塞〕sè 322

congestion

鼻塞〔鼻塞〕*bí sè*, nasal congestion

涩〔澀〕sè 323

astringe, astringent (therapeutic action); rough

涩脉〔澀脈〕*sè mài*, rough pulse

涩肠固脱〔澀腸固脫〕*sè cháng gù tuō*, astringing the intestines and stemming desertion

目干涩〔目乾澀〕*mù gān sè*, dry eyes

山〔山〕shān 324

mountain

烧山火〔燒山火〕*shāo shān huǒ*, burning mountain fire method

闪〔閃〕shǎn 325

flash

疝〔疝〕shàn 326

mounting

寒疝〔寒疝〕*hán shàn*, cold mounting

伤〔傷〕shāng 327

damage

伤津〔傷津〕*shāng jīn*, damage to liquid

烧〔燒〕shāo 328

burn

烧存性〔燒存性〕*shāo cún xìng,* nature-preservative burning

少〔少〕shǎo [329]
scant

小便短少〔小便短少〕*xiǎo biàn duǎn shǎo,* short voidings of scant urine

痰少不易咯〔痰少不易咯〕*tán shǎo bú yì kǎ,* scant phlegm expectorated with difficulty

月经过少〔月經過少〕*yuè jīng guò shǎo,* scant menstruation

少〔少〕shào [330]
lesser

少腹〔少腹〕*shào fù,* lesser abdomen

少阳〔少陽〕*shào yáng,* lesser yáng

舌〔舌〕shé [331]
tongue

心开窍于舌〔心開竅於舌〕*xīn kāi qiào yú shé,* heart opens at the tongue

舌质〔舌質〕*shé zhì,* tongue body

舌体〔舌體〕*shé tǐ,* tongue body

身〔身〕shēn [332]
body

身重〔身重〕*shēn zhòng,* heavy body; generalized heaviness

呻〔呻〕shēn [333]
groan

神〔神〕shén [334]
spirit

心藏神〔心藏神〕*xīn cáng shén,* heart stores the spirit

得神〔得神〕*dé shén,* spiritedness

肾〔腎〕shèn [335]
kidney

肾主水〔腎主水〕*shèn zhǔ shuǐ,* kidney governs water

肾藏精〔腎藏精〕*shèn cáng jīng,* kidney stores essence

肾主开阖〔腎主開闔〕*shèn zhǔ kāi hé,* kidney governs opening and closing

肺肾阴虚〔肺腎陰虛〕*fèi shèn yīn xū,* lung-kidney yīn vacuity

渗〔滲〕shèn [336]
percolate, percolating

利水渗湿〔利水滲濕〕*lì shuǐ shèn shī,* disinhibiting water and percolating dampness

生〔生〕shēng [337]
engender, engendering; raw, crude

过食生冷〔過食生冷〕*guò shí shēng lěng,* excessive consumption of raw and cold foods

相生〔相生〕*xiāng shēng,* engendering

肾生骨髓〔腎生骨髓〕*shèn shēng gǔ suí,* kidney engenders the bone and marrow

热极生风〔熱極生風〕*rè jí shēng fēng,* extreme heat engendering wind

升〔升〕shēng [338]
bearing upward, upbear

脾主升清 〔脾主升清〕 *pí zhǔ sheng qīng*, spleen governs upbearing of the clear

声 〔聲〕 shēng `339`
sound; voice; rale

声音嘶嗄 〔聲音嘶嗄〕 *shēng yīn sī shà*, hoarse voice

咳声重浊 〔咳聲重濁〕 *ké shēng zhòng zhuó*, heavy turbid cough sound

喉中有水鸡声 〔喉中有水雞聲〕 *hóu zhōng yǒu shuǐ jī shēng*, frog rale in the throat

胜 〔勝〕 shèng `340`
prevalent, overcome

祛风胜湿 〔祛風勝濕〕 *qū fēng shèng shī*, dispelling wind and overcoming dampness

盛 〔盛〕 shèng `341`
exuberant

火盛刑金 〔火盛刑金〕 *huǒ shèng xíng jīn*, exuberant fire tormenting metal

心火盛 〔心火盛〕 *xīn huǒ shèng*, exuberant heart fire

失 〔失〕 shī `342`
lose, loss

失精 〔失精〕 *shī jīng*, seminal loss

失神 〔失神〕 *shī shén*, spiritlessness

大便失禁 〔大便失禁〕 *dà biàn shī jìn*, fecal incontinence

失眠 〔失眠〕 *shī mián*, insomnia

月经失调 〔月經失調〕 *yuè jīng shī tiáo*, menstrual irregularities

脾失健运 〔脾失健運〕 *pí shī jiàn yùn*, spleen failing to move and transform

湿 〔濕〕 shī `343`
damp, dampness

水湿 〔水濕〕 *shuǐ shī*, water-damp

食 〔食〕 shí `344`
eat; food

暴饮暴食 〔暴飲暴食〕 *bào yǐn bào shí*, voracious eating and drinking

不思饮食 〔不思飲食〕 *bù sī yǐn shí*, no thought of food and drink

食远服 〔食遠服〕 *shí yuǎn fú*, take between meals

十 〔十〕 shí `345`
ten

十二经 〔十二經〕 *shí èr jīng*, twelve channels

实 〔實〕 shí `346`
repletion, replete

实脉 〔實脈〕 *shí mài*, replete pulse

表实 〔表實〕 *biǎo shí*, exterior repletion

石 〔石〕 shí `347`
stone

石淋 〔石淋〕 *shí lín*, stone strangury

使 〔使〕 shǐ `348`
courier

视 〔視〕 shì `349`
stare

直视〔直視〕*zhí shì*, forward-staring eyes

两目上视〔兩目上視〕*liǎng mù shàng shì*, upward staring eyes

手〔手〕shǒu 350
hand, arm

扬手掷足〔揚手擲足〕*yáng shǒu zhí zú*, flailing of the arms and legs

受〔受〕shòu 351
intake; contract, contraction

胃主受纳〔胃主受納〕*wèi zhǔ shòu nà*, stomach governs intake

感受燥邪〔感受燥邪〕*gǎn shòu zào xié*, contraction of dryness evil

疏〔疏〕shū 352
course, coursing

肝主疏泄〔肝主疏泄〕*gān zhǔ shū xiè*, liver governs free coursing

疏散外风〔疏散外風〕*shū sàn wài fēng*, coursing and dissipating external wind

熟〔熟〕shú 353
ripe, ripen; cooked

胃主腐熟〔胃主腐熟〕*wèi zhǔ fǔ shú*, stomach governs decomposition; stomach governs rotting and ripening

熟〔熟〕*shú*, cooked

暑〔暑〕shǔ 354
summerheat

暑热〔暑熱〕*shǔ rè*, summerheat-heat

衰〔衰〕shuāi 355
debilitated, debilitation

命门火衰〔命門火衰〕*mìng mén huǒ shuāi*, debilitation of the life gate fire

双〔雙〕shuāng 356
double, both

气血双补〔氣血雙補〕*qì xuè shuāng bǔ*, supplementing both qì and blood; dual supplementation of qì and blood

表里双解〔表裡雙解〕*biǎo lǐ shuāng jiě*, resolving both the exterior and interior; exterior-interior resolution

双蛾〔雙蛾〕*shuāng é*, double moth

霜〔霜〕shuāng 357
frost

制霜〔製霜〕*zhì shuāng*, frosting

水〔水〕shuǐ 358
water

水湿〔水濕〕*shuǐ shī*, water-damp

肺主通调水道〔肺主通調水道〕*fèi zhǔ tōng tiáo shuǐ dào*, lung governs regulation of the waterways

肾属水〔腎屬水〕*shèn shǔ shuǐ*, kidney belongs to water

大便水样〔大便水樣〕*dà biàn shuǐ yàng*, watery stool

睡〔睡〕shuì 359
sleep

昏睡〔昏睡〕*hūn shuì*, clouding sleep

瞤〔瞤〕shùn　360

twitching

筋惕肉瞤〔筋惕肉瞤〕*jīn tì ròu shùn*, jerking sinews and twitching flesh

顺〔順〕shùn　361

normalize

顺气化痰〔順氣化痰〕*shùn qì huà tán*, normalizing qì and transforming phlegm

数〔數〕shuò　362

rapid

数脉〔數脈〕*shuò mài*, rapid pulse

思〔思〕sī　363

thought

不思饮食〔不思飲食〕*bù sī yǐn shí*, no thought of food and drink

嘶〔嘶〕sī　364

hoarse

声音嘶嗄〔聲音嘶嗄〕*shēng yīn sī shà*, hoarse voice

宿〔宿〕sù　365

abide

宿食〔宿食〕*sù shí*, abiding food

肃〔肅〕sù　366

depurative

肺主肃降〔肺主肅降〕*fèi zhǔ sù jiàng*, lung governs depurative downbearing

酸〔酸〕suān　367

sour, acid

嗳气酸腐〔噯氣酸腐〕*ài qì suān fǔ*, belching of sour putrid qì (gas)

酸〔痠〕suān　368

ache

腰酸〔腰痠〕*yāo suān*, aching lumbus

髓〔髓〕suǐ　369

marrow

肾生骨髓〔腎生骨髓〕*shèn shēng gǔ suǐ*, kidney engenders the bone and marrow

髓海空虚〔髓海空虚〕*suǐ hǎi kōng xū*, emptiness of the sea of marrow

孙〔孫〕sūn　370

grandchild

孙络〔孫絡〕*sūn luò*, grandchild network vessel

缩〔縮〕suō　371

reduce, reducing

缩尿〔縮尿〕*suō niào*, reducing urine

苔〔苔〕tāi　372

fur

苔厚〔苔厚〕*tāi hòu*, thick fur

苔薄〔苔薄〕*tāi bó*, thin fur

苔垢〔苔垢〕*tāi gòu*, grimy fur

胎〔胎〕tāi　373

fetus

胎动不安 〔胎動不安〕 *tāi dòng bù ān*, stirring fetus

太 〔太〕 tài 374
greater

太阳 〔太陽〕 *tài yáng*, greater yáng

痰 〔痰〕 tán 375
phlegm

痰多清稀 〔痰多清稀〕 *tán duō qīng xī*, copious clear thin phlegm

湿痰 〔濕痰〕 *shī tán*, damp phlegm

炭 〔炭〕 tàn 376
charred

汤 〔湯〕 tāng 377
decoction

溏 〔溏〕 táng 378
sloppy

大便稀溏 〔大便稀溏〕 *dà biàn xī táng*, thin sloppy stool

疼 〔疼〕 téng 379
pain

关节疼痛 〔關節疼痛〕 *guān jié téng tòng*, joint pain

体 〔體〕 tǐ 380
body, constitution

形体肥胖 〔形體肥胖〕 *xíng tǐ féi pàng*, obesity

舌体 〔舌體〕 *shé tǐ*, tongue body

弟 〔涕〕 tì 381
snivel; nasal mucus

鼻流清涕 〔鼻流清涕〕 *bí liú qīng tì*, runny nose with clear snivel (nasal mucus)

嚏 〔嚏〕 tì 382
sneeze

多嚏 〔多嚏〕 *duō tì*, sneezing

甜 〔甜〕 tián 383
sweet, sweetness

口甜 〔口甜〕 *kǒu tián*, sweet taste in the mouth

田 〔田〕 tián 384
field

丹田 〔丹田〕 *dān tián*, cinnabar field

调 〔調〕 tiáo 385
regulate, regulation

肺主通调水道 〔肺主通調水道〕 *fèi zhǔ tōng tiáo shuǐ dào*, lung governs regulation of the waterways

调和肝脾 〔調和肝脾〕 *tiáo hé gān pí*, harmonizing the liver and spleen

月经失调 〔月經失調〕 *yuè jīng shī tiáo*, menstrual irregularities

统 〔統〕 tǒng 386
control; manage, management

脾不统血 〔脾不統血〕 *pí bù tǒng xuè*, spleen failing to control the blood

痛 〔痛〕 tòng 387
ache (in 'headache'), pain

头痛 〔頭痛〕 *tóu tòng*, headache

咽喉肿痛〔咽喉腫痛〕*yān hóu zhǒng tòng*, sore swollen throat

关节疼痛〔關節疼痛〕*guān jié téng tòng*, joint pain

腰痛〔腰痛〕*yāo tòng*, lumbar pain

头〔頭〕tóu [388]
head

正头痛〔正頭痛〕*zhèng tóu tòng*, medial headache

头身困重〔頭身困重〕*tóu shēn kùn zhòng*, heavy cumbersome head and body

头风〔頭風〕*tóu fēng*, head wind

乳头〔乳頭〕*rǔ tóu*, nipple

土〔土〕tǔ [389]
earth (soil)

脾属土〔脾屬土〕*pí shǔ tǔ*, spleen belongs to earth (soil)

吐〔吐〕tù [390]
vomiting

呕吐痰饮〔嘔吐痰飲〕*ǒu tù tán yǐn*, vomiting of phlegm-rheum

吐舌〔吐舌〕*tù shé*, protrusion of the tongue

推〔推〕tuī [391]
push

推罐〔推罐〕*tuī guàn*, push-cupping

腿〔腿〕tuǐ [392]
leg

腰酸腿软〔腰痠腿軟〕*yāo suān tuǐ ruǎn*, aching lumbus and limp legs

退〔退〕tuǐ [393]
retract

退针〔退針〕*tuì zhēn*, needle retraction

吞〔吞〕tūn [394]
swallow

吞酸〔吞酸〕*tūn suān*, swallowing of upflowing acid

豚〔豚〕tún [395]
piglet

奔豚〔奔豚〕*bēn tún*, running piglet

脱〔脫〕tuō [396]
desert, desertion; prolapse; shed, shedding

阳脱〔陽脫〕*yáng tuō*, yáng desertion

气随血脱〔氣隨血脫〕*qì suí xuè tuō*, qì deserting with the blood

脱肛〔脫肛〕*tuō gāng*, prolapse of the rectum

脱肉破䐃〔脫肉破䐃〕*tuō ròu pò jiǒng (jùn)*, shedding of flesh and loss of bulk

唾〔唾〕tuò [397]
spittle

喎〔喎〕wāi [398]
deviated, deviation

口眼喎斜〔口眼喎斜〕*kǒu yǎn wāi xié*, deviated eyes and mouth

外〔外〕wài [399]
external

外因 〔外因〕 *wài yīn*, external cause

丸 〔丸〕 **wán** 400
pill

脘 〔脘〕 **wǎn** 401
stomach duct

脘腹痛喜按 〔脘腹痛喜按〕 *wǎn fù tòng xǐ àn*, pain in the stomach duct and abdomen that likes pressure

腕 〔腕〕 **wàn** 402
wrist

亡 〔亡〕 **wáng** 403
collapse

亡血 〔亡血〕 *wáng xuè*, blood collapse

亡阴 〔亡陰〕 *wáng yīn*, yīn collapse

妄 〔妄〕 **wàng** 404
frenetic

血热妄行 〔血熱妄行〕 *xuè rè wàng xíng*, frenetic movement of hot blood

望 〔望〕 **wàng** 405
inspect

望神 〔望神〕 *wàng shén*, inspecting the spirit

微 〔微〕 **wēi** 406
faint; slight; light

微脉 〔微脈〕 *wēi mài*, faint pulse

目窠上微肿 〔目窠上微腫〕 *mù kē shàng wēi zhǒng*, slight swelling of the eye nest

微炒 〔微炒〕 *wēi chǎo*, light stir-frying

煨 〔煨〕 **wēi** 407
roasting

维 〔維〕 **wéi** 408
linking

阴维脉 〔陰維脈〕 *yīn wéi mài*, yīn linking vessel

痿 〔痿〕 **wěi** 409
wilt, wilting

痿证 〔痿證〕 *wěi zhèng*, wilting pattern

肺痿 〔肺痿〕 *fèi wěi*, lung wilting

阳痿 〔陽痿〕 *yáng wěi*, impotence; yáng wilt

味 〔味〕 **wèi** 410
flavor

性味 〔性味〕 *xìng wèi*, nature and flavor

胃 〔胃〕 **wèi** 411
stomach

胃之大络 〔胃之大絡〕 *wèi zhī dà luò*, great network vessel of the stomach

肠胃积滞 〔腸胃積滯〕 *cháng wèi jī zhì*, gastrointestinal accumulation

卫 〔衛〕 **wèi** 412
defense

卫气 〔衛氣〕 *wèi qì*, defense qì

卫分证 〔衛分證〕 *wèi fēn zhèng*, defense-aspect pattern

温 〔溫〕 **wēn** 413
warm, warming, warmth

四肢欠温 〔四肢欠溫〕 *sì zhī qiàn wēn,* lack of warmth in the limbs

温邪 〔溫邪〕 *wēn xié,* warm evil

腹痛喜温 〔腹痛喜溫〕 *fù tòng xǐ wēn,* abdominal pain that likes warmth

辛温解表 〔辛溫解表〕 *xīn wēn jiě biǎo,* resolving the exterior with warmth and acridity

卧 〔臥〕 **wò** 414

sleep

向里蜷卧 〔向裡踡臥〕 *xiàng lǐ quán wò,* lying in curled-up posture

不得卧 〔不得臥〕 *bù dé wò,* sleeplessness

五 〔五〕 **wǔ** 415

five

五俞穴 〔五兪穴〕 *wǔ shū xué,* five transport points

恶 〔惡〕 **wù** 416

averse to, aversion to

恶寒 〔惡寒〕 *wù hán,* aversion to cold

侮 〔侮〕 **wǔ** 417

rebel, rebellion

膝 〔膝〕 **xī** 418

knee

腰膝软弱 〔腰膝軟弱〕 *yāo xī ruǎn ruò,* limp lumbus and knees

稀 〔稀〕 **xī** 419

thin (phlegm, stool)

痰多清稀 〔痰多清稀〕 *tán duō qīng xī,* copious clear thin phlegm

息 〔息〕 **xī** 420

breathe, breathing

肩息 〔肩息〕 *jiān xī,* raised-shoulder breathing

叹息 〔嘆息〕 *tàn xī,* sighing

熄 〔熄〕 **xī** 421

extinguish, extinguishing

潜阳熄风 〔潛陽熄風〕 *qián yáng xī fēng,* subduing yáng and extinguishing wind

喜 〔喜〕 **xǐ** 422

joy, like

渴喜凉饮 〔渴喜涼飲〕 *kě xǐ liáng yǐn,* thirst with a liking for cool drinks

脘腹痛喜按 〔脘腹痛喜按〕 *wǎn fù tòng xǐ àn,* pain in the stomach duct and abdomen that likes pressure

洗 〔洗〕 **xǐ** 423

wash, washing

细 〔細〕 **xì** 424

fine

细脉 〔細脈〕 *xì mài,* fine pulse

下 〔下〕 **xià** 425

below; lower; down; precipitate, precipitation

心下 〔心下〕 *xīn xià,* [region] below the heart

下合穴 〔下合穴〕 *xià hé xué,* lower uniting point

食不下〔食不下〕*shí bù xià*, inability to get food down

寒下〔寒下〕*hán xià*, cold precipitation

先〔先〕xiān 426
advanced

月经先期〔月經先期〕*yuè jīng xiān qī*, advanced menstruation (early periods)

涎〔涎〕xián 427
drool

口角流涎〔口角流涎〕*kǒu jiǎo liú xián*, drooling from the corners of the mouth

咸〔鹹〕xián 428
salty, saltiness

弦〔弦〕xián 429
stringlike

弦脉〔弦脈〕*xián mài*, stringlike pulse

痫〔癇〕xián 430
epilepsy

癫痫〔癲癇〕*diān xián*, epilepsy

癣〔癬〕xiǎn 431
lichen

陷〔陷〕xiàn 432
fall (center qì); sunken (eyes); depressed (fontanel)

中气下陷〔中氣下陷〕*zhōng qì xià xiàn*, center qì fall

目窠内陷〔目窠內陷〕*mù kē nèi xiàn*, sunken eyes

囟门下陷〔囟門下陷〕*xìn mén xià xiàn*, depressed fontanel gate

相〔相〕xiāng 433
each other

肺与大肠相表里〔肺與大腸相表裡〕*fèi yǔ dà cháng xiāng biǎo lǐ*, lung and large intestine stand in interior-exterior relationship

项〔項〕xiàng 434
nape

颈项强直〔頸項強直〕*jǐng xiàng jiàng zhí*, rigidity of the neck

相〔相〕xiàng 435
ministerial

相火〔相火〕*xiàng huǒ*, ministerial fire

消〔消〕xiāo 436
disperse, dispersing, dispersion

消渴〔消渴〕*xiāo kě*, dispersion-thirst

消食〔消食〕*xiāo shí*, dispersing food

哮〔哮〕xiāo 437
wheezing

哮喘〔哮喘〕*xiāo chuǎn*, wheezing and panting

小〔小〕xiǎo 438
small, smaller

小肠〔小腸〕*xiǎo cháng*, small intestine

小腹〔小腹〕*xiǎo fù*, smaller abdomen

邪〔邪〕xié 439
evil

邪气〔邪氣〕*xié qì*, evil qi

胁〔脅〕xié 440

rib-side

胁痛〔脅痛〕*xié tòng*, rib-side pain

斜〔斜〕xié 441

deviated, deviation

口眼㖞斜〔口眼㖞斜〕*kǒu yǎn wāi xié*, deviated eyes and mouth

泄〔泄〕xiè 442

discharge; diarrhea; ejaculation

疏风泄热〔疏風泄熱〕*shū fēng xiè rè*, coursing wind and discharging heat

泄泻〔泄瀉〕*xiè xiè*, diarrhea

五更泄〔五更泄〕*wǔ gēng xiè*, fifth-watch diarrhea

早泄〔早洩〕*zǎo xiè*, premature ejaculation

肝主疏泄〔肝主疏泄〕*gān zhǔ shū xiè*, liver governs free coursing

泻〔瀉〕xiè 443

drain; diarrhea

泄泻〔泄瀉〕*xiè xiè*, diarrhea

实则泻之〔實則瀉之〕*shí zé xiè zhī*, repletion is treated by draining

辛〔辛〕xīn 444

acrid, acridity

辛温解表〔辛溫解表〕*xīn wēn jiě biǎo*, resolving the exterior with warmth and acridity

心〔心〕xīn 445

heart

心主血脉〔心主血脈〕*xīn zhǔ xuè mài*, heart governs the blood and vessels

囟〔囟〕xìn 446

fontanel

囟门〔囟門〕*xìn mén*, fontanel gate, anterior fontanel

形〔形〕xíng 447

body; physical

形体肥胖〔形體肥胖〕*xíng tǐ féi pàng*, obesity

形寒〔形寒〕*xíng hán*, physical cold

形倦神怠〔形倦神怠〕*xíng juàn shén dài*, physical fatigue and lassitude of spirit

行〔行〕xíng 448

movement; phase

血热妄行〔血熱妄行〕*xuè rè wàng xíng*, frenetic movement of hot blood

五行〔五行〕*wǔ xíng*, five phases

性〔性〕xìng 449

nature

四性〔四性〕*sì xìng*, four natures

胸〔胸〕xiōng 450

chest

胸痛〔胸痛〕*xiōng tòng*, chest pain

虚〔虚〕xū 451

vacuity, vacuous

虚里〔虚里〕*xū lǐ,* vacuous lǐ

虚脉〔虚脈〕*xū mài,* vacuous pulse

表虚〔表虚〕*biǎo xū,* exterior vacuity

宣〔宣〕xuān 452
diffuse

肺气不宣〔肺氣不宣〕*fèi qì bù xuān,* nondiffusion of lung qì

眩〔眩〕xuàn 453
dizzy, dizziness

眩晕〔眩暈〕*xuàn yūn,* dizziness

穴〔穴〕xué 454
acupuncture point

穴道〔穴道〕*xué dào,* acupuncture point

血〔血〕xuè 455
blood

瘀血〔瘀血〕*yū xuè,* static blood

牙〔牙〕yá 456
tooth; dental

牙齿〔牙齒〕*yá chǐ,* tooth (*n.*); dental (*adj.*)

咽〔咽〕yān 457
pharynx, pharyngeal; throat

咽喉肿痛〔咽喉腫痛〕*yān hóu zhǒng tòng,* sore swollen throat

言〔言〕yán 458
speak, speech

懒言〔懶言〕*lǎn yán,* laziness to speak

炎〔炎〕yán 459
flame

心火上炎〔心火上炎〕*xīn huǒ shàng yán,* heart fire flaming upward

眼〔眼〕yǎn 460
eye

口眼㖞斜〔口眼㖞斜〕*kǒu yǎn wāi xié,* deviated eyes and mouth

厌〔厭〕yàn 461
averse, aversion to (food)

厌食〔厭食〕*yàn shí,* aversion to food

阳〔陽〕yáng 462
yáng

太阳〔太陽〕*tài yáng,* greater yáng

养〔養〕yǎng 463
nourish, nourishing

养阴〔養陰〕*yǎng yīn,* nourishing yīn

腰〔腰〕yāo 464
lumbus; lumbar

腰痛〔腰痛〕*yāo tòng,* lumbar pain

摇〔搖〕yáo 465
shaking

头摇〔頭搖〕*tóu yáo,* shaking of the head

药〔藥〕yào 466
medicine, medicinal

药膏〔藥膏〕*yào gāo,* medicinal paste

噎〔噎〕yē 467
dysphagia

噎膈 〔噎膈〕 *yē gé*, dysphagia-occlusion

液 〔液〕 yè 468
humor

五液 〔五液〕 *wǔ yè*, five humors

遗 〔遺〕 yí 469
emission

遗精 〔遺精〕 *yí jīng*, seminal emission

遗尿 〔遺尿〕 *yí niào*, enuresis

益 〔益〕 yì 470
boost, boosting

益气 〔益氣〕 *yì qì*, boosting qì

阴 〔陰〕 yīn 471
yīn

少阴 〔少陰〕 *shào yīn*, lesser yīn

阴虚 〔陰虛〕 *yīn xū*, yīn vacuity

因 〔因〕 yīn 472
cause

三因 〔三因〕 *sān yīn*, three causes (of disease)

音 〔音〕 yīn 473
sound; voice

声音嘶嗄 〔聲音嘶嗄〕 *shēng yīn sī shà*, hoarse voice

龈 〔齦〕 yín 474
gum

齿龈 〔齒齦〕 *chǐ yín*, gum

齿龈结瓣 〔齒齦結瓣〕 *chǐ yín jié bàn*, petaled gums

淫 〔淫〕 yín 475
excess

六淫 〔六淫〕 *liù yín*, six excesses

吟 〔吟〕 yín 476
groan

呻吟 〔呻吟〕 *shēn yín*, groaning

饮 〔飲〕 yǐn 477
drink; fluid intake; rheum

暴饮暴食 〔暴飲暴食〕 *bào yǐn bào shí*, voracious eating and drinking

渴不多饮 〔渴不多飲〕 *kě bù duō yǐn*, thirst without large fluid intake

饮食不节 〔飲食不節〕 *yǐn shí bù jié*, dietary irregularities

痰饮 〔痰飲〕 *tán yǐn*, phlegm-rheum

营 〔營〕 yíng 478
construction

营气 〔營氣〕 *yíng qì*, construction qì

瘿 〔癭〕 yǐng 479
goiter

瘿 〔癭〕 *yǐng*, goiter

痈 〔癰〕 yōng 480
welling-abscess

肺痈 〔肺癰〕 *fèi yōng*, pulmonary welling-abscess

痈 〔癰〕 yōng 481
welling-abscess

忧 〔憂〕 yōu 482
anxiety

瘀 〔瘀〕 yū 483
stasis, static

瘀血〔瘀血〕*yū xuè*, static blood

血瘀〔血瘀〕*xuè yū*, blood stasis

语〔語〕yǔ 484

talk, speak, speech

独语〔獨語〕*dú yǔ*, soliloquy; talking alone

欲〔欲〕yù 485

desire

渴不欲饮〔渴不欲飲〕*kě bù yù yǐn*, thirst with no desire to drink

郁〔鬱〕yù 486

depressed, depression

肝气郁结〔肝氣鬱結〕*gān qì yù jié*, binding depression of liver qì

育〔育〕yù 487

foster, fostering

育阴〔育陰〕*yù yīn*, fostering yīn

元〔元〕yuán 488

origin(al)

真元〔眞元〕*zhēn yuán*, true origin

原〔原〕yuán 489

source

膜原〔膜原〕*mó yuán*, membrane source

月〔月〕yuè 490

month, in 月经 *yuè jīng*, menses, menstruation, menstrual

月经过少〔月經過少〕*yuè jīng guò shǎo*, scant menstruation

晕〔暈〕yūn 491

dizzy; dizziness

眩晕〔眩暈〕*xuàn yūn*, dizziness

晕〔暈〕yùn 492

sickness

晕针〔暈針〕*yùn zhēn*, needle sickness

运〔運〕yùn 493

move, movement

脾主运化〔脾主運化〕*pí zhǔ yùn huà*, spleen governs movement and transformation

孕〔孕〕yùn 494

pregnant, pregnancy

不孕〔不孕〕*bù yùn*, infertility

蕴〔蘊〕yùn 495

brew, brewing

湿热蕴结肝胆〔濕熱蘊結肝膽〕*shī rè yùn jié gān dǎn*, damp-heat brewing in the liver and gallbladder

杂〔雜〕zá 496

miscellaneous

杂病〔雜病〕*zá bìng*, miscellaneous disease

脏〔臟〕zàng 497

viscus, visceral

脏腑之气〔臟腑之氣〕*zàng fǔ zhī qì*, bowel and visceral qì

糟〔糟〕zāo 498

waste

大肠主传化糟粕〔大腸主傳化糟粕〕 *dà cháng zhǔ chuán huà zāo pò*, large intestine governs the conveyance and transformation of waste

早〔早〕zǎo [499]
premature

头发早白〔頭髮早白〕 *tóu fà zǎo bái*, premature graying of the hair

燥〔燥〕zào [500]
dry, drying, dryness

牙齿干燥如枯骨〔牙齒乾燥如枯骨〕 *yá chǐ gān zào rú kū gǔ*, teeth dry as desiccated bones

感受燥邪〔感受燥邪〕 *gǎn shòu zào xié*, contraction of dryness evil

燥湿〔燥濕〕 *zào shī*, drying dampness

躁〔躁〕zào [501]
agitation

憎〔憎〕zēng [502]
abhor, abhorrence

憎寒〔憎寒〕 *zēng hán*, abhorrence of cold

谵〔譫〕zhān [503]
delirious

谵言〔譫言〕 *zhān yán*, delirious speech

战〔戰〕zhàn [504]
shiver

战汗〔戰汗〕 *zhàn hàn*, shiver sweating

胀〔脹〕zhàng [505]
distention

头胀〔頭脹〕 *tóu zhàng*, distention in the head

腹胀〔腹脹〕 *fù zhàng*, abdominal distention

折〔折〕zhé [506]
break, breakage

折针〔折針〕 *zhé zhēn*, needle breakage

真〔眞〕zhēn [507]
true

真元〔眞元〕 *zhēn yuán*, true origin

针〔針〕zhēn [508]
needle

疹〔疹〕zhěn [509]
papules

斑疹〔斑疹〕 *bān zhěn*, maculopapular eruption

诊〔診〕zhěn [510]
examination

四诊〔四診〕 *sì zhěn*, four examinations

望诊〔望診〕 *wàng zhěn*, inspection

镇〔鎭〕zhèn [511]
settle, settling

重镇安神〔重鎭安神〕 *zhòng zhèn ān shén*, quieting the spirit with heavy settlers

蒸〔蒸〕zhēng [512]
steam, steaming

骨蒸潮热 〔骨蒸潮熱〕 *gǔ zhēng cháo rè*, steaming bone tidal heat [effusion]; steaming bone tidal fever

癥 〔癥〕 zhēng ☐513

concretion

癥瘕积聚 〔癥瘕積聚〕 *zhēng jiǎ jī jù*, concretions, conglomerations, accumulations, and gatherings

正 〔正〕 zhèng ☐514

right (qì); straight (treatment); medial (headache)

正气 〔正氣〕 *zhèng qì*, right qì

正头痛 〔正頭痛〕 *zhèng tóu tòng*, medial headache

正治 〔正治〕 *zhèng zhì*, straight treatment

证 〔證〕 zhèng ☐515

sign; pattern

表证 〔表證〕 *biǎo zhèng*, exterior pattern

病证 〔病證〕 *bìng zhèng*, disease pattern

症 〔症〕 zhèng ☐516

pathocondition

肢 〔肢〕 zhī ☐517

limb

肢倦 〔肢倦〕 *zhī juàn*, fatigued limbs

四肢困倦 〔四肢困倦〕 *sì zhī kùn juàn*, fatigued cumbersome limbs

止 〔止〕 zhǐ ☐518

check, checking (vaginal discharge); suppress, suppressing (cough); stanch, stanching (bleeding)

止带 〔止帶〕 *zhǐ dài*, checking vaginal discharge

化痰止咳 〔化痰止咳〕 *huà tán zhǐ ké*, transforming phlegm and suppressing cough

止血 〔止血〕 *zhǐ xuè*, stanching bleeding

止痛 〔止痛〕 *zhǐ tòng*, relieving pain

治 〔治〕 zhì ☐519

treat, treatment; control, controlling

治本 〔治本〕 *zhì běn*, treating the root

反治 〔反治〕 *fǎn zhì*, paradoxical treatment

治风化痰 〔治風化痰〕 *zhì fēng huà tán*, controlling wind and transforming phlegm

滞 〔滯〕 zhì ☐520

stagnation

气滞 〔氣滯〕 *qì zhì*, qì stagnation

炙 〔炙〕 zhì ☐521

mix-fry

制 〔製〕 zhì ☐522

process, processing

水制 〔水製〕 *shuǐ zhì*, water processing

中 〔中〕 zhōng ☐523

center

温中散寒〔溫中散寒〕*wēn zhōng sàn hán*, warming the center and dissipating cold

口中和〔口中和〕*kǒu zhōng hé*, harmony of mouth

肿〔腫〕zhǒng [524]
swelling

水肿〔水腫〕*shuǐ zhǒng*, water swelling

中〔中〕zhòng [525]
strike, stroke

中风〔中風〕*zhòng fēng*, wind stroke; wind strike

重〔重〕zhòng [526]
heavy, heaviness

身重〔身重〕*shēn zhòng*, heavy body; generalized heaviness

周〔周〕zhōu [527]
generalized

周痹〔周痹〕*zhōu bì*, generalized impediment

肘〔肘〕zhǒu [528]
elbow

逐〔逐〕zhú [529]
expel

逐瘀〔逐瘀〕*zhú yū*, expelling stasis

主〔主〕zhǔ [530]
govern

心主血脉〔心主血脈〕*xīn zhǔ xuè mài*, heart governs the blood and vessels

煮〔煮〕zhǔ [531]
boil

注〔注〕zhù [532]
pour

湿热下注大肠〔濕熱下注大腸〕*shī rè xià zhù dà cháng*, damp-heat pouring down into the large intestine

炷〔炷〕zhù [533]
cone

助〔助〕zhù [534]
assist

助阳〔助陽〕*zhù yáng*, assisting yáng

爪〔爪〕zhuǎ [535]
nail

肝，其华在爪〔肝，其華在爪〕*gān, qí huá zài zhǎo*, liver... its bloom is in the nails

转〔轉〕zhuǎn [536]
turn, convert

转胞〔轉胞〕*zhuǎn bāo*, shifted bladder

阴阳转化〔陰陽轉化〕*yīn yáng zhuǎn huà*, yīn and yáng convert into each other

捻转补泻〔捻轉補瀉〕*niǎn zhuǎn bǔ xiè*, twirling supplementation and drainage

壮〔壯〕zhuàng [537]
vigorous

壮热〔壯熱〕*zhuàng rè*, vigorous heat [effusion]; vigorous fever

浊〔濁〕zhuó [538]
turbid, turbidity

胃主降浊〔胃主降濁〕*wèi zhǔ jiàng zhuó*, stomach governs downbearing of the turbid

着〔著〕zhuó 539
fixed

着痹〔著痹〕*zhuó bì*, fixed impediment

滋〔滋〕zī 540
enrich, enriching

滋阴〔滋陰〕*zī yīn*, enriching yīn

膏滋〔膏滋〕*gāo zī*, rich paste

子〔子〕zǐ 541
child

无子〔無子〕*wú zǐ*, childlessness

紫〔紫〕zǐ 542
purple

面色青紫〔面色青紫〕*miàn sè qīng zǐ*, green-blue or purple facial complexion

自〔自〕zì 543
spontaneous

自汗〔自汗〕*zì hàn*, spontaneous sweating

总〔總〕zǒng 544
command

四总穴〔四總穴〕*sì zǒng xué*, four command points

瘲〔瘲〕zòng 545
slackening

瘛瘲〔瘛瘲〕*qì zòng*, tugging and slackening

足〔足〕zú 546
foot; leg

扬手掷足〔揚手擲足〕*yáng shǒu zhí zú*, flailing of the arms and legs

足阳明经〔足陽明經〕*zú yáng míng jīng*, foot yáng brightness channel

阻〔阻〕zǔ 547
obstruct, obstruction

湿阻〔濕阻〕*shī zǔ*, damp obstruction

佐〔佐〕zuǒ 548
assistant

附录四：习题搭案
Appendix IV: Key to Questions

Chapter 1

1. The liver, heart, spleen, lung, kidney; gallbladder, small intestine, stomach, large intestine, bladder, triple burner.
2. Muscles, tendons, and ligaments.
3. Drool is thin and associated with the spleen; spittle is thick and associated with the kidney.
4. Acrid.
5. The upper abdomen is above the umbilicus; the lower abdomen below it.
6. Kidney yáng.
7. The eyes, ears, nostrils, and mouth (clear orifices); the anal and genital orifices (turbid orifices).
8. The kidney.
9. The "grain" of the skin, flesh, and organs or the connective tissue in the skin and flesh.
10. They are difficult to cure.
11. In the chest.
12. Wood.
13. Yellow.
14. Fire is heat in the environment; summerheat is specifically the heat of summer.
15. A thin form of phlegm.
16. Wind.
17. The heart.
18. Dampness.
19. Construction qì.
20. Evil qì.
21. Phlegm.
22. The lumbus.
23. The spirit.
24. Liquid is thin; humor is thick.
25. In the region of the chest or diaphragm (not clearly defined).
26. The bladder.
27. The liver.
28. Anterior fontanel.
29. The spleen.
30. Water.
31. *Páng guāng*; bladder.
32. *Mìng mén*; life gate.
33. *Yuán qì*; original qì.
34. *Xiōng*; chest.
35. *Hóu guān*; throat pass.
36. *Jié hóu*; laryngeal prominence.
37. *Xuán yōng chuí*; uvula.
38. *Yín*; gum.
39. *Xiǎo cháng*; small intestine.
40. *Dǎn*; gallbladder.
41. *Gé*; diaphragm.
42. *Xìn*; fontanel.
43. *Xié*; rib-side.
44. *Nèi shāng qī qíng*; internal damage by the seven affects; affect damage.
45. *Bù nèi wài yīn*; neutral causes.
46. *Zàng fǔ zhī qì*; bowel and visceral qì.
47. *Mó yuán*; membrane source.
48. *Xī*; knee.
49. *Fù*; abdomen.
50. *Jiān*; shoulder.
51. 怒; anger.
52. 头; head.
53. 会厌; epiglottis.
54. 胁; rib-side.
55. 虚里; Vacuous lǐ.
56. 胃脘; stomach duct.
57. 踝; ankle.
58. 肘; elbow.

59. 腠理; interstices.
60. 经络之气; channel and network vessel qì.
61. 大便; stool.
62. 风; wind.
63. 气化; qì transformation.
64. 牙齿; teeth.
65. 心包络; pericardium.
66. 大腹; greater abdomen.
67. 喉核; throat node.
68. 正气; right qì.
69. 津液; liquid and humor (fluids).
70. 神; spirit.
71. 原气; *yuán qì.*
72. 尿、小便; *niào, xiǎo biàn.*
73. 肢; *zhī.*
74. 手; *shǒu.*
75. 心下; *xīn xià.*
76. 大肠; *dà cháng.*
77. 恐; *kǒng.*
78. 三焦. *sān jiāo.*
79. 涕; *tì.*
80. 苦; *kǔ.*
81. 汗; *hàn.*
82. 唇; *chún.*
83. 囟; *xìn.*
84. 少腹; *shào fù.*
85. 窍; *qiào.*
86. 元气; *yuán qì.*
87. 营气; *yíng qì.*
88. 大便; *dà biàn.*
89. 胁; *xié.*
90. 膈; *gé.*

Chapter 2

91. Network vessels.
92. Greater yáng (*tài yáng*) channel (SI, BL); yáng brightness (*yáng míng*) (LI, ST); lesser yáng (*shào yáng*) (TB, GB); greater yīn (*tài yīn*) (LU, SP); lesser yīn (*shào yīn*) (HT, KI); reverting yīn (*jué yīn*) (PC, LR).
93. The controlling, governing, thoroughfare, girdling, yīn springing, yáng springing, yīn linking, and yáng linking vessels.
94. Hand lesser yáng heart channel.
95. ST-36 (*zú sān lǐ,* Leg Three Li), BL-40 (*wěi zhōng,* Bend Center), LU-7 (*liè quē,* Broken Sequence), and LI-4 (*hé gǔ,* Union Valley).
96. Hand lesser yáng (*shào yáng*) triple burner channel.
97. The large intestine and the stomach.
98. The triple burner and the gallbladder.
99. The heart and small intestine.
100. The controlling vessel.
101. The controlling vessel.
102. The yáng springing vessel.
103. The yīn linking vessel.
104. The foot lesser yīn (*shào yīn*) kidney channel.
105. The girdling vessel.
106. The well, brook (spring), stream, channel (river), and uniting points.
107. The foot greater yáng *tài yáng* bladder channel.
108. PC-6 (*nèi guān,* Inner Pass).
109. ST-39 (*xià jù xū,* Lower Great Hollow).
110. Governing vessel.
111. *Yuán xué;* source point.
112. *Tóng shēn cùn;* body inch.
113. *Jiāo huì xué;* intersection point.
114. *Luò xué;* network point.
115. *Tài yīn;* greater yīn.
116. *Shǔ luò;* homing and netting.
117. *mù xué;* alarm point; mustering point.
118. *Sì zǒng xué;* four command points.
119. *Shí èr jīng jīn;* twelve channel sinews.

120. *Jīng luò*; channels and network vessels.
121. *Wèi zhī dà luò*; great network vessel of the stomach.
122. *Yáng míng*; yáng brightness.
123. *Xué dào*; acupuncture point.
124. *yáng qiāo mài*; yáng springing vessel.
125. *shū xué*; transport point.
126. *Xià hé xué*; lower uniting point.
127. *Jué yīn*; reverting yīn.
128. *Rèn mài*; controlling vessel.
129. *Yīn wéi mài*; yīn linking vessel.
130. *Dài mài*; girdling vessel.
131. 十二经; the twelve channels.
132. 十五络; the fifteen network vessels.
133. 浮络; the superficial network vessels.
134. 少阴; lesser yīn.
135. 阴跷（蹻）脉; yīn springing vessel.
136. 背俞; back transport points.
137. 下合穴; lower uniting points.
138. 五俞穴; five transport points.
139. 孙络; grandchild network vessels.
140. 经穴; channel points.
141. 井穴; well points.
142. 十二经筋; twelve channel sinews.
143. 荥穴; brook points.
144. 脾之大络; great network vessel of the spleen.
145. 络脉; network vessel.
146. 太阳; greater yáng.
147. 络穴; network points.
148. 同身寸; body inch.
149. 交会穴; intersection point.
150. 冲脉; thoroughfare vessel.
151. 阴维脉; *yīn wéi mài*.
152. 任脉; *rèn mài*.
153. 冲脉; *chōng mài*.
154. 阳维脉; *yáng wéi mài*.
155. 募穴; *mù xué*.

156. 同身寸; *tóng shēn cùn*.
157. 脾之大络; *pí zhī dà luò*.
158. 十五大络; *shí wǔ dà luò*.
159. 督脉; *dū mài*.
160. 经穴; *jīng xué*.
161. 合穴; *hé xué*.
162. 厥阴; *jué yīn*.
163. 阳明; *yáng míng*.
164. 十二经筋; *shí èr jīng jīn*.
165. 奇经八脉; *qí jīng bā mài*.
166. 五俞穴; *wǔ shū xué*.
167. 四总穴; *sì zǒng xué*.
168. 阴跷（蹻）脉; *yīn qiāo mài*.
169. 浮络; *fú luò*.
170. 拔火罐; *bá huǒ guàn*.

Chapter 3

171. The kidney.
172. The heart.
173. The lung.
174. The stomach.
175. The liver.
176. The small intestine.
177. The small intestine.
178. The kidney.
179. The liver.
180. The liver.
181. The liver.
182. The kidney.
183. The large intestine.
184. The kidney.
185. The kidney.
186. The liver.
187. The brain.
188. The triple burner.
189. Wood.
190. The kidney.
191. The stomach.
192. The kidney.
193. The thoroughfare (*chōng*) and controlling (*rèn*) vessels.
194. The small intestine.
195. The lung.

196. The anal and genital orifices.
197. The spleen.
198. The liver.
199. Metal.
200. They stand in interior-exterior relationship.
201. *Zǐ gōng*; uterus.
202. *Wèi zhǔ shòu nà*; the stomach governs intake.
203. *Sān jiāo*; triple burner.
204. *Shèn cáng jīng*; the kidney stores essence.
205. *Shèn kāi qiào yú ěr*; the kidney opens at the ears.
206. *Nǎo*; brain.
207. *Shèn yǔ páng guāng xiāng biǎo lǐ*; the kidney and bladder stand in interior-exterior relationship.
208. *Fèi zhǔ pí máo*; the lung governs the skin and [body] hair.
209. *Fèi zhǔ qì*; the lung governs qì.
210. *Gān kāi qiào yú mù*; the liver opens at the eyes.
211. *Fèi zhǔ tōng tiáo shuǐ dào*; the lung governs regulation of the waterways.
212. *Xīn kāi qiào yú shé*; the heart opens at the tongue.
213. *Gān zhǔ jīn*; the liver governs the sinews.
214. *Pí shǔ tǔ*; the spleen governs earth.
215. *Gān cáng xuè*; the liver stores blood.
216. *Shèn zhǔ kāi hé*; the kidney governs opening and closing.
217. *Pí zhǔ yùn huà*; the spleen governs movement and transformation.
218. *Gān shǔ mù*; the liver belongs to wood.
219. *Sān jiāo zhǔ jué dú*; the triple burner governs the sluices.

220. *Xīn zhǔ xuè mài*; the heart governs the blood and vessels.
221. 肾开窍于二阴; the kidney opens at the two yīn.
222. 肝主疏泻; the liver governs free coursing.
223. 大肠主传化糟粕; the large intestine governs the conveyance and transformation of waste.
224. 女子胞; uterus.
225. 大肠主津; the large intestine governs liquid.
226. 胃主降浊; the stomach governs the downbearing of the turbid.
227. 肾主骨; the kidney governs the bone.
228. 小肠主液; the small intestine governs humor.
229. 肾，其充在骨; the kidney... its fullness is in the bone.
230. 胃主腐熟; the stomach governs rotting and ripening (decomposition).
231. 脾属土; the spleen belongs to earth.
232. 肝属木; the liver belongs to wood.
233. 小肠主分别清浊; the small intestine governs separation of the clear and turbid.
234. 脾，其华在唇四白; the spleen... its bloom is in the four whites of the lips.
235. 脾开窍于口; the spleen opens at the mouth.
236. 肝主筋; *gān zhǔ jīn*.
237. 运化; *yùn huà*.
238. 心开窍于舌; *xīn kāi qiào yú shé*.
239. 肺主肃降; *fèi zhǔ sù jiàng*.
240. 脾主肌肉、四肢; *pí zhǔ jī ròu, sì zhī*.
241. 肺开窍于鼻; *fèi kāi qiào yú bí*.
242. 脾主升清; *pí zhǔ shēng qīng*.

243. 大肠主传化糟粕; *dà chǎng zhǔ chuán huà zāo pò.*
244. 心主血脉; *xīn zhǔ xuè mài.*
245. 肝属木; *gān shǔ mù.*
246. 三焦主决渎; *sān jiāo zhǔ jué dú.*
247. 心藏神; *xīn cáng shén.*
248. 小肠主液; *xiǎo cháng zhǔ yè.*
249. 肺主气; *fèi zhǔ qì.*
250. 肾，其充在骨; *shèn qí chōng zài gǔ.*
251. 女子胞; *nǚ zǐ bāo.*
252. 脾开窍于口; *pí kāi qiào yú kǒu.*
253. 肾开窍于二阴; *shèn kāi qiào yú èr yīn.*
254. 肺属金; *fèi shǔ jīn.*
255. 肝主疏泄; *gān zhǔ shū xiè.*
256. 肾属水; *shèn shǔ shuǐ.*
257. 心与小肠相表里; *xīn yǔ xiǎo cháng xiāng biǎo lǐ.*
258. 四肢; *sì zhī.*
259. 肾藏精; *shèn cáng jīng.*
260. 胃主降浊; *wèi zhǔ jiàng zhuó.*

Chapter 4

261. Jaundice.
262. Goiter due to exuberant liver fire; wheezing.
263. Deviation of the mouth; facial paralysis.
264. Desiccation of kidney yīn.
265. Heat patterns.
266. An external evil that has passed from the exterior into the interior of the body.
267. Yīn vacuity.
268. Aversion to wind.
269. Resolution.
270. False spiritedness.
271. Common cold.
272. Spleen-kidney yáng vacuity.
273. Qì vacuity.
274. Rapid breathing with short breaths.

275. Severe panting.
276. Binding depression of liver qì (and in qì vacuity).
277. Stomach qì ascending counterflow.
278. Rumbling intestines.
279. Muttering.
280. Stirred pulse.
281. Skipping pulse.
282. Heat [effusion].
283. Binding depression of liver qì.
284. Agitation.
285. Yīn patterns and cold patterns.
286. External dampness, wind contending with water, or yáng vacuity water flood.
287. Wind stroke.
288. Alternating tensing and relaxing of the muscles.
289. Qì vacuity or water-damp.
290. A moderate pulse has 4 beats per respiration; a slow pulse 3 beats or less.
291. Bright, pale, and somber white.
292. Red.
293. Green-blue or purple color or stasis speckles.
294. Damage to yīn by intense heat.
295. Exuberant heat.
296. Dampness trapping deep-lying heat.
297. White.
298. Infants.
299. Kidney yīn vacuity or blood heat with yīn-blood failing to nourish the hair.
300. Head heavy as if swathed.
301. Kidney vacuity, external injury.
302. Yes.
303. No.
304. Children.
305. Spleen-kidney yáng vacuity, center qì fall, exuberant heat toxin.

306. Dysentery.
307. Blood stasis.
308. A tongue fur that is disappearing.
309. Ungratifying defecation.
310. Yes.
311. Voracious eating.
312. Clamoring stomach.
313. Swallowing of upflowing acid.
314. Kidney.
315. Hyperactivity of ministerial fire, insecurity of kidney qi, heart-spleen depletion, liver channel damp-heat, binding depression of liver qì.
316. Clouding sleep is more severe.
317. Menstruation at irregular intervals.
318. Heart qì vacuity, congealing cold and stagnant qì, heart blood stasis obstruction, dual vacuity of qì and yīn, phlegm turbidity obstruction, pulmonary welling-abscess.
319. Fearful throbbing.
320. Repletion.
321. Impaired hearing, not as severe as deafness.
322. Insufficiency of lung yīn with vacuity fire flaming upward, liver-kidney yīn depletion, insufficiency of liver blood.
323. Abdominal fullness is subjective; abdominal distention is objective.
324. Yes.
325. Tinnitus.
326. Seminal loss.
327. Stirring fetus.
328. Bound.
329. Floating.
330. Slow.
331. Large.
332. Heat.
333. Rough.
334. Surging.
335. Surging.

336. Dissipated.
337. A tight pulse is forceful.
338. No.
339. Reversal.
340. Heat that is palpable.
341. Inch, bar, cubit.
342. Delayed menstruation.
343. After childbirth.
344. Yīn protrusion.
345. Impotence.
346. Cold.
347. Liver and gallbladder.
348. The heart.
349. Seminal efflux.
350. Blood vacuity, kidney vacuity, and qì stagnation and blood stasis.
351. Spleen qì vacuity, phlegm-damp.
352. Yīn vacuity fire.
353. Worms.
354. Stomach.
355. Children and elderly.
356. Fifth-watch diarrhea.
357. Qì vacuity, insufficiency of center qì, bladder damp-heat.
358. Yīn vacuity.
359. Yáng qì vacuity.
360. Vexing heat in the five hearts.
361. *Sì zhī qiàn wēn*; lack of warmth in the limbs.
362. *Wǔ xīn fán rè*; vexing heat in the five hearts.
363. *Sì zhī nì lěng*; counterflow cold of the limbs.
364. *Dài mài*; intermittent pulse.
365. *Dòng mài*; stirred pulse.
366. *Xián mài*; stringlike pulse.
367. *Yuè jīng guò shǎo*; scant menstruation.
368. *Shī jīng*; seminal loss.
369. *Bù mèng ér yí*; seminal emission without dreaming.
370. *Hūn shuì*; clouded sleep.
371. *Mù tòng*; eye pain.

372. *Shào fù tòng*; lesser abdominal pain.
373. *Wăn fù tòng jù àn*; pain in the stomach duct and abdomen that rejects pressure.
374. *Zhòng tīng*; hardness of hearing.
375. *Jīng jì*; fright palpitations.
376. *Láo mài*. Firm pulse.
377. *Ě xīn*; nausea.
378. *Xiōng măn*; fullness in the chest.
379. *Nà gŭ bù xiāng*; no pleasure in food.
380. *Dà biàn bù shuăng*; ungratifying defecation.
381. *Tuō gāng*; prolapse of the rectum.
382. *Wŭ gēng xiè*; fifth-watch diarrhea.
383. *Yè jiān duō niào*; profuse urination at night.
384. *Xiăo biàn duăn chì*; short voidings of reddish urine.
385. *Yāo tòng*; lumbar pain.
386. *Jiàn wàng*; forgetfulness.
387. *Yāo xī ruăn ruò*; limp lumbus and knees.
388. *Xīn fán*; heart vexation.
389. *Zēng hán*; abhorrence of cold.
390. *Dào hán*; night sweating.
391. *Qì cù*; hasty breathing.
392. *Dà biàn xī táng*; thin sloppy stool.
393. *Kă xuè*; expectoration of blood.
394. *Bí sè*; nasal congestion.
395. *Chĭ yín jiē bàn*; petaled gums.
396. *Kŏu chún gān jiāo*; parched lips.
397. *Fă kū*; dry hair.
398. *Tāi gòu*; grimy fur.
399. *Tù shé*; protrusion of the tongue.
400. *Shé pàng dà*; enlarged tongue.
401. *Jīn tì ròu shùn*; jerking sinews and twitching flesh.
402. *Jīn mài jū jí*; tension of the sinews.
403. *Kŏu yăn wāi xié*; deviation of the eyes and mouth.

404. *Tóu shēn kùn zhòng*; heavy cumbersome head and body.
405. *Jī ròu shòu xuè*; emaciation.
406. *Yŏu shén*; spiritedness.
407. *Sì zhī kùn juàn*; fatigued cumbersome limbs.
408. *Kuáng zào*; mania and agitation.
409. *Yì nù*; irascibility.
410. *Cuō kōng lĭ xiàn*; groping in the air and pulling [invisible] strings.
411. 沉脉; sunken pulse (deep pulse).
412. 疾脉; racing pulse.
413. 四肢厥冷; counterflow cold of the limbs.
414. 短脉; short pulse.
415. 促脉; skipping pulse.
416. 小便清长; long voidings of clear urine.
417. 战汗; shiver sweating.
418. 潮热; tidal fever.
419. 面色白; white facial complexion
420. 苔厚; thick tongue fur.
421. 腰酸膝软; aching lumbus and limp knees.
422. 口噤; clenched jaw.
423. 残灯复明; last flicker of the lamp.
424. 舌卷; curled tongue.
425. 自汗; spontaneous sweating.
426. 扬手掷足; flailing of the arms and legs.
427. 面色青紫; green-blue or purple facial complexion.
428. 颈项强直; rigidity of the neck.
429. 角弓反张; arched-back rigidity.
430. 舌边齿痕; dental impression on the margins of the tongue.
431. 黄苔; yellow fur.
432. 头摇; shaking of the head.
433. 发落; hair loss.
434. 两目上视; upward staring eyes.
435. 目赤; red eyes.
436. 口角流涎; drooling from the corners of the mouth.

437. 耳轮枯焦; withered helices.
438. 咳痰黄稠; coughing of thick yellow phlegm.
439. 大便如羊屎; stool like sheep's droppings.
440. 痰中带血; phlegm streaked with blood.
441. 声音重浊; heavy turbid voice.
442. 喉中有水鸡声; frog rale in the throat.
443. 懒言; laziness to speak.
444. 肩息; raised-shoulder breathing.
445. 谵言; delirious speech.
446. 肠鸣; rumbling intestines.
447. 郑语; muttering (mussitation).
448. 发热; heat effusion (fever).
449. 头重如裹; head heavy as if swathed.
450. 眩晕; dizziness.
451. 脐周窜痛; scurrying pain around the umbilicus.
452. 不得卧; sleeplessness.
453. 月经失调; menstrual irregularities.
454. 早泄; premature ejaculation.
455. 关节疼痛; joint pain.
456. 腰酸; aching lumbus.
457. 小便短赤; short voidings of reddish urine.
458. 泻泄; diarrhea.
459. 口渴; thirst.
460. 大渴引饮; great thirst with fluid intake.
461. 食欲不振; poor appetite.
462. 口干; dry mouth.
463. 心悸; heart palpitations.
464. 吐血; blood ejection.
465. 切脉; take the pulse.
466. 食候困顿; drowsiness after eating.
467. 月经先期; advanced menstruation.
468. 恶露不绝; persistent flow of the lochia.
469. 把脉; take the pulse.
470. 身热不外扬; unsurfaced heat.
471. 午后潮热; postmeridian tidal fever.
472. 头痛如掣; headache with pulling sensation.
473. 寸口; wrist pulse (inch opening).
474. 数脉; rapid pulse.
475. 迟脉; slow pulse.
476. 洪脉; surging pulse.
477. 结脉; bound pulse.
478. 浮肿; puffy swelling.
479. 形寒; physical cold.
480. 痞块; glomus lump.
481. 向里蜷卧; xiàng lǐ quán wò.
482. 口噤; kǒu jìn.
483. 短气; duǎn qì.
484. 骨蒸潮热; gǔ zhēng cháo rè.
485. 面色黑; miàn sè hēi.
486. 恶风; wù fēng.
487. 舌瘦瘪; shé shòu biě.
488. 头重; tóu zhòng.
489. 口中和; kǒu zhōng hé.
490. 口苦; kǒu kǔ.
491. 镜面舌; jìng miàn shé.
492. 小便不利; xiǎo biàn bù lì.
493. 呃逆; è nì.
494. 尿有余沥; niào yǒu yú lì.
495. 化苔; huà tāi.
496. 遗尿; yí niào.
497. 小便失禁; xiǎo biàn shī jìn.
498. 革脉; gé mài.
499. 厌食; yàn shí.
500. 下利清谷; xià lì qīng gǔ.
501. 微脉; wéi mài.
502. 便难; biàn nán.
503. 不思饮食; bù sī yǐn shí.
504. 不食; bù shí.
505. 涩脉; sè mài.
506. 泛酸; fàn suan.
507. 胸闷; xiōng mèn.
508. 缓脉; huǎn mài.
509. 耳聋; ěr lóng.

510. 腹满; *fù mǎn.*
511. 乱经; *luàn jīng.*
512. 实脉; *shí mài.*
513. 腹痛喜按; *fù tòng xǐ àn.*
514. 耳鸣; *ěr míng.*
515. 失眠; *shī mián.*
516. 恶光羞明; *wù guāng xiū míng.*
517. 目干涩; *mù gān sè.*
518. 月经过多; *yuè jīng guò duō.*
519. 梦遗; *mèng yí.*
520. 促脉; *cù mài.*
521. 嗜睡; *shì shuì.*
522. 胎动不安; *tāi dòng bù ān.*
523. 寸口; *cùn kǒu.*
524. 芤脉; *kōu mài.*
525. 长脉; *cháng mài.*
526. 泛恶; *fàn ě.*
527. 有力; *yǒu lì.*
528. 浮肿; *fú zhǒng.*
529. 不寐、不得卧; *bù mèi, bù dé wò.*
530. 循衣摸床; *xún yī mō chuáng.*

Chapter 5

531. Exterior pattern.
532. Binding depression of liver qì.
533. Liver yang transforming into wind, extreme heat engendering wind, blood vacuity engendering wind.
534. a).
535. Stomach duct pain, vomiting of sour fluid, torpid intake, aversion to food.
536. Distention and diarrhea.
537. Insufficiency of kidney essence.
538. Fatigue and lack of strength, spontaneous sweating at the slightest movement, bright white facial complexion, dizziness, faint voice, shortness of breath, weak fine soft pulse.
539. Distention and fullness and oppression in the affected area, pain of unfixed location, scurrying pain, belching and passing of flatus.
540. Blood stasis is associated with pain of fixed location and qì stagnation with pain of unfixed location.
541. Lung, stomach, liver.
542. Pale white or withered yellow.
543. Bleeding (expectoration of blood, retching of blood, bloody stool or urine, nosebleed, menstrual irregularities).
544. Qì deserting with the blood.
545. Cold.
546. Heart yīn vacuity.
547. Heart impediment.
548. Midstage penetration (half-exterior half-interior).
549. Nondiffusion of lung qì.
550. Lung qì vacuity.
551. Spleen failing to move and transform, insufficiency of center qì, center qì fall, spleen failing to control the blood.
552. Bleeding.
553. Binding depression of liver qì.
554. Ascendant hyperactivity of liver yáng.
555. Liver blood vacuity.
556. Exterior repletion.
557. Kidney vacuity.
558. Insecurity of kidney qì.
559. Liver fire flaming upward.
560. Dual vacuity of qì and blood.
561. Qì deserting with the blood.
562. Heart blood vacuity, heart yīn vacuity, heart fire flaming upward.
563. Heart qì vacuity, heart yáng vacuity, heart blood vacuity, and heart yīn vacuity.
564. Heart-kidney yīn vacuity.
565. Nondiffusion of lung qì.

566. *Yīn xū huǒ wàng*; effulgent yīn vacuity fire.
567. *Shī rè xià zhù dà cháng*; damp-heat pouring down into the large intestine.
568. *Shāng shí*; food damage.
569. *Pí shèn yáng xū*; spleen-kidney yáng vacuity.
570. *Xià yuán xū bèi*; exhaustion of the lower origin.
571. *Yíng fèn zhèng*; construction-aspect pattern.
572. *Yáng xū shuǐ fàn*; yáng vacuity water flood.
573. *Bàn biǎo bàn lǐ*; half-exterior half-interior pattern.
574. *Rè rù xīn bāo*; heat entering the pericardium.
575. *Fèi qì bù lì*; inhibition of lung qì.
576. *Gān yáng shàng kàng*; hyperactivity of liver yáng.
577. *Shèn qì bù gù*; insecurity of kidney qì.
578. *Fēng hán*; wind-cold.
579. *Tán zhuó shàng rǎo*; phlegm turbidity harassing the upper body.
580. *Biǎo shí*; exterior repletion.
581. *Qì xuè jù xū*; dual vacuity of qì and blood.
582. *Pí fèi liǎng xū*; dual vacuity of the spleen and stomach.
583. *Shī zǔ*; damp obstruction.
584. *Hán shān*; cold mounting.
585. *Wèi fèn zhèng*; defense-aspect pattern.
586. 热极生风; extreme heat engendering wind.
587. 肝气郁结; binding depression of liver qì.
588. 命门火衰; debilitation of the life gate fire.
589. 肾精不足; insufficiency of kidney essence.
590. 外感寒邪; external contraction of cold evil.
591. 湿热留恋气分; damp-heat lodged in the qì aspect.
592. 太阳病; greater yáng (*tài yáng*) disease.
593. 痰饮; phlegm-rheum.
594. 痰蒙心包; phlegm clouding the pericardium.
595. 血热妄行; frenetic movement of hot blood.
596. 气闭; qì block.
597. 痰浊蒙蔽心包; phlegm turbidity clouding the pericardium.
598. 卫分证; defense-aspect patterns.
599. 气逆; qì counterflow.
600. 中气下陷; center qì fall.
601. 亡血; blood collapse.
602. 里证; interior patterns.
603. 气滞; qì stagnation.
604. 气随血脱; qì deserting with the blood.
605. 肝火上炎; liver fire flaming upward.
606. 肠胃积滞; *cháng wèi jī zhì*.
607. 伤津; *shāng jīn*.
608. 痰迷心窍; *tán mí xīn qiào*.
609. 太阳病; *tài yáng bìng*.
610. 寒证; *hán zhèng*.
611. 虚证; *xū zhèng*.
612. 辨证; *biàn zhèng*.
613. 气滞血瘀; *qì zhì xuè yū*.
614. 心气虚; *xīn qì xū*.
615. 心血虚; *xīn xuè xū*.
616. 心火上炎; *xīn huǒ shàng yán*.
617. 真阳不足; *zhēn yáng bù zú*.
618. 心火移热于小肠; *xīn huǒ yí rè yú xiǎo cháng*.
619. 肺失肃降; *fèi shī sù jiàng*.
620. 脾阳不振; *pí yáng bù zhèn*.
621. 脾失健运; *pí shī jiàn yùn*.
622. 心痹; *xīn bì*.
623. 肝气犯脾; *gān qì fàn pí*.

624. 肾阴虚; *shèn yīn xū.*
625. 肾不纳气; *shèn bù nà qì.*
626. 风邪入经; *fēng xié rù jīng.*
627. 暑热; *shǔ rè.*
628. 湿热阻滞脾胃; *shī rè zǔ zhì pí wèi.*
629. 厥阴病; *jué yīn bìng.*
630. 痰蒙心包; *tán méng xīn bāo.*

Chapter 6

631. Diphtheria.
632. Nipple moth (baby moth).
633. Cholera (sudden turmoil).
634. Running piglet.
635. Concretions, conglomerations, accumulations, and gatherings.
636. Mounting.
637. Wind-stroke.
638. Epilepsy.
639. Profuse and scant non-menstrual bleeding.
640. Malign obstruction.
641. Cinnabar toxin (erysipelas).
642. Clove sore.
643. Scrofula.
644. Welling abscess is raised above the surface.
645. Lichen.
646. Suppuration deep in the body that moves from one location to another.
647. Goiter.
648. Malaria.
649. Dispersion-thirst.
650. Tetany.
651. Crick in the neck.
652. Stomach reflux.
653. Plum-pit qì.
654. Wilting.
655. Consumption.
656. Panting.
657. Deep-source nasal congestion.
658. Miscellaneous disease.
659. Measles.
660. Head wind.
661. *Yē gé*; dysphagia-occlusion.
662. *Bì zhèng*; impediment pattern.
663. *Wěi zhèng*; wilting pattern.
664. *Lín zhèng*; strangury pattern.
665. *Gān*; gān.
666. *Gǔ zhàng*; drum distention.
667. *Shàn*; mounting.
668. *Lóng bì*; dribbling urinary block.
669. *Cháng yōng*; intestinal welling-abscess.
670. *Gāo lín*; unctuous strangury.
671. *Jié*; boil.
672. *Jū*; flat-abscess.
673. *Tiān huā*; smallpox.
674. *Bǎi rì ké*; whooping cough.
675. *Zhēng jiǎ jī jù*; concretions, conglomerations, accumulations, and gatherings.
676. *Lào zhěn*; crick in the neck.
677. *Xiāo chuǎn*; panting.
678. *Tóu fēng*; head wind.
679. *Shuǐ zhǒng*; water swelling.
680. *Pò shāng fēng*; lockjaw.
681. 石淋; stone strangury.
682. 崩漏; flooding and spotting.
683. 肺痿; lung wilting.
684. 肺痈; pulmonary welling-abscess.
685. 瘰疬; scrofula.
686. 疮疡; sores.
687. 瘿; goiter.
688. 痰核; phlegm node.
689. 癣; lichen.
690. 癫狂; mania and withdrawal.
691. 黄疸; jaundice.
692. 痉病; tetanic disease.
693. 乳蛾; nipple moth (baby moth).
694. 疳; gān.
695. 痢疾; dysentery.
696. 惊风; fright wind.
697. 霍乱; cholera (sudden turmoil).
698. 疝气; mounting qì.
699. 痘; pox.

700. 反胃; stomach reflux.
701. 淋证; *lín zhèng.*
702. 肺痈; *fèi yōng.*
703. 转胞; *zhuǎn bāo.*
704. 恶阻; *è zǔ.*
705. 肺痿; *fèi wěi.*
706. 丹毒; *dān dú.*
707. 疔疮; *dīng chuāng.*
708. 痈; *yōng.*
709. 崩漏; *bēng lòu.*
710. 中风; *zhòng fēng.*
711. 消渴; *xiāo kě.*
712. 奔豚; *bēn tún.*
713. 痘; *dòu.*
714. 百日咳; *bǎi rì ké.*
715. 肩息; *jiān xī.*
716. 喘逆; *chuǎn nì.*
717. 痿躄; *wěi bì.*
718. 刚痉; *gāng jìng.*
719. 赤白痢; *chì bái lì.*
720. 山岚瘴气; *shān lán zhàng qì.*

Chapter 7

721. Transforming dampness.
722. Constraining the lung and suppressing cough.
723. Treating the root.
724. Paradoxical treatment (coacting treatment).
725. Disinhibiting water and percolating dampness.
726. Astringing the intestines and stemming desertion.
727. Reducing urine.
728. Resolving the exterior with coolness and acridity.
729. Exterior resolution without necessarily making the patient sweat.
730. Clearing heat and resolving toxin.
731. Clearing heat and disinhibiting dampness.

732. Clearing construction and cooling the blood.
733. Cold, warm, and moist precipitation.
734. Harmonizing the lesser yáng (*shào yáng*).
735. Transforming, drying, and disinhibiting.
736. Stanching bleeding.
737. Calming the liver and extinguishing wind.
738. Moistening dryness by light diffusion.
739. Supplementing yīn.
740. Harmonizing the liver and stomach.
741. Returning yáng and stemming counterflow.
742. Harmonizing the stomach and rectifying qì.
743. Dispersing food and abducting stagnation.
744. Softening hardness.
745. Downbearing qì and calming panting.
746. stemming flooding and checking (vaginal) discharge.
747. Supplementing qì.
748. None.
749. Supplementing yáng.
750. Quieting the spirit with heavy settlers.
751. *Suō niào*; reducing urination.
752. *Zào shī*; drying dampness.
753. *Yù yīn*; fostering yīn.
754. *Qū shī*; dispelling dampness.
755. *Wēn jīng sàn hán*; warming the channels and dissipating cold.
756. *Zhèng zhì*; straight treatment.
757. *Jiàng nì zhǐ ǒu*; Downbearing counterflow and checking vomiting.
758. *Huí yáng jiù nì*; returning yáng and stemming counterflow.

759. *Tiáo hé gān pí*; harmonizing the liver and spleen.
760. *Ruǎn jiān*; softening hardness.
761. *Shí zé xiè zhī*; repletion is treated by draining.
762. *Jiě biǎo*; resolving the exterior.
763. *Pò qì*; breaking qì.
764. *Shū biǎo*; coursing the exterior.
765. *Qīng fǎ*; clearing.
766. icXiāo dǎo; abductive dispersion.
767. *Qīng rè qū shī*; clearing heat and dispelling dampness.
768. *Zhù yáng*; assisting yáng.
769. *Wēn xià*; warm precipitation.
770. *Sè cháng gù tuō*; astringing the intestine and stemming desertion.
771. 清气分热; clearing qì-aspect heat.
772. 清利湿热; clearing heat and disinhibiting dampness.
773. 和法; harmonization.
774. 逐水; expelling water.
775. 重镇安神; quieting the spirit with heavy settlers.
776. 补阴; supplement yīn.
777. 滋阴解表; enriching yīn and resolving the exterior.
778. 治标; treating the tip.
779. 驱虫; expelling worms.
780. 豁痰开窍; sweeping phlegm and opening the orifices.
781. 利湿; disinhibiting dampness.
782. 清血热; clearing blood heat.
783. 助阳; assisting yáng.
784. 宣肺化痰; diffusing the lung and transforming phlegm.
785. 调和肠胃; harmonizing the stomach and intestines.
786. 活血化瘀; quickening the blood and transforming stasis.
787. 止血; stanching bleeding.
788. 敛汗固表; constraining sweat and securing the exterior.

789. 清热开窍; clearing heat and opening the orifices.
790. 化痰; transforming phlegm.
791. 治本; *zhì běn*.
792. 和解半表半里; *hé jiě bàn biǎo bàn lǐ*.
793. 化痰止咳; *huà tán zhǐ ké*.
794. 治法; *zhì fǎ*.
795. 吐法; *tù fǎ*.
796. 温肺化饮; *wēn fèi huà yǐn*.
797. 治则; *zhì zé*.
798. 固精; *gù jīng*.
799. 燥湿; *zào shī*.
800. 清利湿热; *qīng lì shī rè*.
801. 助阳; *zhù yáng*.
802. 开窍; *kāi qiào*.
803. 调和肝脾; *tiáo hé gān pí*.
804. 利湿; *lì shī*.
805. 固涩法; *gù sè fǎ*.
806. 润下; *rùn xià*.
807. 豁痰开窍; *huò tán kāi qiào*.
808. 回阳救逆; *huí yáng jiù nì*.
809. 攻痰; *gōng tán*.
810. 益气; *yì qì*.

Chapter 8

811. A medicinal paste mounted on cloth.
812. A beverage that can be taken at any time.
813. Glue.
814. Beverage.
815. Swallow pills, powders, or glue mixed with fluid.
816. Take in one go.
817. A rich paste.
818. Sovereign.
819. Distillate.
820. Pills.
821. *sǎn*; powder.
822. *shǐ*; courier.
823. *zhēng*; steaming.
824. *jiǔ jì*; wine preparation.

825. *gāo zī*; rich paste.
826. *rè yùn*; hot pack.
827. *shāo cún xìng*; nature-preservative burning.
828. *jiāo*; glue.
829. *piàn*; tablet.
830. *lín shuì qián fú*; take before sleeping.
831. *dùn fú*; quaff.
832. 调敷; apply mixed.
833. 药膏; Medicinal paste.
834. 闷润; covered moistening.
835. 片; tablet.
836. 送服; Swallow with fluid.
837. 制霜; frosting.
838. 佐; Assistant.
839. 汤; Decoction.
840. 冲服; take drenched.
841. 臣; minister.
842. 剂型; *jì xíng*.
843. 炖; *dùn*.
844. 水丸; *shuǐ wán*.
845. 煅淬; *duàn cuì*.
846. 炒炭; *chǎo tàn*.
847. 归经; *guī jīng*.
848. 升降浮沉; *shēng jiàng fú chén*.
849. 炮炙; *páo zhì*.
850. 捣碎; *dǎo suì*.
851. 水制; *shuǐ zhì*.

Chapter 9

852. Flash cupping.
853. Moxa cone.
854. Warm needling.
855. Scarring and nonscarring.
856. Three-edged needle.
857. Stationary cupping.
858. Fire needling.
859. The filiform needle.
860. Thumbtack needle.

861. Pricking and cupping.
862. *Wú bān hén jiǔ*; nonscarring moxibustion.
863. *Liú zhēn*; needle retention.
864. *Jiān jiē jiǔ*; indirect moxibustion.
865. *Ài tiáo jiǔ*; poling.
866. *Shāo shān huǒ*; burning mountain method.
867. *Kāi hé bǔ xiè*; open and closed supplementation and drainage.
868. *Dé qì*; obtaining qì.
869. *Dǎo zhēn*; needle pounding.
870. *Tuì zhēn*; needle retraction.
871. *gé suàn jiǔ*; moxibustion on garlic.
872. *zhí jiē jiǔ*; direct moxibustion.
873. 进针; needle insertion.
874. 迎随补泻; directional supplementation and drainage.
875. 透天凉; heaven-penetrating cooling method.
876. 捻转补泻; twirling supplementation and drainage.
877. 针刺; Acupuncture needling.
878. 出针; needle removal.
879. 开阖补泻; open and closed supplementation and drainage.
880. 回阳九针; nin needles for returning yáng.
881. 得气; obtaining qì.
882. 艾绒; moxa floss.
883. 呼吸补泻; *hū xī bǔ xiè*.
884. 艾灸; *ài jiǔ*.
885. 温针; *wēn zhēn*.
886. 提插补泻; *tí chá bǔ xiè*.
887. 气至; *qì zhì*.
888. 疾徐补泻; *jí xú bǔ xiè*.
889. 电针; *diàn zhēn*.
890. 艾条; *ài tiáo*.
891. 梅花针; *méi huā zhēn*.
892. 隔盐灸; *gé yán jiǔ*.

附录五：名词表
Appendix V: Term List

1 Basic Concepts

1. 阴 [陰] *yīn*, yīn

2. 阳 [陽] *yáng*, yáng

3. 阴阳互根 [陰陽互根] *yīn yáng hù gēn*, yīn and yáng are rooted in each other

4. 阴阳制约 [陰陽制約] *yīn yáng zhì yuē*, yīn and yáng counterbalance each other

5. 阴阳消长 [陰陽消長] *yīn yáng xiāo zhǎng*, waxing and waning of yīn and yáng

6. 阴阳转化 [陰陽轉化] *yīn yáng zhuǎn huà*, yīn and yáng convert into each other

7. 阳胜则热 [陽勝則熱] *yáng shèng zé rè*, when yáng prevails, there is heat

8. 阴胜则寒 [陰勝則寒] *yīn shèng zé hán*, when yīn prevails, there is cold

9. 木 [木] *mù*, wood

10. 火 [火] *huǒ*, fire

11. 土 [土] *tǔ*, earth (soil)

12. 金 [金] *jīn*, metal

13. 水 [水] *shuǐ*, water

14. 相生 [相生] *xiāng shēng*, engendering

15. 相克 [相剋] *xiāng kè*, restraining

16. 相侮 [相侮] *xiāng wǔ*, rebellion

17. 相乘 [相乘] *xiāng chéng*, overwhelming

18. 木火刑金 [木火刑金] *mù huǒ xíng jīn*, wood fire tormenting metal

19. 火盛刑金 [火盛刑金] *huǒ shèng xíng jīn*, exuberant fire tormenting metal

20. 木郁化火 [木鬱化火] *mù yù huà huǒ*, depressed wood transforming into fire

21. 水火相济 [水火相濟] *shuǐ huǒ xiāng jì*, fire and water help each other

22. 水亏火旺 [水虧火旺] *shuǐ kuī huǒ wàng*, depleted water and effulgent fire

23. 火不生土 [火不生土] *huǒ bù shēng tǔ*, fire failing to engender earth

24. 母病及子 [母病及子] *mǔ bìng jí zǐ*, disease of the mother affects the child

25. 肝 [肝] *gān*, liver

26. 心 [心] *xīn*, heart

27. 脾 [脾] *pí*, spleen

28. 肺 [肺] *fèi*, lung

29. 肾 [腎] *shèn*, kidney

30. 筋 [筋] *jīn*, sinew

31. 脉 [脈] *mài*, vessel

32. 肌肉 [肌肉] *jī ròu*, flesh

33. 皮毛 [皮毛] *pí máo*, skin and [body] hair

34. 骨 [骨] *gǔ*, bone

35. 目 [目] *mù*, eye

36. 舌 [舌] *shé*, tongue

37. 唇 [唇] *chún*, lips

38. 鼻［鼻］*bí*, nose
39. 耳［耳］*ěr*, ear
40. 青［青］*qīng*, green-blue
41. 赤［赤］*chì*, red
42. 黄［黃］*huáng*, yellow
43. 白［白］*bái*, white
44. 黑［黑］*hēi*, black
45. 泪［淚］*lèi*, tears
46. 汗［汗］*hàn*, sweat
47. 涎［涎］*xián*, drool
48. 涕［涕］*tì*, snivel; nasal mucus
49. 唾［唾］*tuò*, spittle
50. 酸［酸］*suān*, sour, sourness
51. 苦［苦］*kǔ*, bitter, bitterness
52. 甘［甘］*gān*, sweet, sweetness
53. 辛［辛］*xīn*, acrid, acridity
54. 咸［鹹］*xián*, salty, saltiness
55. 怒［怒］*nù*, anger
56. 喜［喜］*xǐ*, joy
57. 思［思］*sī*, thought
58. 忧［憂］*yōu*, anxiety
59. 恐［恐］*kǒng*, fear
60. 七情［七情］*qī qíng*, seven affects
61. 情志［情志］*qíng zhì*, affect-mind
62. 悲［悲］*bēi*, sorrow
63. 惊［驚］*jīng*, fright
64. 心包络［心包絡］*xīn bāo luò*, pericardiac network
65. 胃［胃］*wèi*, stomach
66. 小肠［小腸］*xiǎo cháng*, small intestine
67. 大肠［大腸］*dà cháng*, large intestine
68. 胆［膽］*dǎn*, gallbladder
69. 膀胱［膀胱］*páng guāng*, bladder
70. 三焦［三焦］*sān jiāo*, triple burner
71. 身［身］*shēn*, body
72. 形［形］*xíng*, body
73. 体［體］*tǐ*, body; constitution
74. 头［頭］*tóu*, head
75. 额［額］*é*, forehead
76. 面［面］*miàn*, face (*n.*); facial (*adj.*)
77. 囟［囟］*xìn*, fontanel
78. 囟门［囟門］*xìn mén*, fontanel gate, anterior fontanel
79. 口［口］*kǒu*, mouth (*n.*); oral (*adj.*)
80. 齿［齒］*chǐ*, tooth (*n.*); dental (*adj.*)
81. 牙［牙］*yá*, tooth (*n.*); dental (*adj.*)
82. 牙齿［牙齒］*yá chǐ*, tooth (*n.*); dental (*adj.*)
83. 齿牙［齒牙］*chǐ yá*, tooth (*n.*); dental (*adj.*)
84. 龈［齦］*yín*, gum
85. 齿龈［齒齦］*chǐ yín*, gum
86. 颈［頸］*jǐng*, neck
87. 项［項］*xiàng*, nape
88. 咽［咽］*yān*, pharynx (*n.*), pharyngeal (*adj.*); throat (*n.*)
89. 喉［喉］*hóu*, throat, larynx
90. 喉核［喉核］*hóu hé*, throat node
91. 喉关［喉關］*hóu guān*, throat pass
92. 悬雍垂［懸雍垂］*xuán yōng chuí*, uvula
93. 会厌［會厭］*huì yàn*, epiglottis
94. 结喉［結喉］*jié hóu*, laryngeal prominence

95. 胸 [胸] *xiōng*, chest

96. 胁 [脅] *xié*, rib-side

97. 乳 [乳] *rŭ*, breast

98. 乳头 [乳頭] *rŭ tóu*, nipple

99. 虚里 [虛里] *xū lĭ*, vacuous lĭ

100. 心下 [心下] *xīn xià*, [region] below the heart

101. 胃脘 [胃脘] *wèi wăn*, stomach duct

102. 脘 [脘] *wăn*, stomach duct

103. 腹 [腹] *fù*, abdomen (*n.*); abdominal (*adj.*)

104. 脐 [臍] *qí*, umbilicus (*n.*); umbilical (*adj.*)

105. 大腹 [大腹] *dà fù*, greater abdomen

106. 小腹 [小腹] *xiăo fù*, smaller abdomen

107. 少腹 [少腹] *shào fù*, lesser abdomen

108. 肩 [肩] *jiān*, shoulder

109. 背 [背] *bèi*, back

110. 膈 [膈] *gé*, diaphragm (*n.*); diaphragmatic (*adj.*)

111. 腰 [腰] *yāo*, lumbus (*n.*); lumbar (*adj.*)

112. 肢 [肢] *zhī*, limb

113. 手 [手] *shŏu*, hand

114. 手（臂）[手（臂）] *shŏu (bèi)*, arm

115. 足 [足] *zú*, foot

116. 足 [足] *zú*, leg

117. 手足 [手足] *shŏu zú*, extremities

118. 腿 [腿] *tuĭ*, leg

119. 膝 [膝] *xī*, knee

120. 肘 [肘] *zhŏu*, elbow

121. 踝 [踝] *huái*, ankle

122. 腕 [腕] *wàn*, wrist

123. 腠理 [腠理] *còu lĭ*, interstices

124. 窍 [竅] *qiào*, orifice

125. 命门 [命門] *mìng mén*, life gate

126. 精关 [精關] *jīng guān*, essence gate

127. 真元 [眞元] *zhēn yuán*, true origin

128. 膏肓 [膏肓] *gāo huāng*, gāo-huāng

129. 膜原 [膜原] *mó yuán*, membrane source

130. 丹田 [丹田] *dān tián*, cinnabar field

131. 血室 [血室] *xuè shì*, blood chamber

132. 气海 [氣海] *qì hăi*, sea of qì

133. 气 [氣] *qì*, qì

134. 阳气 [陽氣] *yáng qì*, yáng qì

135. 阴气 [陰氣] *yīn qì*, yīn qì

136. 原气 [原氣] *yuán qì*, source qì

137. 营气 [營氣] *yíng qì*, construction qì

138. 卫气 [衛氣] *wèi qì*, defense qì

139. 正气 [正氣] *zhèng qì*, right qì

140. 邪气 [邪氣] *xié qì*, evil qì

141. 元气 [元氣] *yuán qì*, original qì

142. 宗气 [宗氣] *zōng qì*, ancestral qì

143. 脏腑之气 [臟腑之氣] *zàng fŭ zhī qì*, bowel and visceral qì

144. 经络之气 [經絡之氣] *jīng luò zhī qì*, channel and network vessel qì

145. 气化 [氣化] *qì huà*, qì transformation

146. 血 [血] *xuè*, blood

147. **阴血** [陰血] *yīn xuè*, yīn-blood
148. **精** [精] *jīng*, essence
149. **津液** [津液] *jīn yè*, liquid and humor (fluids)
150. **君火** [君火] *jūn huǒ*, sovereign fire
151. **神** [神] *shén*, spirit
152. **相火** [相火] *xiàng huǒ*, ministerial fire
153. **大便** [大便] *dà biàn*, stool (*n.*); fecal (*adj.*); defecation (*n.*)
154. **小便** [小便] *xiǎo biàn*, urine (*n.*), urinary (*adj.*); urination, voiding (*n.*)
155. **尿** [尿] *niào*, urine (*n.*), urinary (*adj.*); urination (*n.*)
156. **三因** [三因] *sān yīn*, three causes (of disease):
157. **内因** [內因] *nèi yīn*, internal cause:
158. **内伤七情** [內傷七情] *nèi shāng qī qíng*, internal damage by the seven affects; affect damage
159. **外因** [外因] *wài yīn*, external cause:
160. **不内外因** [內因外因] *bù nèi wài yīn*, neutral cause:
161. **六淫** [六淫] *liù yín*, six excesses:
162. **风** [風] *fēng*, wind
163. **寒** [寒] *hán*, cold
164. **暑** [暑] *shǔ*, summerheat
165. **湿** [濕] *shī*, damp, dampness
166. **燥** [燥] *zào*, dryness
167. **火** [火] *huǒ*, fire
168. **温邪** [溫邪] *wēn xié*, warm evil
169. **疠气** [癘氣] *lì qì*, pestilential qì

170. **毒** [毒] *dú*, toxin
171. **瘀血** [瘀血] *yū xuè*, static blood
172. **血瘀** [血瘀] *xuè yū*, blood stasis
173. **痰** [痰] *tán*, phlegm
174. **饮** [飲] *yǐn*, rheum
175. **水湿** [水濕] *shuǐ shī*, water-damp
176. **饮食不节** [飲食不節] *yǐn shí bù jié*, dietary irregularities
177. **暴饮暴食** [暴飲暴食] *bào yǐn bào shí*, voracious eating and drinking
178. **过食生冷** [過食生冷] *guò shí shēng lěng*, excessive consumption of raw and cold foods
179. **过食肥甘** [過食肥甘] *guò shí féi gān*, excessive consumption of sweet and fatty foods
180. **偏嗜油腻厚味** [偏嗜油腻厚味] *piān shì yóu nì hòu wèi*, predilection for greasy and rich foods
181. **过食辛辣** [過食辛辣] *guò shí xīn là*, excessive consumption of hot-spicy acrid foods
182. **跌打** [跌打] *dié dǎ*, knocks and falls
183. **虫兽伤** [蟲獸傷] *chóng shòu shāng*, animal and insect wounds
184. **房室不节** [房室不節] *fáng shì bù jié*, sexual intemperance
185. **劳倦** [勞倦] *láo juàn*, taxation fatigue

2 Channels and Network Ve

186. **经络** [經絡] *jīng luò*, channels and network vessels

187. 十二经 [十二經] *shí èr jīng*, twelve channels

188. 十二经筋 [十二經筋] *shí èr jīng jīn*, twelve channel sinews

189. 络脉 [絡脈] *luò mài*, network vessel

190. 十五络 [十五絡] *shí wǔ luò*, fifteen network vessels

191. 浮络 [浮絡] *fú luò*, superficial network vessel

192. 孙络 [孫絡] *sūn luò*, grandchild network vessel

193. 脾之大络 [脾之大絡] *pí zhī dà luò*, great network vessel of the spleen

194. 胃之大络 [胃之大絡] *wèi zhī dà luò*, great network vessel of the stomach

195. 太阳 [太陽] *tài yáng*, greater yáng

196. 阳明 [陽明] *yáng míng*, yáng brightness

197. 少阳 [少陽] *shào yáng*, lesser yáng

198. 太阴 [太陰] *tài yīn*, greater yīn

199. 少阴 [少陰] *shào yīn*, lesser yīn

200. 厥阴 [厥陰] *jué yīn*, reverting yīn

201. 任脉 [任脈] *rèn mài*, controlling vessel

202. 督脉 [督脈] *dū mài*, governing vessel

203. 冲脉 [衝脈] *chōng mài*, thoroughfare vessel

204. 带脉 [帶脈] *dài mài*, girdling vessel

205. 阴跷（蹻）脉 [陰蹻（蹻）脈] *yīn qiāo mài*, yīn springing vessel

206. 阳跷（蹻）脉 [陽蹻（蹻）脈] *yáng qiāo mài*, yáng springing vessel

207. 阴维脉 [陰維脈] *yīn wéi mài*, yīn linking vessel

208. 阳维脉 [陽維脈] *yáng wéi mài*, yáng linking vessel

209. 穴道 [穴道] *xué dào*, acupuncture point

210. 同身寸 [同身寸] *tóng shēn cùn*, body inch

211. 属络 [屬絡] *shǔ luò*, homing and netting

212. 交会穴 [交會穴] *jiāo huì xué*, intersection point

213. 背俞 [背俞] *bèi shū*, back transport [point]

214. 募穴 [募穴] *mù xué*, alarm point; mustering point

215. 原穴 [原穴] *yuán xué*, source point

216. 络穴 [絡穴] *luò xué*, network point; connecting point

217. 下合穴 [下合穴] *xià hé xué*, lower uniting point

218. 五俞穴 [五俞穴] *wǔ shū xué*, five transport points

219. 四总穴 [四總穴] *sì zǒng xué*, four command points

3 Five Viscera and Six Bowels

220. 心属火 [心屬火] *xīn shǔ huǒ*, heart belongs to fire

221. 心与小肠相表里 [心與小腸相表裡] *xīn yǔ xiǎo cháng xiāng biǎo lǐ*, heart and small intestine stand in interior-exterior relationship

222. **心主血脉** [心主血脈] *xīn zhǔ xuè mài*, heart governs the blood and vessels

223. **心藏神** [心藏神] *xīn cáng shén*, heart stores the spirit

224. **心开窍于舌** [心開竅於舌] *xīn kāi qiào yú shé*, heart opens at the tongue

225. **肺属金** [肺屬金] *fèi shǔ jīn*, lung belongs to metal

226. **肺与大肠相表里** [肺與大腸相表裡] *fèi yǔ dà cháng xiāng biǎo lǐ*, lung and large intestine stand in interior-exterior relationship

227. **肺主气** [肺主氣] *fèi zhǔ qì*, lung governs qì

228. **肺主肃降** [肺主肅降] *fèi zhǔ sù jiàng*, lung governs depurative downbearing

229. **肺主通调水道** [肺主通調水道] *fèi zhǔ tōng tiáo shuǐ dào*, lung governs regulation of the waterways

230. **肺主皮毛** [肺主皮毛] *fèi zhǔ pí máo*, lung governs the skin and [body] hair

231. **肺开窍于鼻** [肺開竅於鼻] *fèi kāi qiào yú bí*, lung opens at the nose

232. **脾属土** [脾屬土] *pí shǔ tǔ*, spleen belongs to earth (soil)

233. **脾与胃相表里** [脾與胃相表裡] *pí yǔ wèi xiāng biǎo lǐ*, spleen and stomach stand in interior-exterior relationship

234. **脾主运化** [脾主運化] *pí zhǔ yùn huà*, spleen governs movement and transformation

235. **脾主升清** [脾主升清] *pí zhǔ shēng qīng*, spleen governs upbearing of the clear

236. **脾主肌肉、四肢** [脾主肌肉、四肢] *pí zhǔ jī ròu, sì zhī*, spleen governs the flesh and limbs

237. **脾，其华在唇四白** [脾，其華在唇四白] *pí, qí huá zài chún sì bái*, spleen... its bloom is in the four whites of the lips

238. **脾开窍于口** [脾開竅於口] *pí kāi qiào yú kǒu*, spleen opens at the mouth

239. **胃主受纳** [胃主受納] *wèi zhǔ shòu nà*, stomach governs intake

240. **胃主腐熟** [胃主腐熟] *wèi zhǔ fǔ shú*, stomach governs decomposition; stomach governs rotting and ripening

241. **胃主降浊** [胃主降濁] *wèi zhǔ jiàng zhuó*, stomach governs downbearing of the turbid

242. **小肠主分别清浊** [小腸主分別清濁] *xiǎo cháng zhǔ fēn bié qīng zhuó*, small intestine governs separation of the clear and turbid

243. **小肠主液** [小腸主液] *xiǎo cháng zhǔ yè*, small intestine governs humor

244. **大肠主传化糟粕** [大腸主傳化糟粕] *dà cháng zhǔ chuán huà zāo pò*, large intestine governs the conveyance and transformation of waste

245. **大肠主津** [大腸主津] *dà cháng zhǔ jīn*, large intestine governs liquid

246. **肝与胆相表里** [肝與膽相表裡] *gān yǔ dǎn xiāng biǎo lǐ*, liver and gallbladder stand in interior-exterior relationship

247. **肝属木** [肝屬木] *gān shǔ mù*, liver belongs to wood

248. 肝主疏泄 [肝主疏泄] *gān zhǔ shū xiè*, liver governs free coursing

249. 肝藏血 [肝藏血] *gān cáng xuè*, liver stores blood

250. 肝主筋 [肝主筋] *gān zhǔ jīn*, liver governs the sinews

251. 肝，其华在爪 [肝，其華在 爪] *gān, qí huá zài zhǎo*, liver... its bloom is in the nails

252. 肝开窍于目 [肝開竅於目] *gān kāi qiào yú mù*, liver opens at the eyes

253. 肝为刚脏 [肝爲剛臟] *gān wéi gāng zàng*, liver is the unyielding viscus

254. 肾属水 [腎屬水] *shèn shǔ shuǐ*, kidney belongs to water

255. 肾主水 [腎主水] *shèn zhǔ shuǐ*, kidney governs water

256. 肾与膀胱相表里 [腎與膀胱 相表裡] *shèn yǔ páng guāng xiāng biǎo lǐ*, kidney and bladder stand in interior-exterior relationship

257. 肾藏精 [腎藏精] *shèn cáng jīng*, kidney stores essence

258. 肾主开阖 [腎主開闔] *shèn zhǔ kāi hé*, kidney governs opening and closing

259. 肾开窍于耳 [腎開竅於耳] *shèn kāi qiào yú ěr*, kidney opens at the ears

260. 肾开窍于二阴 [腎開竅於二 陰] *shèn kāi qiào yú èr yīn*, kidney opens at the two yīn

261. 肾，其华在发 [腎，其華在 髮] *shèn, qí huá zài fà*, kidney... its bloom is in the hair (of the head)

262. 肾生骨髓 [腎生骨髓] *shèn shēng gǔ suí*, kidney engenders the bone and marrow

263. 肾主骨 [腎主骨] *shèn zhǔ gǔ*, kidney governs the bones

264. 肾，其充在骨 [腎，其充在 骨] *shèn, qí chōng zài gǔ*, kidney... its fullness is in the bone

265. 脑 [腦] *nǎo*, brain

266. 子宫 [子宮] *zǐ gōng*, uterus

267. 女子胞 [女子胞] *nǔ zǐ bāo*, uterus

268. 三焦主决渎 [三焦主決瀆] *sān jiāo zhǔ jué dú*, triple burner governs the sluices

4 Four Examinations

269. 证（候）[證（候）] *zhèng hòu*, sign

270. 得神 [得神] *dé shén*, spiritedness

271. 失神 [失神] *shī shén*, spiritlessness

272. 假神 [假神] *jiǎ shén*, false spiritedness

273. 神昏 [神昏] *shén hūn*, clouded spirit

274. 形体肥胖 [形體肥胖] *xíng tǐ féi pàng*, obesity

275. 肌肉瘦削 [肌肉瘦削] *jī ròu shòu xuè*, emaciation

276. 脱肉破䐃 [脱肉破䐃] *tuō ròu pò jiǒng (jùn)*, shedding of flesh and loss of bulk

277. 向里蜷卧 [向裡踡臥] *xiàng lǐ quán wò*, lying in curled-up posture

278. 身重 [身重] *shēn zhòng*, heavy body; generalized heaviness

279. **四肢困倦** [四肢困倦] *sì zhī kùn juàn*, fatigued cumbersome limbs

280. **头身困重** [頭身困重] *tóu shēn kùn zhòng*, heavy cumbersome head and body

281. **身重不易转侧** [身重不易轉側] *shēn zhòng bù yì zhuǎn cè*, heavy body with difficulty in turning sides

282. **扬手掷足** [揚手擲足] *yáng shǒu zhí zú*, flailing of the arms and legs

283. **躁** [躁] *zào*, agitation

284. **易怒** [易怒] *yì nù*, irascibility

285. **狂躁** [狂躁] *kuáng zào*, mania and agitation

286. **循衣摸床** [循衣摸床] *xún yī mō chuáng*, picking at bedclothes

287. **撮空理线** [撮空理線] *cuō kōng lǐ xiàn*, groping in the air and pulling [invisible] strings

288. **口眼喎斜** [口眼喎斜] *kǒu yǎn wāi xié*, deviated eyes and mouth

289. **瘛瘲** [瘛瘲] *qì zòng*, tugging and slackening

290. **四肢抽搐** [四肢抽搐] *sì zhī chōu chù*, convulsion of the limbs

291. **抽风** [抽風] *chōu fēng*, tugging wind

292. **痉厥** [痙厥] *jìng jué*, tetanic reversal

293. **抽动** [抽動] *chōu dòng*, jerking

294. **筋惕肉瞤** [筋惕肉瞤] *jīn tì ròu shùn*, jerking sinews and twitching flesh

295. **筋脉拘急** [筋脈拘急] *jīn mài jū jí*, tension of the sinews

296. **筋脉拘挛** [筋脈拘攣] *jīn mài jū luán*, hypertonicity of the sinews

297. **颈项强直** [頸項強直] *jǐng xiàng jiàng zhí*, rigidity of the neck

298. **角弓反张** [角弓反張] *jiǎo gōng fǎn zhāng*, arched-back rigidity

299. **口噤** [口噤] *kǒu jìn*, clenched jaw

300. **昏倒** [昏倒] *hūn dǎo*, clouding collapse

301. **半身不遂** [半身不遂] *bàn shēn bù suì*, hemiplegia

302. **头摇** [頭搖] *tóu yáo*, shaking of the head

303. **面色白** [面色白] *miàn sè bái*, white facial complexion

304. **面色淡白** [面色淡白] *miàn sè dàn bái*, pale white facial complexion

305. **面色苍白** [面色蒼白] *miàn sè cāng bái*, somber white facial complexion

306. **面色㿠白** [面色㿠白] *miàn sè huǎng bái*, bright white facial complexion

307. **面色黄** [面色黃] *miàn sè huáng*, yellow facial complexion

308. **面色萎黄** [面色萎黃] *miàn sè wěi huáng*, withered-yellow facial complexion

309. **面色无华** [面色無華] *miàn sè wú huá*, lusterless facial complexion

310. **面色青紫** [面色青紫] *miàn sè qīng zǐ*, green-blue or purple facial complexion

311. **面色红** [面色紅] *miàn sè hóng*, red facial complexion

312. **面赤** [面赤] *miàn chì*, red fac

313. 面色黑 [面色黑] *miàn sè hēi,* black facial complexion

314. 斑疹 [斑疹] *bān zhěn,* maculopapular eruption

315. 舌质 [舌質] *shé zhì,* tongue body

316. 舌体 [舌體] *shé tǐ,* tongue body

317. 舌胖大 [舌胖大] *shé pàng dà,* enlarged tongue

318. 舌淡胖嫩 [舌淡胖嫩] *shé dàn pàng nèn,* pale tender-soft enlarged tongue

319. 舌边齿痕 [舌邊齒痕] *shé biān chǐ hén,* dental impressions on the margins of the tongue

320. 舌瘦瘪 [舌瘦瘪] *shé shòu biě,* shrunken tongue

321. 舌起芒刺 [舌起芒刺] *shé qǐ máng cì,* prickly tongue

322. 舌裂 [舌裂] *shé liè,* fissured tongue

323. 舌卷 [舌卷] *shé juǎn,* curled tongue

324. 吐弄舌 [吐弄舌] *tù nòng shé,* protrusion and worrying of the tongue

325. 吐舌 [吐舌] *tù shé,* protrusion of the tongue

326. 弄舌 [弄舌] *nòng shé,* worrying of the tongue

327. 舌强 [舌強] *shé jiàng,* stiff tongue

328. 舌强语謇 [舌強語謇] *shé jiàng yǔ jiǎn,* stiff tongue and impeded speech

329. 舌淡 [舌淡] *shé dàn,* pale tongue

330. 舌红 [舌紅] *shé hóng,* red tongue

331. 舌绛 [舌絳] *shé jiàng,* crimson tongue

332. 镜面舌 [鏡面舌] *jìng miàn shé,* mirror tongue

333. 舌光红 [舌光紅] *shé guāng hóng,* smooth, bare red tongue

334. 舌紫 [舌紫] *shé zǐ,* purple tongue

335. 瘀点 [瘀點] *yū diǎn,* stasis speckles

336. 瘀斑 [瘀斑] *yū bān,* stasis macules

337. 苔厚 [苔厚] *tāi hòu,* thick fur

338. 苔薄 [苔薄] *tāi bó,* thin fur

339. 舌苔干燥 [舌苔乾燥] *shé tāi gān zào,* dry tongue fur

340. 舌净 [舌淨] *shé jìng,* clean tongue

341. 苔垢 [苔垢] *tāi gòu,* grimy fur

342. 苔腻 [苔膩] *tāi nì,* slimy fur

343. 苔剥 [苔剝] *tāi bō,* peeling fur

344. 舌苔白如积粉 [舌苔白如積粉] *shé tāi bái rú jī fěn,* mealy white tongue fur

345. 白苔 [白苔] *bái tāi,* white fur

346. 黄苔 [黃苔] *huáng tāi,* yellow fur

347. 黑苔 [黑苔] *hēi tāi,* black fur

348. 苔化 [苔化] *tāi huà,* transforming fur

349. 囟门高突 [囟門高突] *xìn mén gāo tú,* bulging fontanel gate

350. 囟门下陷 [囟門下陷] *xìn mén xià xiàn,* depressed fontanel gate

351. 囟门迟闭 [囟門遲閉] *xìn mén chí bì,* retarded closure of the fontanel gate

352. 头摇 [頭搖] *tóu yáo,* shaking of the head

353. 头发早白 [頭髮早白] *tóu fà zǎo bái*, premature graying of the hair

354. 发枯 [髮枯] *fà kū*, dry hair

355. 发落 [髮落] *fà luò*, hair loss

356. 眼无光彩 [眼無光彩] *yǎn wú guāng cǎi*, dull eyes

357. 直视 [直視] *zhí shì*, forward-staring eyes

358. 两目上视 [兩目上視] *liǎng mù shàng shì*, upward staring eyes

359. 目上视 [目上視] *mù shàng shì*, upward staring eyes

360. 斜视 [斜視] *xié shì*, squint

361. 目赤 [目赤] *mù chì*, red eyes

362. 目黄 [目黃] *mù huáng*, yellow eyes

363. 目窠上微肿 [目窠上微腫] *mù kē shàng wēi zhǒng*, slight swelling of the eye nest

364. 目窠内陷 [目窠內陷] *mù kē nèi xiàn*, sunken eyes

365. 眼球外突 [眼球外突] *yǎn qiú wài tú*, bulging eyes

366. 鼻翼煽动 [鼻翼煽動] *bí yì shān dòng*, flaring nostrils

367. 口唇淡白 [口唇淡白] *kǒu chún dàn bái*, pale lips

368. 口唇青紫 [口唇青紫] *kǒu chún qīng zǐ*, green-blue or purple lips

369. 口唇干焦 [口唇乾焦] *kǒu chún gān jiāo*, parched lips

370. 口角不闭 [口角不閉] *kǒu jiǎo bù bì*, gaping corners of the mouth

371. 口角流涎 [口角流涎] *kǒu jiǎo liú xián*, drooling from the corners of the mouth

372. 喉中有痰声 [喉中有痰聲] *hóu zhōng yǒu tán shēng*, sound of phlegm in the throat

373. 咽喉肿痛 [咽喉腫痛] *yān hóu zhōng tòng*, sore swollen throat

374. 牙齿干燥如枯骨 [牙齒乾燥如枯骨] *yá chǐ gān zào rú kū gǔ*, teeth dry as desiccated bones

375. 齿龈结瓣 [齒齦結瓣] *chǐ yín jié bàn*, petaled gums

376. 齿龈虚浮 [齒齦虛浮] *chǐ yín xū fú*, vacuous puffy gums

377. 齿牙松动 [齒牙鬆動] *chǐ yá sōng dòng*, loosening of the teeth

378. 耳轮枯焦 [耳輪枯焦] *ěr lún kū jiāo*, withered helices

379. 痰多清稀 [痰多清稀] *tán duō qīng xī*, copious clear thin phlegm

380. 咳痰黄稠 [咳痰黃稠] *ké tán huáng chóu*, cough with thick yellow phlegm

381. 痰少不易咯 [痰少不易咯] *tán shǎo bú yì kǎ*, scant phlegm expectorated with difficulty

382. 痰中带血 [痰中帶血] *tán zhōng dài xuè*, phlegm containing blood

383. 咯血 [咯血] *kǎ xuè*, expectoration of blood

384. 鼻流清涕 [鼻流清涕] *bí liú qīng tì*, runny nose with clear snivel (nasal mucus)

385. 鼻塞 [鼻塞] *bí sè*, nasal congestion

386. 多嚏 [多嚏] *duō tì*, sneezing

387. 呕吐痰饮 [嘔吐痰飲] *ǒu tù tán yǐn*, vomiting of phlegm-rheum

388. 大便稀溏 [大便稀溏] *dà biàn xī táng*, thin sloppy stool

389. 便血 [便血] *biàn xuè*, bloody stool

390. 大便下血 [大便下血] *dà biàn xià xuè*, precipitation of blood with the stool

391. 大便黑色 [大便黑色] *dà biàn hēi sè*, black stool

392. 下利清谷 [下利清穀] *xià lì qīng gǔ*, clear-grain diarrhea; clear-food diarrhea

393. 大便水样 [大便水樣] *dà biàn shuǐ yàng*, watery stool

394. 大便如羊屎 [大便如羊屎] *dà biàn rú yáng shǐ*, stool like sheep's droppings

395. 喉中有水鸡声 [喉中有水雞聲] *hóu zhōng yǒu shuǐ jī shēng*, frog rale in the throat

396. 咳声重浊 [咳聲重濁] *ké shēng zhòng zhuó*, heavy turbid cough sound

397. 懒言 [懶言] *lǎn yán*, laziness to speak

398. 气粗 [氣粗] *qì cū*, rough breathing

399. 气促 [氣促] *qì cù*, hasty breathing

400. 短气 [短氣] *duǎn qì*, shortness of breath

401. 气急 [氣急] *qì jí*, rapid breathing

402. 肩息 [肩息] *jiān xī*, raised-shoulder breathing

403. 少气 [少氣] *shǎo qì*, shortage of qi

404. 叹息 [嘆息] *tàn xī*, sighing

405. 声音嘶嗄 [聲音嘶嗄] *shēng yīn sī shà*, hoarse voice

406. 谵言 [譫言] *zhān yán*, delirious speech

407. 骂詈无常 [罵詈無常] *mà lì wú cháng*, abnormal chiding and cursing

408. 呻吟 [呻吟] *shēn yín*, groaning

409. 独语 [獨語] *dú yǔ*, soliloquy; talking alone

410. 郑语 [鄭語] *zhèng yǔ*, muttering; mussitation

411. 肠鸣 [腸鳴] *cháng míng*, rumbling intestines

412. 呃逆 [呃逆] *è nì*, hiccup

413. 嗳气酸腐 [噯氣酸腐] *ài qì suān fǔ*, belching of sour putrid qì (gas)

414. 腹泻秽臭 [腹瀉穢臭] *fù xiè huì chòu*, foul-smelling diarrhea

415. 发热 [發熱] *fā rè*, heat effusion; fever

416. 壮热 [壯熱] *zhuàng rè*, vigorous heat [effusion]; vigorous fever

417. 身热 [身熱] *shēn rè*, generalized heat [effusion]; generalized fever

418. 身热不扬 [身熱不揚] *shēn rè bù yáng*, unsurfaced heat; unsurfaced fever

419. 潮热 [潮熱] *cháo rè*, tidal heat [effusion]; tidal fever

420. 午后潮热 [午後潮熱] *wǔ hòu cháo rè*, postmeridian tidal heat [effusion]; postmeridian tidal fever

421. 骨蒸潮热 [骨蒸潮熱] *gǔ zhēng cháo re=4*, steaming bone tidal heat [effusion]; steaming bone tidal fever

422. 五心烦热 [五心煩熱] *wǔ xīn fán rè*, vexing heat in the five hearts

423. **手足心热** [手足心熱] *shǒu zú xīn rè*, heat in the (hearts of the) palms and soles

424. **恶寒** [惡寒] *wù hán*, aversion to cold

425. **寒热往来** [寒熱往來] *hán rè wǎng lái*, alternating [aversion to] cold and heat [effusion]; alternating fever and chills

426. **恶风** [惡風] *wù fēng*, aversion to wind

427. **憎寒** [憎寒] *zēng hán*, abhorrence of cold

428. **自汗** [自汗] *zì hàn*, spontaneous sweating

429. **盗汗** [盜汗] *dào hàn*, night sweating; thief sweating

430. **战汗** [戰汗] *zhàn hàn*, shiver sweating

431. **头痛** [頭痛] *tóu tòng*, headache

432. **正头痛** [正頭痛] *zhèng tóu tòng*, medial headache

433. **偏头痛** [偏頭痛] *piān tóu tòng*, hemilateral headache

434. **头重** [頭重] *tóu zhòng*, heavy-headedness

435. **头重如裹** [頭重如裹] *tóu zhòng rú guǒ*, head heavy as if swathed

436. **头胀** [頭脹] *tóu zhàng*, distention in the head

437. **头痛如掣** [頭痛如掣] *tóu tòng rú chè*, headache with pulling sensation

438. **眩晕** [眩暈] *xuàn yūn*, dizziness

439. **头晕** [頭暈] *tóu yūn*, dizzy head

440. **健忘** [健忘] *jiàn wàng*, forgetfulness

441. **目眩** [目眩] *mù xuàn*, dizzy vision

442. **心烦** [心煩] *xīn fán*, heart vexation

443. **易惊** [易驚] *yì jīng*, susceptibility to fright

444. **关节疼痛** [關節疼痛] *guān jié téng tòng*, joint pain

445. **腰痛** [腰痛] *yāo tòng*, lumbar pain

446. **腰酸** [腰痠] *yāo suān*, aching lumbus

447. **腰膝软弱** [腰膝軟弱] *yāo xī ruǎn ruò*, limp lumbus and knees

448. **腰酸腿软** [腰痠腿軟] *yāo suān tuǐ ruǎn*, aching lumbus and limp legs

449. **腰酸膝软** [腰痠膝軟] *yāo suān xī ruǎn*, aching lumbus and limp knees

450. **四肢麻木** [四肢麻木] *sì zhī má mù*, numbness (and tingling) of the limbs

451. **倦怠乏力** [倦怠乏力] *juàn dài fá lì*, fatigue and lack of strength

452. **形倦神怠** [形倦神怠] *xíng juàn shén dài*, physical fatigue and lassitude of spirit

453. **肢倦** [肢倦] *zhī juàn*, fatigued limbs

454. **小便短赤** [小便短赤] *xiǎo biàn duǎn chì*, short voidings of reddish urine

455. **小便短少** [小便短少] *xiǎo biàn duǎn shǎo*, short voidings of scant urine

456. **小便清长** [小便清長] *xiǎo biàn qīng cháng*, long voidings of clear urine

457. 夜间多尿 [夜間多尿] *yè jiān duō niào*, profuse urination at night; nocturia

458. 小便频数 [小便頻數] *xiǎo biàn pín shuò*, frequent urination

459. 小便不利 [小便不利] *xiǎo biàn bù lì*, inhibited urination

460. 尿有余沥 [尿有餘瀝] *niào yǒu yú lì*, dribble after voiding

461. 遗尿 [遺尿] *yí niào*, enuresis

462. 小便失禁 [小便失禁] *xiǎo biàn shī jìn*, urinary incontinence

463. 便秘 [便秘] *biàn bì*, constipation

464. 大便干结 [大便乾結] *dà biàn gān jié*, dry bound stool

465. 便难 [便難] *biàn nán*, difficult defecation

466. 泄泻 [泄瀉] *xiè xiè*, diarrhea

467. 大便失禁 [大便失禁] *dà biàn shī jìn*, fecal incontinence

468. 五更泄 [五更泄] *wǔ gēng xiè*, fifth-watch diarrhea

469. 里急后重 [裡急後重] *lǐ jí hòu zhòng*, tenesmus; abdominal urgency and rectal heaviness

470. 大便不爽 [大便不爽] *dà biàn bù shuǎng*, ungratifying defecation

471. 久泄 [久泄] *jiǔ xiè*, enduring diarrhea

472. 脱肛 [脱肛] *tuō gāng*, prolapse of the rectum

473. 口渴 [口渴] *kǒu kě*, thirst

474. 口干 [口乾] *kǒu gān*, dry mouth

475. 渴不欲饮 [渴不欲飲] *kě bù yù yǐn*, thirst with no desire to drink

476. 渴不多饮 [渴不多飲] *kě bù duō yǐn*, thirst without large fluid intake

477. 渴喜凉饮 [渴喜涼飲] *kě xǐ liáng yǐn*, thirst with a liking for cool drinks

478. 渴喜热饮 [渴喜熱飲] *kě xǐ rè yǐn*, thirst with a liking for hot drinks

479. 大渴引饮 [大渴引飲] *dà kě yǐn yǐn*, great thirst with fluid intake

480. 漱口不欲饮 [漱口不欲飲] *shù kǒu bù yù yǐn*, washing the mouth with water without desire to swallow it

481. 食欲不振 [食欲不振] *shí yù bù zhèn*, poor appetite

482. 不思饮食 [不思飲食] *bù sī yǐn shí*, no thought of food and drink

483. 饮食少思 [飲食少思] *yǐn shí shǎo sī*, little thought of food and drink

484. 纳谷不香 [納穀不香] *nà gǔ bù xiāng*, no pleasure in eating

485. 纳谷不馨 [納穀不馨] *nà gǔ bù xīn*, no pleasure in eating

486. 食不下 [食不下] *shí bù xià*, inability to get food down

487. 不食 [不食] *bù shí*, inability to eat

488. 厌食 [厭食] *yàn shí*, aversion to food

489. 贪食 [貪食] *tān shí*, rapacious eating

490. 纳呆 [納呆] *nà dāi*, torpid intake

491. 嘈杂 [嘈雜] *cáo zá*, clamoring stomach

492. 口中和 [口中和] *kǒu zhōng hé*, harmony of mouth

493. 口甜 [口甜] *kǒu tián*, sweet taste in the mouth

494. 口酸 [口酸] *kǒu suān*, sour taste in the mouth

495. 口苦 [口苦] *kǒu kǔ*, bitter taste in the mouth

496. 呕吐 [嘔吐] *ǒu tù*, (retching and) vomiting

497. 恶心 [惡心] *ě xīn*, nausea

498. 泛酸 [泛酸] *fàn suān*, acid upflow

499. 吞酸 [吞酸] *tūn suān*, swallowing of upflowing acid

500. 吐酸 [吐酸] *tù suān*, vomiting of acid

501. 吐血 [吐血] *tù xuè*, blood ejection

502. 泛恶 [泛惡] *fàn ě*, upflow nausea

503. 胸痛 [胸痛] *xiōng tòng*, chest pain

504. 胸满 [胸滿] *xiōng mǎn*, fullness in the chest

505. 胸闷 [胸悶] *xiōng mèn*, oppression in the chest

506. 胸痞 [胸痞] *xiōng pǐ*, glomus in the chest

507. 胁痛 [脅痛] *xié tòng*, rib-side pain

508. 胸胁苦满 [胸脅苦滿] *xiōng xié kǔ mǎn*, chest and rib-side fullness

509. 心悸 [心悸] *xīn jì*, heart palpitations

510. 惊悸 [驚悸] *jīng jì*, fright palpitations

511. 怔忡 [怔忡] *zhēng chōng*, fearful throbbing

512. 心下痞 [心下痞] *xīn xià pǐ*, glomus below the heart

513. 脘腹痛喜按 [脘腹痛喜按] *wǎn fù tòng xǐ àn*, pain in the stomach duct and abdomen that likes pressure

514. 脘腹痛拒按 [脘腹痛拒按] *wǎn fù tòng jù àn*, pain in the stomach duct and abdomen that refuses pressure

515. 腹满 [腹滿] *fù mǎn*, abdominal fullness

516. 腹痛 [腹痛] *fù tòng*, abdominal pain

517. 腹痛喜温 [腹痛喜溫] *fù tòng xǐ wēn*, abdominal pain that likes warmth

518. 腹痛拒按 [腹痛拒按] *fù tòng jù àn*, abdominal pain that refuses pressure

519. 脐周窜痛 [臍周竄痛] *qí zhōu cuàn tòng*, scurrying pain around the umbilicus

520. 少腹痛 [少腹痛] *shào fù tòng*, lesser-abdominal pain

521. 小腹痛 [小腹痛] *xiǎo fù tòng*, smaller-abdominal pain

522. 耳聋 [耳聾] *ěr lóng*, deafness

523. 重听 [重聽] *zhòng tīng*, hardness of hearing; hearing impairment

524. 耳鸣 [耳鳴] *ěr míng*, tinnitus; ringing in the ears

525. 耳鸣如蝉声 [耳鳴如蟬聲] *ěr míng rú chán shēng*, ringing in the ears like the sound of cicadas

526. 目痛 [目痛] *mù tòng*, eye pain

527. 目花 [目花] *mù huā*, flowery vision

528. 目糊 [目糊] *mù hú*, blurred vision

529. 目干涩 [目乾澀] *mù gān sè*, dry eyes

530. 恶光羞明 [惡光羞明] *wù guāng xiū míng*, aversion to light

531. 失眠 [失眠] *shī mián*, insomnia

532. 不得卧 [不得臥] *bù dé wò*, sleeplessness

533. 不寐 [不寐] *bù mèi*, sleeplessness

534. 多梦 [多夢] *duō mèng*, profuse dreaming

535. 昏睡 [昏睡] *hūn shuì*, clouding sleep

536. 嗜眠 [嗜眠] *shì mián*, somnolence

537. 食后困顿 [食後困頓] *shí hòu kùn dùn*, drowsiness after eating

538. 失精 [失精] *shī jīng*, seminal loss

539. 遗精 [遺精] *yí jīng*, seminal emission

540. 滑精 [滑精] *huá jīng*, seminal efflux

541. 不梦而遗 [不夢而遺] *bù mèng ér yí*, seminal emission without dreaming

542. 梦遗 [夢遺] *mèng yí*, dream emission

543. 阳痿 [陽痿] *yáng wěi*, impotence; yáng wilt

544. 早泄 [早洩] *zǎo xiè*, premature ejaculation

545. 卵缩 [卵縮] *luǎn suō*, retracted testicles

546. 月经失调 [月經失調] *yuè jīng shī tiáo*, menstrual irregularities

547. 月经过多 [月經過多] *yuè jīng guò duō*, profuse menstruation

548. 月经过少 [月經過少] *yuè jīng guò shǎo*, scant menstruation

549. 月经不利 [月經不利] *yuè jīng bù lì*, inhibited menstruation

550. 月经先期 [月經先期] *yuè jīng xiān qī*, advanced menstruation (early periods)

551. 月经后期 [月經後期] *yuè jīng hòu qī*, delayed menstruation (late periods)

552. 经行先后无定期 [經行先後無定期] *jīng xíng xiān hòu wú dìng qī*, menstruation at irregular intervals

553. 乱经 [亂經] *luàn jīng*, chaotic menstruation

554. 闭经 [閉經] *bì jīng*, menstrual block; amenorrhea

555. 带下 [帶下] *dài xià*, vaginal discharge

556. 子宫下垂 [子宮下垂] *zǐ gōng xià chuí*, prolapse of the uterus

557. 胎动不安 [胎動不安] *tāi dòng bù ān*, stirring fetus

558. 恶露不绝 [惡露不絕] *è lù bù jué*, persistent flow of the lochia

559. 寸口 [寸口] *cùn kǒu*, wrist pulse; inch opening

560. 把脉 [把脈] *bǎ mài*, take the pulse

561. 切脉 [切脈] *qiè mài*, take the pulse

562. 寸 [寸] *cùn*, inch

563. 关 [關] *guān*, bar

564. 尺 [尺] *chǐ*, cubit

565. 浮脉 [浮脈] *fú mài*, floating pulse

566. 沉脉 [沉脈] *chén mài*, sunken pulse; deep pulse

567. 迟脉 [遲脈] *chí mài*, slow pulse

568. 数脉 [數脈] *shuò mài*, rapid pulse

569. 虚脉 [虛脈] *xū mài*, vacuous pulse

570. 实脉 [實脈] *shí mài*, replete pulse

571. 滑脉 [滑脈] *huá mài*, slippery pulse

572. 涩脉 [澀脈] *sè mài*, rough pulse

573. 弦脉 [弦脈] *xián mài*, stringlike pulse

574. 濡脉 [濡脈] *rú mài*, soggy pulse

575. 洪脉 [洪脈] *hóng mài*, surging pulse

576. 微脉 [微脈] *wēi mài*, faint pulse

577. 细脉 [細脈] *xì mài*, fine pulse

578. 弱脉 [弱脈] *ruò mài*, weak pulse

579. 大脉 [大脈] *dà mài*, large pulse

580. 散脉 [散脈] *sàn mài*, dissipated pulse

581. 紧脉 [緊脈] *jǐn mài*, tight pulse

582. 芤脉 [芤脈] *kōu mài*, scallion-stalk pulse

583. 革脉 [革脈] *gé mài*, drumskin pulse

584. 牢脉 [牢脈] *láo mài*, firm pulse; confined pulse

585. 疾脉 [疾脈] *jí mài*, racing pulse

586. 动脉 [動脈] *dòng mài*, stirred pulse

587. 伏脉 [伏脈] *fú mài*, hidden pulse

588. 缓脉 [緩脈] *huǎn mài*, moderate pulse

589. 促脉 [促脈] *cù mài*, skipping pulse

590. 结脉 [結脈] *jié mài*, bound pulse

591. 代脉 [代脈] *dài mài*, intermittent pulse

592. 长脉 [長脈] *cháng mài*, long pulse

593. 短脉 [短脈] *duǎn mài*, short pulse

594. 有力 [有力] *yǒu lì*, forceful

595. 无力 [無力] *wú lì*, forceless

596. 肢冷 [肢冷] *zhī lěng*, cold limbs

597. 四肢欠温 [四肢欠溫] *sì zhī qiàn wēn*, lack of warmth in the limbs

598. 四肢不温 [四肢不溫] *sì zhī bù wēn*, lack of warmth in the limbs

599. 四肢厥冷 [四肢厥冷] *sì zhī jué lěng*, reversal cold of the limbs

600. 四肢逆冷 [四肢逆冷] *sì zhī nì lěng*, counterflow cold of the limbs

601. 厥逆 [厥逆] *jué nì*, reverse-flow

602. 形寒 [形寒] *xíng hán*, physical cold

603. 五心烦热 [五心煩熱] *wǔ xīn fán rè*, vexing heat in the five hearts

604. 痞块 [痞塊] *pǐ kuài*, glomus lump

605. 腹胀 ［腹脹］ *fù zhàng*, abdominal distention

606. 浮肿 ［浮腫］ *fú zhǒng*, puffy swelling

607. 灼热 ［灼熱］ *zhuó rè*, scorching heat

5 Diseases

608. 外感 ［外感］ *wài gǎn*, external contraction

609. 杂病 ［雜病］ *zá bìng*, miscellaneous disease

610. 内伤杂病 ［內傷雜病］ *nèi shāng zá bìng*, miscellaneous internal damage disease

611. 鼻渊 ［鼻淵］ *bí yuān*, deep-source nasal congestion

612. 头风 ［頭風］ *tóu fēng*, head wind

613. 痨瘵 ［癆瘵］ *láo zhài*, consumption

614. 喘 ［喘］ *chuǎn*, panting

615. 哮 ［哮］ *xiāo*, wheezing

616. 哮喘 ［哮喘］ *xiāo chuǎn*, wheezing and panting

617. 百日咳 ［百日咳］ *bǎi rì ké*, whooping cough

618. 白喉 ［白喉］ *bái hóu*, diphtheria

619. 喉痹 ［喉痹］ *hóu bì*, throat impediment

620. 乳蛾 ［乳蛾］ *rǔ é*, nipple moth; baby moth

621. 单蛾 ［單蛾］ *dān é*, single moth

622. 双蛾 ［雙蛾］ *shuāng é*, double moth

623. 解颅 ［解顱］ *jiě lú*, ununited skull

624. 麻疹 ［麻疹］ *má zhěn*, measles

625. 痄腮 ［痄腮］ *zhà sāi*, mumps

626. 天花 ［天花］ *tiān huā*, smallpox

627. 痘 ［痘］ *dòu*, pox

628. 痹 ［痹］ *bì*, impediment

629. 行痹 ［行痹］ *xíng bì*, moving impediment

630. 周痹 ［周痹］ *zhōu bì*, generalized impediment

631. 着痹 ［著痹］ *zhuó bì*, fixed impediment

632. 热痹 ［熱痹］ *rè bì*, heat impediment

633. 历节风 ［歷節風］ *lì jié fēng*, joint-running wind

634. 鹤膝风 ［鶴膝風］ *hè xī fēng*, crane's-knee wind

635. 落枕 ［落枕］ *lào zhěn*, crick in the neck

636. 痿 ［痿］ *wěi*, wilting

637. 梅核气 ［梅核氣］ *méi hé qì*, plum-pit qì

638. 噎膈 ［噎膈］ *yē gé*, dysphagia-occlusion

639. 反胃 ［反胃］ *fǎn wèi*, stomach reflux

640. 霍乱 ［霍亂］ *huò luàn*, cholera; sudden turmoil

641. 痢疾 ［痢疾］ *lì jí*, dysentery

642. 黄疸 ［黃疸］ *huáng dǎn*, jaundice

643. 痉病 ［痙病］ *jìng bìng*, tetany

644. 小儿惊风 ［小兒驚風］ *xiǎo ér jīng fēng*, child fright wind

645. 惊风 ［驚風］ *jīng fēng*, fright wind

646. 疳 ［疳］ *gān*, gān

647. 疟疾 ［瘧疾］ *nüè jí*, malaria

648. 心痹 ［心痹］ *xīn bì*, heart impediment

649. 奔豚 [奔豚] *bēn tún*, running piglet

650. 鼓胀 [鼓脹] *gǔ zhàng*, drum distention

651. 消渴 [消渴] *xiāo kě*, dispersion-thirst

652. 癥瘕积聚 [癥瘕積聚] *zhēng jiǎ jī jù*, concretions, conglomerations, accumulations, and gatherings

653. 疝 [疝] *shàn*, mounting

654. 疝气 [疝氣] *shàn qì*, mounting qì

655. 中风 [中風] *zhòng fēng*, wind stroke; wind strike

656. 癫痫 [癲癇] *diān xián*, epilepsy

657. 癫狂 [癲狂] *diān kuáng*, mania and withdrawal

658. 破伤风 [破傷風] *pò shāng fēng*, lockjaw

659. 癃闭 [癃閉] *lóng bì*, dribbling urinary block

660. 水肿 [水腫] *shuǐ zhǒng*, water swelling

661. 淋证 [淋證] *lín zhèng*, strangury pattern

662. 血淋 [血淋] *xuè lín*, blood strangury

663. 膏淋 [膏淋] *gāo lín*, unctuous strangury

664. 气淋 [氣淋] *qì lín*, qì strangury

665. 石淋 [石淋] *shí lín*, stone strangury

666. 劳淋 [勞淋] *láo lín*, taxation strangury

667. 淋浊 [淋濁] *lín zhuó*, strangury-turbidity

668. 转胞 [轉胞] *zhuǎn bāo*, shifted bladder

669. 茄子病 [茄子病] *qié zi bìng*, eggplant disease

670. 崩漏 [崩漏] *bēng lòu*, flooding and spotting

671. 遏阻 [遏阻] *è zǔ*, malign obstruction; morning sickness

672. 恶露不行 [惡露不行] *è lù bù xíng*, retention of the lochia

673. 恶露不断 [惡露不斷] *è lù bù duàn*, persistent flow of the lochia

674. 无子 [無子] *wú zǐ*, childlessness

675. 不孕 [不孕] *bù yùn*, infertility

676. 阴挺 [陰挺] *yīn tǐng*, yīn protrusion

677. 肺痈 [肺癰] *fèi yōng*, pulmonary welling-abscess

678. 肠痈 [腸癰] *cháng yōng*, intestinal welling-abscess

679. 肺痿 [肺痿] *fèi wěi*, lung wilting

680. 衄 [衄] *nǜ*, spontaneous external bleeding

681. 瘿 [癭] *yǐng*, goiter

682. 脚气 [腳氣] *jiǎo qì*, leg qì

683. 疮疡 [瘡瘍] *chuāng yáng*, sore

684. 痈 [癰] *yōng*, welling-abscess

685. 疽 [疽] *jū*, flat-abscess

686. 疖 [癤] *jié*, boil

687. 疔疮 [疔瘡] *dīng chuāng*, clove sore

688. 瘰疬 [瘰癧] *luǒ lì*, scrofula

689. 痰核 [痰核] *tán hé*, phlegm node

690. 流注 [流注] *liú zhù*, streaming sore

691. 疥 [疥] *jiè*, scab

692. 癞 [癩] *lài*, lài

693. 癣［癬］*xiǎn,* lichen

694. 口（中生）疮［口（中生）瘡］*kǒu (zhōng shēng) chuāng,* mouth sore

695. 口舌生疮［口舌生瘡］*kǒu shé shēng chuāng,* sores of the mouth and tongue

696. 冻疮［凍瘡］*dòng chuāng,* frostbite

697. 丹毒［丹毒］*dān dú,* erysipelas; cinnabar toxin [sore]

698. 扭伤［扭傷］*niǔ shāng,* sprain

6 Patterns

699. 证（候）［證（候）］*zhèng hòu,* pattern

700. 病证［病證］*bìng zhèng,* disease pattern

701. 症［症］*zhèng,* pathocondition

702. 八纲辨证［八綱辨證］*bā gāng biàn zhèng,* eight-principle pattern identification

703. 表证［表證］*biǎo zhèng,* exterior pattern

704. 表寒［表寒］*biǎo hán,* exterior cold

705. 表热［表熱］*biǎo rè,* exterior heat

706. 表虚［表虛］*biǎo xū,* exterior vacuity

707. 表实［表實］*biǎo shí,* exterior repletion

708. 里证［裡證］*lǐ zhèng,* interior pattern

709. 半表半里证［半表半裡證］*bàn biǎo bàn lǐ zhèng,* midstage pattern; half-interior half-exterior pattern

710. 寒证［寒證］*hán zhèng,* cold pattern

711. 热证［熱證］*rè zhèng,* heat pattern

712. 虚证［虛證］*xū zhèng,* vacuity pattern

713. 虚损［虛損］*xū sǔn,* vacuity detriment

714. 虚劳［虛勞］*xū láo,* vacuity taxation

715. 实证［實證］*shí zhèng,* repletion pattern

716. 阴证［陰證］*yīn zhèng,* yīn pattern

717. 阳证［陽證］*yáng zhèng,* yáng pattern

718. 阴虚［陰虛］*yīn xū,* yīn vacuity

719. 阳虚［陽虛］*yáng xū,* yáng vacuity

720. 亡阴［亡陰］*wáng yīn,* yīn collapse

721. 阴脱［陰脱］*yīn tuō,* yīn desertion

722. 阴液暴脱［陰液暴脱］*yīn yè bào tuō,* fulminant desertion of yīn humor

723. 亡阳［亡陽］*wáng yáng,* yáng collapse

724. 阳脱［陽脱］*yáng tuō,* yáng desertion

725. 脱证［脱證］*tuō zhèng,* desertion pattern

726. 气虚［氣虛］*qì xū,* qì vacuity

727. 气滞［氣滯］*qì zhì,* qì stagnation

728. 气逆［氣逆］*qì nì,* qì counterflow

729. 气闭［氣閉］*qì bì,* qì block

730. 血瘀［血瘀］*xuè yū,* blood stasis

731. 血虚 [血虚] *xuè xū*, blood vacuity

732. 阴血不足 [陰血不足] *yīn xuè bù zú*, insufficiency of yīn-blood

733. 亡血 [亡血] *wáng xuè*, blood collapse

734. 血热 [血熱] *xuè rè*, blood heat

735. 血热妄行 [血熱妄行] *xuè rè wàng xíng*, frenetic movement of hot blood

736. 血寒 [血寒] *xuè hán*, blood cold

737. 气滞血瘀 [氣滯血瘀] *qì zhì xuè yū*, qì stagnation and blood stasis

738. 气血俱虚 [氣血俱虛] *qì xuè jù xū*, dual vacuity of qì and blood

739. 气随血脱 [氣隨血脫] *qì suí xuè tuō*, qì deserting with the blood

740. 心气虚 [心氣虛] *xīn qì xū*, heart qì vacuity

741. 心阳虚 [心陽虛] *xīn yáng xū*, heart yáng vacuity

742. 心血虚 [心血虛] *xīn xuè xū*, heart blood vacuity

743. 心阴虚 [心陰虛] *xīn yīn xū*, heart yīn vacuity

744. 心火上炎 [心火上炎] *xīn huǒ shàng yán*, heart fire flaming upward

745. 心火亢盛 [心火亢盛] *xīn huǒ kàng shèng*, hyperactive heart fire

746. 心火炽盛 [心火熾盛] *xīn huǒ chì shèng*, intense heart fire

747. 心火盛 [心火盛] *xīn huǒ shèng*, exuberant heart fire

748. 心血瘀阻 [心血瘀阻] *xīn xuè yū zǔ*, heart blood stasis obstruction

749. 心神不安 [心神不安] *xīn shén bù ān*, disquieted heart spirit

750. 心火移热于小肠 [心火移熱於小腸] *xīn huǒ yí rè yú xiǎo cháng*, heart fire spreading heat to the small intestine

751. 水气凌心 [水氣凌心] *shuǐ qì líng xīn*, water qì intimidating the heart

752. 肺气不宣 [肺氣不宣] *fèi qì bù xuān*, nondiffusion of lung qì

753. 肺失肃降 [肺失肅降] *fèi shī sù jiàng*, impaired depurative downbearing of the lung

754. 肺气不利 [肺氣不利] *fèi qì bù lì*, inhibition of lung qì

755. 肺气虚 [肺氣虛] *fèi qì xū*, lung qì vacuity

756. 肺阴虚 [肺陰虛] *fèi yīn xū*, lung yīn vacuity

757. 肺肾阴虚 [肺腎陰虛] *fèi shèn yīn xū*, lung-kidney yīn vacuity

758. 脾虚 [脾虛] *pí xū*, spleen vacuity

759. 脾气虚 [脾氣虛] *pí qì xū*, spleen qì vacuity

760. 脾失健运 [脾失健運] *pí shī jiàn yùn*, spleen failing to move and transform

761. 脾虚湿困 [脾虛濕困] *pí xū shī kùn*, spleen vacuity damp encumbrance

762. 中气不足 [中氣不足] *zhōng qì bù zú*, insufficiency of center qì

763. 脾不统血 [脾不統血] *pí bù tǒng xuè*, spleen failing to control the blood

764. 脾阴虚 [脾陰虛] *pí yīn xū*, spleen yīn vacuity

765. **脾阳虚** [脾陽虛] *pí yáng xū*, spleen yáng vacuity

766. **脾阳不振** [脾陽不振] *pí yáng bù zhèn*, devitalized spleen yáng

767. **脾肺两虚** [脾肺兩虛] *pí fèi liǎng xū*, dual vacuity of the spleen and lung

768. **脾肺气虚** [脾肺氣虛] *pí fèi qì xū*, spleen-lung qì vacuity

769. **心脾两虚** [心脾兩虛] *xīn pí liǎng xū*, dual vacuity of the heart and spleen

770. **胃气虚寒** [胃氣虛寒] *wèi qì xū hán*, stomach qì vacuity cold

771. **胃虚寒** [胃虛寒] *wèi xū hán*, stomach vacuity cold

772. **胃阴虚** [胃陰虛] *wèi yīn xū*, stomach yīn vacuity

773. **胃阴不足** [胃陰不足] *wèi yīn bù zú*, insufficiency of stomach yīn

774. **胃热** [胃熱] *wèi rè*, stomach heat

775. **胃气上逆** [胃氣上逆] *wèi qì shàng nì*, counterflow ascent of stomach qì

776. **胃火** [胃火] *wèi huǒ*, stomach fire

777. **大肠液亏** [大腸液虧] *dà cháng yè kuī*, large intestinal humor depletion

778. **肠液亏耗** [腸液虧耗] *cháng yè kuī hào*, intestinal humor depletion

779. **心肾阴虚** [心腎陰虛] *xīn shèn yīn xū*, heart-kidney yīn vacuity

780. **心脾血虚** [心脾血虛] *xīn pí xuè xū*, heart-spleen blood vacuity

781. **肝气郁结** [肝氣鬱結] *gān qì yù jié*, binding depression of liver qì

782. **肝郁** [肝鬱] *gān yù*, liver depression

783. **肝郁化火** [肝鬱化火] *gān yù huà huǒ*, liver depression transforming into fire

784. **肝火上炎** [肝火上炎] *gān huǒ shàng yán*, liver fire flaming upward

785. **肝阳上亢** [肝陽上亢] *gān yáng shàng kàng*, ascendant hyperactivity of liver yáng; ascendant liver yáng

786. **肝血虚** [肝血虛] *gān xuè xū*, liver blood vacuity

787. **肝风内动** [肝風內動] *gān fēng nèi dòng*, liver wind stirring internally

788. **肝阳化风** [肝陽化風] *gān yáng huà fēng*, liver yáng transforming into wind

789. **热极生风** [熱極生風] *rè jí shēng fēng*, extreme heat engendering wind

790. **血虚生风** [血虛生風] *xuè xū shēng fēng*, blood vacuity engendering wind

791. **肝经湿热** [肝經濕熱] *gān jīng shī rè*, liver channel damp-heat

792. **肝胆湿热** [肝膽濕熱] *gān dǎn shī rè*, liver-gallbladder damp-heat

793. **肝气犯胃** [肝氣犯胃] *gān qì fàn wèi*, liver qì invading the stomach

794. **肝气犯脾** [肝氣犯脾] *gān qì fàn pí*, liver qì invading the spleen

795. 胆热 [膽熱] *dǎn rè*, gallbladder heat

796. 胆火 [膽火] *dǎn huǒ*, gallbladder fire

797. 胆虚 [膽虛] *dǎn xū*, gallbladder vacuity

798. 胆虚气怯 [膽虛氣怯] *dǎn xū qì qiè*, gallbladder vacuity and qì timidity

799. 胆气不足 [膽氣不足] *dǎn qì bù zú*, insufficiency of gallbladder qì

800. 心虚胆怯 [心虛膽怯] *xīn xū dǎn qiè*, heart vacuity and gallbladder timidity

801. 心胆虚怯 [心膽虛怯] *xīn dǎn xū qiè*, heart-gallbladder vacuity timidity

802. 肾阴虚 [腎陰虛] *shèn yīn xū*, kidney yīn vacuity

803. 肾阴枯涸 [腎陰枯涸] *shèn yīn kū hé*, desiccation of kidney yīn

804. 肾阳虚 [腎陽虛] *shèn yáng xū*, kidney yáng vacuity

805. 肾阳虚衰 [腎陽虛衰] *shèn yáng xū shuāi*, debilitation of kidney yáng

806. 真阳不足 [眞陽不足] *zhēn yáng bù zú*, insufficiency of true yáng

807. 真元不足 [眞元不足] *zhēn yuán bù zú*, insufficiency of the true origin

808. 下元虚惫 [下元虛憊] *xià yuán xū bèi*, exhaustion of the lower origin

809. 阳虚水泛 [陽虛水泛] *yáng xū shuǐ fàn*, yáng vacuity water flood

810. 肾虚水泛 [腎虛水泛] *shèn xū shuǐ fàn*, kidney vacuity water flood

811. 命门火衰 [命門火衰] *mìng mén huǒ shuāi*, debilitation of the life gate fire

812. 肾精不足 [腎精不足] *shèn jīng bù zú*, insufficiency of kidney essence

813. 髓海空虚 [髓海空虛] *suǐ hǎi kōng xū*, emptiness of the sea of marrow

814. 肾不纳气 [腎不納氣] *shèn bù nà qì*, kidney failing to absorb qì

815. 肾气虚 [腎氣虛] *shèn qì xū*, kidney qì vacuity

816. 肾气不固 [腎氣不固] *shèn qì bù gù*, insecurity of kidney qì

817. 肾虚 [腎虛] *shèn xū*, kidney vacuity

818. 心肾不交 [心腎不交] *xīn shèn bù jiāo*, noninteraction of the heart and kidney

819. 心肾阳虚 [心腎陽虛] *xīn shèn yáng xū*, heart-kidney yáng vacuity

820. 脾肾阳虚 [脾腎陽虛] *pí shèn yáng xū*, spleen-kidney yáng vacuity

821. 肝肾阴亏 [肝腎陰虧] *gān shèn yīn kuī*, liver-kidney yīn depletion

822. 外感风邪 [外感風邪] *wài gǎn fēng xié*, external contraction of wind evil

823. 风寒 [風寒] *fēng hán*, wind-cold

824. 风热 [風熱] *fēng rè*, wind-hea

825. 风热犯肺 [風熱犯肺] *fēng rè fàn fèi*, wind-heat invading the lung

826. 风寒束肺 [風寒束肺] *fēng hán shù fèi*, wind-cold fettering the lung

827. 风邪入经 [風邪入經] *fēng xié rù jīng*, wind evil entering the channels

828. 外感寒邪 [外感寒邪] *wài gǎn hán xié*, external contraction of cold evil

829. 寒痹 [寒痹] *hán bì*, cold impediment

830. 寒疝 [寒疝] *hán shàn*, cold mounting

831. 寒气凝滞 [寒氣凝滯] *hán qì níng zhì*, congealing cold and stagnant qì

832. 阴盛内寒 [陰盛內寒] *yīn shèng nèi hán*, exuberant internal yīn cold

833. 寒滞肝脉 [寒滯肝脈] *hán zhì gān mài*, cold stagnating in the liver vessel

834. 实热 [實熱] *shí rè*, repletion heat

835. 虚热 [虛熱] *xū rè*, vacuity heat

836. 虚火 [虛火] *xū huǒ*, vacuity fire

837. 阴虚火旺 [陰虛火旺] *yīn xū huǒ wàng*, effulgent yīn vacuity fire

838. 暑热 [暑熱] *shǔ rè*, summerheat-heat

839. 暑湿 [暑濕] *shǔ shī*, summerheat-damp

840. 湿阻 [濕阻] *shī zǔ*, damp obstruction

841. 寒湿 [寒濕] *hán shī*, cold-damp

842. 湿热 [濕熱] *shī rè*, damp-heat

843. 湿遏热伏 [濕遏熱伏] *shī è rè fú*, dampness trapping hidden (deep-lying) heat

844. 湿热留恋气分 [濕熱留戀氣分] *shī rè liú liàn qì fēn*, damp-heat lodged in the qì aspect

845. 湿热阻滞脾胃 [濕熱阻滯脾胃] *shī rè zǔ zhì pí wèi*, damp-heat obstructing the spleen and stomach

846. 湿热蕴结肝胆 [濕熱蘊結肝膽] *shī rè yùn jié gān dǎn*, damp-heat brewing in the liver and gallbladder

847. 湿热下注大肠 [濕熱下注大腸] *shī rè xià zhù dà cháng*, damp-heat pouring down into the large intestine

848. 大肠湿热 [大腸濕熱] *dà cháng shī rè*, large intestinal damp-heat

849. 湿热下注膀胱 [濕熱下注膀胱] *shī rè xià zhù páng guāng*, damp-heat pouring down into the bladder

850. 膀胱湿热 [膀胱濕熱] *páng guāng shī rè*, bladder damp-heat

851. 感受燥邪 [感受燥邪] *gǎn shòu zào xié*, contraction of dryness evil

852. 伤津 [傷津] *shāng jīn*, damage to liquid

853. 伤阴 [傷陰] *shāng yīn*, damage to yīn

854. 伤食 [傷食] *shāng shí*, food damage

855. 宿食 [宿食] *sù shí*, abiding food

856. **肠胃积滞** [腸胃積滯] *cháng wèi jī zhì*, gastrointestinal accumulation

857. **脾虚夹食** [脾虛夾食] *pí xū jiā shí*, spleen vacuity with food damage

858. **伤酒** [傷酒] *shāng jiǔ*, liquor damage

859. **湿痰** [濕痰] *shī tán*, damp phlegm

860. **寒痰** [寒痰] *hán tán*, cold phlegm

861. **热痰** [熱痰] *rè tán*, heat phlegm

862. **痰浊上扰** [痰濁上擾] *tán zhuó shàng rǎo*, phlegm turbidity harassing the upper body

863. **痰迷心窍** [痰迷心竅] *tán mí xīn qiào*, phlegm confounding the orifices of the heart

864. **痰浊蒙蔽心包** [痰濁蒙蔽心包] *tán zhuó méng bì xīn bāo*, phlegm turbidity clouding the pericardium

865. **痰火** [痰火] *tán huǒ*, phlegm-fire

866. **痰热** [痰熱] *tán rè*, phlegm-heat

867. **痰留经络** [痰留經絡] *tán liú jīng luò*, phlegm lodged in the channels

868. **痰火扰心** [痰火擾心] *tán huǒ rǎo xīn*, phlegm-fire harassing the heart

869. **痰饮** [痰飲] *tán yǐn*, phlegm-rheum

870. **痰湿** [痰濕] *tán shī*, phlegm-damp

871. **痰浊** [痰濁] *tán zhuó*, phlegm turbidity

872. **风痰** [風痰] *fēng tán*, wind-phlegm

873. **外感热病** [外感熱病] *wài gǎn rè bìng*, externally contracted heat (febrile) disease

874. **六经辨证** [六經辨證] *liù jīng biàn zhèng*, six-channel pattern identification

875. **太阳病** [太陽病] *tài yáng bìng*, greater yáng disease

876. **阳明病** [陽明病] *yáng míng bìng*, yáng brightness disease

877. **少阳病** [少陽病] *shào yáng bìng*, lesser yáng disease

878. **太阴病** [太陰病] *tài yīn bìng*, greater yīn disease

879. **少阴病** [少陰病] *shào yīn bìng*, lesser yīn disease

880. **厥阴病** [厥陰病] *jué yīn bìng*, reverting yīn disease

881. **卫分证** [衛分證] *wèi fèn zhèng*, defense-aspect pattern

882. **气分证** [氣分證] *qì fèn zhèng*, qì-aspect pattern

883. **营分证** [營分證] *yíng fèn zhèng*, construction-aspect pattern

884. **血分证** [血分證] *xuè fèn zhèng*, blood-aspect pattern

885. **热入营血** [熱入營血] *rè rù yíng xuè*, heat entering construction-blood

886. **心包证** [心包證] *xīn bāo zhèng*, pericardiac patterns

887. **热入心包** [熱入心包] *rè rù xīn bāo*, heat entering the pericardium:

888. **痰蒙心包** [痰蒙心包] *tán méng xīn bāo*, phlegm clouding the pericardium:

889. **风温** [風溫] *fēng wēn*, wind warmth

890. 湿温 ［濕溫］ *shī wēn*, damp warmth

891. 气阴两虚 ［氣陰兩虛］ *qì yīn liǎng xū*, dual vacuity of qì and yīn

892. 实则泻之 ［實則瀉之］ *shí zé xiè zhī*, repletion is treated by draining

893. 虚则补之 ［虛則補之］ *xū zé bǔ zhī*, vacuity is treated by supplementing

7 Methods of Treatment

894. 治本 ［治本］ *zhì běn*, treating the root

895. 治标 ［治標］ *zhì biāo*, treating the tip

896. 正治 ［正治］ *zhèng zhì*, straight treatment

897. 反治 ［反治］ *fǎn zhì*, paradoxical treatment

898. 八法 ［八法］ *bā fǎ*, eight methods

899. 解表 ［解表］ *jiě biǎo*, resolving the exterior

900. 汗法 ［汗法］ *hàn fǎ*, sweating

901. 辛温解表 ［辛溫解表］ *xīn wēn jiě biǎo*, resolving the exterior with warmth and acridity

902. 辛凉解表 ［辛涼解表］ *xīn liáng jiě biǎo*, resolving the exterior with coolness and acridity

903. 疏表 ［疏表］ *shū biǎo*, coursing the exterior

904. 疏风泄热 ［疏風泄熱］ *shū fēng xiè rè*, coursing wind and discharging heat

905. 滋阴解表 ［滋陰解表］ *zī yīn jiě biǎo*, enriching yīn and resolving the exterior

906. 助阳解表 ［助陽解表］ *zhù yáng jiě biǎo*, reinforcing yáng and resolving the exterior

907. 益气解表 ［益氣解表］ *yì qì jiě biǎo*, boosting qì and resolving the exterior

908. 表里双解 ［表裡雙解］ *biǎo lǐ shuāng jiě*, resolving both the exterior and interior; exterior-interior resolution

909. 清气分热 ［清氣分熱］ *qīng qì fēn rè*, clearing qì-aspect heat

910. 清营凉血 ［清營涼血］ *qīng yíng liáng xuè*, clearing construction and cooling the blood

911. 凉血 ［涼血］ *liáng xuè*, cooling the blood

912. 清热解暑 ［清熱解暑］ *qīng rè jiě shǔ*, clearing heat and resolving summerheat

913. 清热解毒 ［清熱解毒］ *qīng rè jiě dú*, clearing heat and resolving toxin

914. 清脏腑热 ［清臟腑熱］ *qīng zàng fǔ rè*, clearing bowel and visceral heat

915. 清虚热 ［清虛熱］ *qīng xū rè*, clearing vacuity heat

916. 寒下 ［寒下］ *hán xià*, cold precipitation

917. 温下 ［溫下］ *wēn xià*, warm precipitation

918. 润下 ［潤下］ *rùn xià*, moist precipitation

919. 增液润下 ［增液潤下］ *zēng yè rùn xià*, humor-increasing moist precipitation

920. 逐水 ［逐水］ *zhú shuǐ*, expelling water

921. **和解少阳** [和解少陽] *hé jiě shào yáng*, harmonizing (and resolving) the lesser yáng

922. **和解半表半里** [和解半表半裡] *hé jiě bàn biǎo bàn lǐ*, harmonizing (and resolving) midstage patterns; harmonizing (and resolving) half-exterior half-interior patterns

923. **调和肝脾** [調和肝脾] *tiáo hé gān pí*, harmonizing the liver and spleen

924. **调和肝胃** [調和肝胃] *tiáo hé gān wèi*, harmonizing the liver and stomach

925. **调和肠胃** [調和腸胃] *tiáo hé cháng wèi*, harmonizing the stomach and intestines

926. **祛湿** [祛濕] *qū shī*, dispelling dampness

927. **燥湿和胃** [燥濕和胃] *zào shī hé wèi*, drying dampness and harmonizing the stomach

928. **清热祛湿** [清熱祛濕] *qīng rè qū shī*, clearing heat and dispelling dampness

929. **清利湿热** [清利濕熱] *qīng lì shī rè*, clearing heat and disinhibiting dampness

930. **利水渗湿** [利水滲濕] *lì shuǐ shèn shī*, disinhibiting water and percolating dampness

931. **温化水湿** [溫化水濕] *wēn huà shuǐ shī*, warming and transforming water-damp

932. **祛风胜湿** [祛風勝濕] *qū fēng shèng shī*, dispelling wind and overcoming dampness

933. **健脾利水** [健脾利水] *jiàn pí lì shuǐ*, fortifying the spleen and disinhibiting water

934. **健脾利湿** [健脾利濕] *jiàn pí lì shī*, fortifying the spleen and disinhibiting dampness

935. **润燥** [潤燥] *rùn zào*, moistening dryness

936. **轻宣润燥** [輕宣潤燥] *qīng xuān rùn zào*, moistening dryness by light diffusion

937. **滋阴润燥** [滋陰潤燥] *zī yīn rùn zào*, enriching yīn and moistening dryness

938. **温中散寒** [溫中散寒] *wēn zhōng sàn hán*, warming the center and dissipating cold

939. **回阳救逆** [回陽救逆] *huí yáng jiù nì*, returning yáng and stemming counterflow

940. **温经散寒** [溫經散寒] *wēn jīng sàn hán*, warming the channels and dissipating cold

941. **理气** [理氣] *lǐ qì*, rectifying qì

942. **行气** [行氣] *xíng qì*, moving qì

943. **疏郁理气** [疏鬱理氣] *shū yù lǐ qì*, coursing depression and rectifying qì

944. **降逆止呕** [降逆止嘔] *jiàng nì zhǐ ǒu*, downbearing counterflow and checking vomiting

945. **和胃理气** [和胃理氣] *hé wèi lǐ qì*, harmonizing the stomach and rectifying qì

946. **降气平喘** [降氣平喘] *jiàng qì píng chuǎn*, downbearing qì and calming panting

947. **破气** [破氣] *pò qì*, breaking qì

948. **消导化积** [消導化積] *xiāo dǎo huà jī*, abductive dispersion and transforming accumulations

949. 消食导滞 [消食導滯] *xiāo shí dǎo zhì*, dispersing food and abducting stagnation

950. 消食 [消食] *xiāo shí*, dispersing food

951. 消瘿瘰痰核 [消癭瘰痰核] *xiāo yǐng luó tán hé*, dispersing goiter, scrofula, and phlegm nodes

952. 消癥瘕积聚 [消癥瘕積聚] *xiāo zhēng jiǎ jī jù*, dispersing concretions, conglommerations, accumulations, and gatherings

953. 软坚 [軟堅] *ruǎn jiān*, softening hardness

954. 驱虫 [驅蟲] *qū chóng*, expelling worms

955. 理血 [理血] *lǐ xuè*, rectifying the blood

956. 祛瘀活血 [祛瘀活血] *qū yū huó xuè*, dispelling stasis and quickening the blood

957. 活血化瘀 [活血化瘀] *huó xuè huà yū*, quickening the blood and transforming stasis

958. 破血 [破血] *pò xuè*, breaking blood

959. 止血 [止血] *zhǐ xuè*, stanching bleeding

960. 祛痰 [祛痰] *qū tán*, dispelling phlegm

961. 燥湿化痰 [燥濕化痰] *zào shī huà tán*, drying dampness and transforming phlegm

962. 宣肺化痰 [宣肺化痰] *xuān fèi huà tán*, diffusing the lung and transforming phlegm

963. 温肺化饮 [溫肺化飲] *wēn fèi huà yǐn*, warming the lung and transforming rheum

964. 润肺化痰 [潤肺化痰] *rùn fèi huà tán*, moistening the lung and transforming phlegm

965. 治风化痰 [治風化痰] *zhì fēng huà tán*, controlling wind and transforming phlegm

966. 顺气化痰 [順氣化痰] *shùn qì huà tán*, normalizing qì and transforming phlegm

967. 攻痰 [攻痰] *gōng tán*, attacking phlegm

968. 安神 [安神] *ān shén*, quieting the spirit

969. 养心安神 [養心安神] *yǎng xīn ān shén*, nourishing the heart and quieting the spirit

970. 重镇安神 [重鎮安神] *zhòng zhèn ān shén*, quieting the spirit with heavy settlers

971. 祛风 [祛風] *qū fēng*, dispelling wind

972. 疏散外风 [疏散外風] *shū sàn wài fēng*, coursing and dissipating external wind

973. 平息内风 [平息內風] *píng xī nèi fēng*, calming and extinguishing internal wind

974. 平肝息风 [平肝息風] *píng gān xī fēng*, calming the liver and extinguishing wind

975. 滋阴息风 [滋陰息風] *zī yīn xī fēng*, enriching yīn and extinguishing wind

976. 祛风解痉 [祛風解痙] *qū fēng jiě jìng*, dispelling wind and resolving tetany

977. 清热开窍 [清熱開竅] *qīng rè kāi qiào*, clearing heat and opening the orifices

978. **清心开窍** ［清心開竅］ *qīng xīn kāi qiào*, clearing the heart and opening the orifices

979. **凉开** ［涼開］ *liáng kāi*, cool opening

980. **逐寒开窍** ［逐寒開竅］ *zhú hán kāi qiào*, expelling cold and opening the orifices

981. **温开** ［溫開］ *wēn kāi*, warm opening

982. **化痰开窍** ［化痰開竅］ *huà tán kāi qiào*, transforming phlegm and opening the orifices

983. **豁痰开窍** ［豁痰開竅］ *huò tán kāi qiào*, sweeping phlegm and opening the orifices

984. **补气** ［補氣］ *bǔ qì*, supplementing qì

985. **益气** ［益氣］ *yì qì*, boosting qì

986. **补血** ［補血］ *bǔ xuè*, supplementing the blood

987. **气血双补** ［氣血雙補］ *qì xuè shuāng bǔ*, supplementing both qì and blood; dual supplementation of qì and blood

988. **补阴** ［補陰］ *bǔ yīn*, supplementing yīn

989. **养阴** ［養陰］ *yǎng yīn*, nourishing yīn

990. **滋阴** ［滋陰］ *zī yīn*, enriching yīn

991. **育阴** ［育陰］ *yù yīn*, fostering yīn

992. **补阳** ［補陽］ *bǔ yáng*, supplementing yáng

993. **助阳** ［助陽］ *zhù yáng*, assisting yáng

994. **固涩** ［固澀］ *gù sè*, securing and astriction

995. **敛汗固表** ［斂汗固表］ *liǎn hàn gù biǎo*, constraining sweat and securing the exterior

996. **涩肠固脱** ［澀腸固脫］ *sè cháng gù tuō*, astringing the intestines and stemming desertion

997. **涩精止遗** ［澀精止遺］ *sè jīng zhǐ yí*, astringing essence and checking (seminal) emission and enuresis

998. **缩尿** ［縮尿］ *suō niào*, reducing urine

999. **固崩止带** ［固崩止帶］ *gù bēng zhǐ dài*, stemming flooding and checking (vaginal) discharge

1000. **敛肺止咳** ［斂肺止咳］ *liǎn fèi zhǐ ké*, constraining the lung and suppressing cough

1001. **涌吐** ［湧吐］ *yǒng tù*, ejection

8 Chinese Pharmaceutics

1002. **性味** ［性味］ *xìng wèi*, nature and flavor

1003. **四性** ［四性］ *sì xìng*, four natures

1004. **四气** ［四氣］ *sì qì*, four qì

1005. **五味** ［五味］ *wǔ wèi*, five flavors

1006. **归经** ［歸經］ *guī jīng*, channel entry

1007. **升降浮沉** ［升降浮沉］ *shēng jiàng fú chén*, upbearing, downbearing, floating, and sinking

1008. **炮炙** ［炮炙］ *páo zhì*, processing of medicinals

1009. **饮片** ［飲片］ *yǐn piàn*, decocting pieces

1010. **切** ［切］ *qiē*, cutting

1011. **切片** ［切片］ *qiē piàn*, slicing

1012. **捣碎** ［搗碎］ *dǎo suì*, crushing

1013. 为末 [爲末] *wéi mò*, grinding to a powder

1014. 为细末 [爲細末] *wéi xì mò*, grinding to a fine powder

1015. 生 [生] *shēng*, raw

1016. 生 [生] *shēng*, crude

1017. 熟 [熟] *shú*, cooked

1018. 制霜 [製霜] *zhì shuāng*, frosting

1019. 水制 [水製] *shuǐ zhì*, water processing

1020. 洗 [洗] *xǐ*, washing

1021. 浸泡 [浸泡] *jìn pào*, steeping

1022. 闷润 [悶潤] *mèn rùn*, covered moistening

1023. 漂 [漂] *piǎo*, long-rinsing

1024. 水飞 [水飛] *shuǐ fēi*, water grinding

1025. 火制 [火製] *huǒ zhì*, fire processing

1026. 炒 [炒] *chǎo*, stir-frying

1027. 清炒 [清炒] *qīng chǎo*, plain stir-frying

1028. 炒焦 [炒焦] *chǎo jiāo*, scorch-frying

1029. 微炒 [微炒] *wēi chǎo*, light stir-frying

1030. 炒黄 [炒黃] *chǎo huáng*, stir-frying until yellow

1031. 炮 [炮] *páo*, blast-frying

1032. 炒炭 [炒炭] *chǎo tàn*, char-fry

1033. 烧存性 [燒存性] *shāo cún xìng*, nature-preservative burning

1034. 炙 [炙] *zhì*, mix-fry

1035. 焙 [焙] *bèi*, stone-baking

1036. 煨 [煨] *wēi*, roasting

1037. 煅 [煅] *duàn*, calcine (*v.*); calcination (*n.*)

1038. 水火制 [水火製] *shuǐ huǒ zhì*, fire and water processing

1039. 煮 [煮] *zhǔ*, boiling

1040. 蒸 [蒸] *zhēng*, steaming:

1041. 炖 [燉] *dùn*, double-boiling

1042. 煅淬 [煅淬] *duàn cuì*, calcining and quenching

1043. 剂型 [劑型] *jì xíng*, preparation

1044. 汤 [湯] *tāng*, decoction

1045. 煎 [煎] *jiān*, decoct (*v.*); brew (*v.*)

1046. 饮 [飲] *yǐn*, beverage

1047. 饮子 [飲子] *yǐn zi*, drink

1048. 丸 [丸] *wán*, pill

1049. 水丸 [水丸] *shuǐ wán*, water pill

1050. 散 [散] *sǎn*, powder

1051. 酒剂 [酒劑] *jiǔ jì*, wine preparation

1052. 膏 [膏] *gāo*, paste

1053. 膏滋 [膏滋] *gāo zī*, rich paste

1054. 药膏 [藥膏] *yào gāo*, medicinal paste

1055. 膏药 [膏藥] *gāo yào*, plaster

1056. 露 [露] *lù*, distillate

1057. 露 [露] *lù*, dew

1058. 锭 [錠] *dìng*, lozenge

1059. 片 [片] *piàn*, tablet

1060. 热熨 [熱熨] *rè yùn*, hot pack

1061. 胶 [膠] *jiāo*, glue

1062. 服 [服] *fú*, take

1063. 冲服 [沖服] *chōng fú*, take drenched

1064. 送服 [送服] *sòng fú*, swallow with fluid

1065. 频服 [頻服] *pín fú*, take in frequent small doses

1066. **顿服** [頓服] *dùn fú*, quaff

1067. **食远服** [食遠服] *shí yuǎn fú*, take between meals

1068. **饭前服** [飯前服] *fàn qián fú*, take before meals

1069. **临睡前服** [臨睡前服] *lín shuì qián fú*, take before sleeping

1070. **调敷** [調敷] *tiáo fū*, apply mixed

1071. **君** [君] *jūn*, sovereign

1072. **臣** [臣] *chén*, minister

1073. **佐** [佐] *zuǒ*, assistant

1074. **使** [使] *shǐ*, courier

9 Acumoxatherapy

1075. **毫针** [毫針] *háo zhēn*, filiform needle

1076. **火针** [火針] *huǒ zhēn*, fire needle

1077. **电针** [電針] *diàn zhēn*, electroacupuncture

1078. **三棱针** [三棱針] *sān léng zhēn*, three-edged needle

1079. **皮肤针** [皮膚針] *pí fū zhēn*, cutaneous needle

1080. **梅花针** [梅花針] *méi huā zhēn*, plum-blossom needle

1081. **七星针** [七星針] *qī xīng zhēn*, seven-star needle

1082. **揿针** [撳針] *qìn zhēn*, thumbtack needle

1083. **艾绒** [艾絨] *ài róng*, moxa floss

1084. **艾条** [艾條] *ài tiáo*, moxa pole

1085. **艾炷** [艾炷] *ài zhù*, moxa cone

1086. **进针** [進針] *jìn zhēn*, needle insertion

1087. **出针** [出針] *chū zhēn*, needle removal

1088. **留针** [留針] *liú zhēn*, needle retention

1089. **退针** [退針] *tuì zhēn*, needle retraction

1090. **捣针** [搗針] *dǎo zhēn*, needle pounding

1091. **捻针** [捻針] *niǎn zhēn*, needle twirling

1092. **刮针** [刮針] *guā zhēn*, needle scratching

1093. **摇针** [搖針] *yáo zhēn*, needle waggling

1094. **得气** [得氣] *dé qì*, obtaining qì

1095. **气至** [氣至] *qì zhì*, arrival of qì

1096. **针感** [針感] *zhēn gǎn*, needle sensation

1097. **循摄法** [循攝法] *xún shè fǎ*, channel-freeing manipulation

1098. **弹针** [彈針] *tán zhēn*, needle flicking

1099. **呼吸补泻** [呼吸補瀉] *hū xī bǔ xiè*, respiratory supplementation and drainage

1100. **迎随补泻** [迎隨補瀉] *yíng suí bǔ xiè*, directional supplementation and drainage

1101. **疾徐补泻** [疾徐補瀉] *jí xú bǔ xiè*, quick and slow supplementation and drainage

1102. **捻转补泻** [捻轉補瀉] *niǎn zhuǎn bǔ xiè*, twirling supplementation and drainage

1103. **提插补泻** [提插補瀉] *tí chā bǔ xiè*, lift-and-thrust supplementation and drainage

1104. 开阖补泻 [開闔補瀉] *kāi hé bǔ xiè*, open and closed supplementation and drainage

1105. 透天凉 [透天涼] *tòu tiān liáng*, heaven-penetrating cooling method

1106. 烧山火 [燒山火] *shāo shān huǒ*, burning mountain fire method

1107. 回阳九针 [回陽九針] *huí yáng jiǔ zhēn*, nine needles for returning yáng

1108. 火针 [火針] *huǒ zhēn*, fire needling

1109. 晕针 [暈針] *yùn zhēn*, needle sickness

1110. 滞针 [滯針] *zhì zhēn*, stuck needle

1111. 折针 [折針] *zhé zhēn*, needle breakage

1112. 艾灸 [艾灸] *ài jiǔ*, moxibustion

1113. 艾条灸 [艾條灸] *ài tiáo jiǔ*, poling

1114. 温针 [溫針] *wēn zhēn*, warm needling

1115. 直接灸 [直接灸] *zhí jiē jiǔ*, direct moxibustion

1116. 瘢痕灸 [瘢痕灸] *bān hén jiǔ*, scarring moxibustion

1117. 无瘢痕灸 [無瘢痕灸] *wú bān hén jiǔ*, nonscarring moxibustion

1118. 艾炷灸 [艾炷灸] *ài zhù jiǔ*, cone moxibustion

1119. 壮数 [壯數] *zhuàng shù*, number of cones

1120. 间接灸 [間接灸] *jiān jiē jiǔ*, indirect moxibustion

1121. 隔附子灸 [隔附子灸] *gé fù zǐ jiǔ*, moxibustion on aconite

1122. 隔姜灸 [隔薑灸] *gé jiāng jiǔ*, moxibustion on ginger

1123. 隔蒜灸 [隔蒜灸] *gé suàn jiǔ*, moxibustion on garlic

1124. 隔盐灸 [隔鹽灸] *gé yán jiǔ*, moxibustion on salt

1125. 拔火罐 [拔火罐] *bá huǒ guàn*, fire cupping

1126. 坐罐法 [坐罐法] *zuò guàn fǎ*, stationary cupping

1127. 推罐 [推罐] *tuī guàn*, push-cupping

1128. 闪罐 [閃罐] *shǎn guàn*, flash cupping

1129. 刺络拔罐 [刺絡拔罐] *cì luò bá guàn*, pricking and cupping

Index

fèi yǔ dà cháng xiāng biǎo lǐ 肺与大肠
相表里 lung and large intestine
stand in interior-exterior
relationship, 44, 279, 311
fèi zhǔ pí máo 肺主皮毛 lung governs
the skin and [body] hair, 44
fèi zhǔ qì 肺主气 lung governs qì, 44
fèi zhǔ sù jiàng 肺主肃降 lung governs
depurative downbearing, 44, 290,
306
fèi zhǔ tōng tiáo shuǐ dào 肺主通调水
道 lung governs regulation of the
waterways, 44, 282, 305, 307
fēn bié 分别 separate, separation, 47
fěn 粉 meal(y), 66, 284
fēng 风 wind, 21, 115, 150, 157, 184,
195, 207–209, 285
fēng hán 风寒 wind-cold, 158
fēng hán shù fèi 风寒束肺 wind-cold
fettering the lung, 158
fēng rè 风热 wind-heat, 158
fēng rè fàn fèi 风热犯肺 wind-heat
invading the lung, 158
fēng tán 风痰 wind-phlegm, 167
fēng wēn 风温 wind warmth, 175
fēng xié rù jīng 风邪入经 wind evil
entering the channels, 158, 301
fermented soybean 淡豆豉 *dàn dòu chǐ*
(Sojae Semen Praeparatum), 184
fetus 胎 *tāi*, 91, 306
fever 热 *rè*, 74, 75, 301
see heat effusion
field 田 *tián*, 15, 307
field thistle 小蓟 *xiǎo jì* (Cirsii Herba),
203, 204
fifteen network vessels 十五络 *shí wǔ
luò*, 34
fifth-watch diarrhea 五更泄 *wǔ gēng
xiè*, 80, 312
filiform needle 毫针 *háo zhēn*, 241
fine 细 *xì*, 94, 226, 310
fine pulse 细脉 *xì mài*, 94, 310
fire 火 *huǒ*, 5, 19, 23, 43, 155, 159, 241,
247, 248, 251, 289

fire and water help each other 水火相济
shuǐ huǒ xiāng jì, 7, 290
fire and water processing 水火制 *shuǐ
huǒ zhì*, 230
fire cupping 拔火罐 *bá huǒ guàn*, 252,
277, 286
fire failing to engender earth 火不生土
huǒ bù shēng tǔ, 8
fire needle 火针 *huǒ zhēn*, 241
fire needling, 248
fire processing 火制 *huǒ zhì*, 228
firm 牢 *láo*, 95, 294
firm pulse; confined pulse 牢脉 *láo mài*,
95, 294
Fish Poison Yam Clear-Turbid
Separation Beverage 萆薢分清饮
bì xiè fēn qīng yǐn, 195
fissured 裂 *liè*, 64, 295
fissured tongue 舌裂 *shé liè*, 64, 295
five 五 *wǔ*, 5, 8–10, 34, 39, 310
five colors 五色 *wǔ sè*, 9, 302
five flavors 五味 *wǔ wèi*, 10, 223
five humors 五液 *wǔ yè*, 10, 314
Five Kernels Pill 五仁丸 *wǔ rén wán*,
190
five minds 五志 *wǔ zhì*, 10
five offices 五官 *wǔ guān*, 9
five phases 五行 *wǔ xíng*, 5, 312
five transport points 五俞穴 *wǔ shū xué*,
39, 310
five viscera 五脏 *wǔ zàng*, 8
fixed 着 *zhuó*, 112, 319
fixed impediment 着痹 *zhuó bì*, 112, 319
flailing of the arms and legs 扬手掷足
yáng shǒu zhí zú, 61, 305, 319
flame 炎 *yán*, 141, 149, 313
flaring nostrils 鼻翼煽动 *bí yì shān
dòng*, 69, 278
flash 闪 *shǎn*, 252, 302
flash cupping 闪罐 *shǎn guàn*, 253
flat-abscess 疽 *jū*, 122, 292
flavor 味 *wèi*, 223, 309
flesh 肌 *jī*, 46, 289
肉 *ròu*, 8, 46, 60, 61, 301

gān huǒ shàng yán 肝火上炎 liver fire flaming upward, 149, 285

gān jiāng 干姜 dried ginger (Zingiberis Rhizoma), 193, 196, 197, 214, 229

gān jīng shī rè 肝经湿热 liver channel damp-heat, 152

gān kāi qiào yú mù 肝开窍于目 liver opens at the eyes, 50, 298

gān lù xiāo dú dān 甘露消毒丹 Sweet Dew Toxin-Dispersing Elixir, 194

gān qì fàn pí 肝气犯脾 liver qì invading the spleen, 152, 284, 299

gān qì fàn wèi 肝气犯胃 liver qì invading the stomach, 152, 284

gān qì yù jié 肝气郁结 binding depression of liver qì, 149, 291, 315

gān shèn yīn kuī 肝肾阴亏 liver-kidney yīn depletion, 157, 294

gān shǔ mù 肝属木 liver belongs to wood, 48, 285, 298

gān suì 甘遂 kansui (Kansui Radix), 191, 230

gān wéi gāng zàng 肝为刚脏 liver is the unyielding viscus, 50

gān xuè xū 肝血虚 liver blood vacuity, 150

gān yáng huà fēng 肝阳化风 liver yáng transforming into wind, 151, 285

gān yáng shàng kàng 肝阳上亢 ascendant (hyperactivity of) liver yáng; ascendant liver yáng,

gān yǔ dǎn xiāng biǎo lǐ 肝与胆相表里 liver and gallbladder stand in interior-exterior relationship, 48, 282, 295

gān yù 肝郁 liver depression, 149

gān yù huà huǒ 肝郁化火 liver depression transforming into fire, 149

gān zhǔ jīn 肝主筋 liver governs the sinews, 49, 291

gān zhǔ shū xiè 肝主疏泄 liver governs free coursing, 48, 305, 312

gǎn 感 contract, contraction, 109, 157, 162, 285

gǎn shòu zào xié 感受燥邪 contraction of dryness evil, 162, 305, 316

gāng 肛 anus, 80, 285

gāo 膏 gāo (as in 'gāo-huāng'), 15, 286

gāo 膏 paste, 233, 286

gāo 膏 unctuous (strangury), 119, 286

gāo (as in 'gāo-huāng') 膏 gāo, 15, 286

gāo-huāng 膏肓 *gāo huāng*, 15, 286, 289

gāo huāng 膏肓 gāo-huāng, 15, 286, 289

gāo liáng jiāng 高良姜 lesser galangal (Alpiniae Officinarum Rhizoma), 196

gāo lín 膏淋 unctuous strangury, 119, 286

gāo yào 膏药 plaster, 234

gāo zī 膏滋 rich paste, 234, 286, 319

gaping corners of the mouth 口角不闭 *kǒu jiǎo bù bì*, 69

gardenia 山栀子 *shān zhī zǐ* (Gardeniae Fructus), 186, 188, 194, 226

Gardenia and Fermented Soybean Decoction 栀子豉汤 *zhī zǐ chǐ tāng*, 186

Gardeniae Fructus 山栀子 *shān zhī zǐ* (gardenia), 186, 188, 194, 226

gastro- 胃 *wèi*, 163, 309

gastrodia 天麻 *tiān má* (Gastrodiae Rhizoma), 208, 224

Gastrodiae Rhizoma 天麻 *tiān má* (gastrodia), 208, 224

gastrointestinal accumulation 肠胃积滞 *cháng wèi jī zhì*, 163, 289, 309

gate 门 *mén*, 14, 67, 297

gate (essence) 关 *guān*, 15, 286

gather, gathering 聚 *jù*, 116, 293

gé 膈 diaphragm; diaphragmatic, 14, 286 occlusion, 113, 286

gé 革 drumskin, 95, 286

gé 隔 separate, 250, 251

gé fù zǐ jiǔ 隔附子灸 moxibustion on aconite, 250

gé gēn 葛根 pueraria (Puerariae Radix), 184, 185

patterns 和解半表半里 *hé jiě bàn biǎo bàn lǐ*, 191, 287

harmonizing (and resolving) the lesser yáng 和解少阳 *hé jiě shào yáng*, 191

harmonizing the liver and spleen 调和肝脾 *tiáo hé gān pí*, 191, 307

harmonizing the liver and stomach 调和肝胃 *tiáo hé gān wèi*, 192

harmonizing the stomach and intestines 调和肠胃 *tiáo hé cháng wèi*, 192

harmonizing the stomach and rectifying qì 和胃理气 *hé wèi lǐ qì*, 198

harmony of mouth 口中和 *kǒu zhōng hé*, 83, 287, 318

hasty 促 *cù*, 72, 281

hasty breathing 气促 *qì cù*, 72, 281

hē 呵 yawn, yawning, 112, 287

hē qiàn 呵欠 yawning, 287

hē zǐ 诃子 chebule (Chebulae Fructus), 216

hé hé 核 node (as in 'phlegm node'), 12, 123, 287

hé hé 核 pit (plum-pit), 113, 287

hé 合 uniting, 38

hé 阖 close, closing, 52, 287

hé 和 harmonize, harmonizing, harmonization, harmony, 83, 191–193, 198, 287

hé fǎ 和法 harmonization, 191

hé jiě bàn biǎo bàn lǐ 和解半表半里 harmonizing (and resolving) midstage patterns; harmonizing (and resolving) half-exterior half-interior patterns, 191, 287

hé jiě shào yáng 和解少阳 harmonizing (and resolving) the lesser yáng, 191

hé shǒu wū 何首乌 flowery knotweed (Polygoni Multiflori Radix), 211

hé wèi lǐ qì 和胃理气 harmonizing the stomach and rectifying qì, 198

hé yè 荷叶 lotus leaf (Nelumbinis Folium), 203, 204

hè shī 鹤虱 carpesium seed (Carpesii Fructus), 202

hè xī fēng 鹤膝风 crane's-knee wind, 113

head 头 *tóu*, 11, 60, 62, 67, 68, 76, 77, 109, 308

head heavy as if swathed 头重如裹 *tóu zhòng rú guǒ*, 77

head wind 头风 *tóu fēng*, 109, 308

headache 头痛 *tóu tòng*, 76, 307

headache with pulling sensation 头痛如掣 *tóu tòng rú chè*, 77

heart 心 *xīn*, 8, 11, 13, 43, 210, 312

heart-gallbladder vacuity timidity 心胆虚怯 *xīn dǎn xū qiè*, 153

heart-kidney yáng vacuity 心肾阳虚 *xīn shèn yáng xū*, 157

heart-kidney yīn vacuity 心肾阴虚 *xīn shèn yīn xū*, 148

heart-spleen blood vacuity 心脾血虚 *xīn pí xuè xū*, 149

heart and small intestine stand in interior-exterior relationship 心与小肠相表里 *xīn yǔ xiǎo cháng xiāng biǎo lǐ*, 43

heart belongs to fire 心属火 *xīn shǔ huǒ*, 43

heart blood stasis obstruction 心血瘀阻 *xīn xuè yū zǔ*, 142

heart blood vacuity 心血虚 *xīn xuè xū*, 140

heart fire flaming upward 心火上炎 *xīn huǒ shàng yán*, 141, 313

heart fire spreading heat to the small intestine 心火移热于小肠 *xīn huǒ yí rè yú xiǎo cháng*, 142

heart governs the blood and vessels 心主血脉 *xīn zhǔ xuè mài*, 43, 312, 318

heart impediment 心痹 *xīn bì*, 116, 278

heart opens at the tongue 心开窍于舌 *xīn kāi qiào yú shé*, 43, 293, 300, 303

heart palpitations 心悸 *xīn jì*, 85, 290

heart qì vacuity 心气虚 *xīn qì xū*, 140

jīng guān 精关 essence gate, 15, 286

jīng jì 惊悸 fright palpitations, 85, 292

jīng jiè 荆芥 schizonepeta
(Schizonepetae Herba), 183, 208

jīng luò 经络 channels and network
vessels, 33, 292

jīng luò zhī qì 经络之气 channel and
network vessel qì, 17

jīng xíng xiān hòu wú dìng qí 经行
先后无定期 menstruation at
irregular intervals, 90

jǐng 颈 neck, 12, 62, 292

jǐng xiàng jiàng zhí 颈项强直 rigidity of
the neck, 62, 291, 292, 311

jìng 镜 mirror, 65, 292

jìng 净 clean, 66, 292

jìng 痉 tetany, tetanic, 61, 114, 292

jìng bìng 痉病 tetany, 114, 292

jìng jué 痉厥 tetanic reversal, 61, 292,
293

jìng miàn shé 镜面舌 mirror tongue, 65,
292

jiǔ 酒 wine, 233, 292

jiǔ 九 nine, 247, 292

jiǔ 灸 moxa, 249–251, 292

jiǔ jì 酒剂 wine preparation, 233

jiǔ qiào 九窍 nine orifices, 292

jiǔ xiān sǎn 九仙散 Nine Immortals
Powder, 216

jiǔ xiè 久泄 enduring diarrhea, 80, 292

jiù 救 stem, stemming, 196, 197, 292

joint 节 *jié*, 77, 291

joint-running wind 历节风 *lì jié fēng*,
112

joint pain 关节疼痛 *guān jié téng tòng*,
77, 286, 291, 307, 308

joy 喜 *xǐ*, 10, 310

jū 疽 flat-abscess, 122, 292

jú hóng 橘红 red tangerine peel (Citri
Reticulatae Pericarpium Rubrum),
216

jú huā 菊花 chrysanthemum
(Chrysanthemi Flos), 208

jù 拒 refuse, 86, 292

jù 聚 gather, gathering, 116, 293

juǎn 卷 curled, 64, 293

juàn 倦 fatigued, fatigue, 27, 60, 78, 29?

juàn dài fá lì 倦怠乏力 fatigue and lack
of strength, 78, 281, 295

jué 厥 reverse, reversal, reverting, 35,
61, 97, 293

jué nì 厥逆 reverse-flow, 97

jué yīn 厥阴 reverting yīn, 35

jué yīn bìng 厥阴病 reverting yīn
disease, 171

Jujubae Fructus 大枣 *dà zǎo* (jujube),
185, 191, 216

jujube 大枣 *dà zǎo* (Jujubae Fructus),
185, 191, 216

jūn 君 sovereign, 19, 237, 293

jūn huǒ 君火 sovereign fire, 19, 289, 29

Junci Medulla 灯心草 *dēng xīn cǎo*
(juncus), 230

juncus 灯心草 *dēng xīn cǎo* (Junci
Medulla), 230

kǎ 咯 expectorate, hack, 70, 293

kǎ xuè 咯血 expectoration of blood, 70

kāi 开 open, opening, 52, 209, 210, 293

kāi hé bǔ xiè 开阖补泻 open and close
supplementation and drainage, 246

kāi qiào fǎ 开窍法 opening the orifices,
209

Kaki Fructus Exsiccatus 柿饼 *shì bǐng*
(dried persimmon), 226

Kaki Saccharum 柿霜 *shì shuāng*
(persimmon frost), 226

kàng 亢 hyperactive, 149, 293

kansui 甘遂 *gān suì* (Kansui Radix),
191, 230

Kansui Radix 甘遂 *gān suì* (kansui),
191, 230

Katsumada's galangal seed 草豆蔻 *cǎo
dòu kòu* (Alpiniae Katsumadai
Semen), 226

kē 窠 nest, 69, 293

ké 咳 cough, 70, 110, 216, 293

kǒu suān 口酸 sour taste in the mouth, 83

kǒu tián 口甜 sweet taste in the mouth, 83, 307

kǒu yǎn wāi xié 口眼喎斜 deviated eyes and mouth, 61, 294, 308, 312, 313

kǒu zhōng hé 口中和 harmony of mouth, 83, 287, 318

kū 枯 desiccated, 69, 294
 dry, 68, 294

kǔ 苦 bitter, bitterness, 10, 83, 294

kǔ liàn pí 苦楝皮 chinaberry bark (Meliae Cortex), 201

kǔ xìng rén 苦杏仁 bitter apricot kernel (Armeniacae Semen Amarum), 233

kuài 块 lump, 97, 294

kuǎn dōng huā 款冬花 coltsfoot (Farfarae Flos), 216, 224

kuáng 狂 mania, 61, 294

kuáng zào 狂躁 mania and agitation, 61, 294

kuī 亏 depletion, 7, 157, 294

kūn bù 昆布 kelp (Laminariae/Eckloniae Thallus), 201

kùn 困 cumbersome, encumbrance, 60, 88, 144, 294

Lablab Flos 扁豆花 *biǎn dòu huā* (lablab flower), 187

lablab flower 扁豆花 *biǎn dòu huā* (Lablab Flos), 187

lack 欠 *qiàn*, 96, 300

lack of warmth in the limbs 四肢不温 *sì zhī bù wēn*, 97

lack of warmth in the limbs 四肢欠温 *sì zhī qiàn wēn*, 96, 300, 309

lái fú zǐ 莱菔子 radish seed (Raphani Semen), 200

lài 癞 *lài*, 123

lài 癫 *lài*, 123

Laminariae/Eckloniae Thallus 昆布 *kūn bù* (kelp), 201

lǎn 懒 lazy, laziness, 72, 294

lǎn yán 懒言 laziness to speak, 72, 294, 313

láo 劳 taxation, 119, 294

láo 牢 firm, 95, 294

láo juàn 劳倦 taxation fatigue, 27, 293

láo lín 劳淋 taxation strangury, 119, 294

láo mài 牢脉 firm pulse; confined pulse, 95, 294

láo zhài 痨瘵 consumption, 109

lǎo huáng 老黄 old yellow, 67, 294

lào zhěn 落枕 crick in the neck, 113

large (pulse, intestine) 大 *dà*, 11, 94, 281

large gentian 秦艽 *qín jiāo* (Gentianae Macrophyllae Radix), 189, 195

large intestinal damp-heat 大肠湿热 *dà cháng shī rè*, 162

large intestinal humor depletion 大肠液亏 *dà cháng yè kuī*, 148

large intestine 大肠 *dà cháng*, 11, 279, 281

large intestine governs liquid 大肠主津 *dà cháng zhǔ jīn*, 48

large intestine governs the conveyance and transformation of waste 大肠主传化糟粕 *dà cháng zhǔ chuán huà zāo pò*, 48, 315

large pulse 大脉 *dà mài*, 94

laryngeal prominence 结喉 *jié hóu*, 12, 288, 291

larynx, laryngeal; throat 喉 *hóu*, 12, 72, 288

Lasiosphaera seu Calvatia 马勃 *mǎ bó* (puffball), 188

later 后 *hòu*, 19, 288

laziness to speak 懒言 *lǎn yán*, 72, 294, 313

lazy, laziness 懒 *lǎn*, 72, 294

leech 水蛭 *shuǐ zhì* (Hirudo), 203

leg 足 *zú*, 14, 60, 319

leg 腿 *tuǐ*, 14, 76, 78, 308

leg qì 脚气 *jiǎo qì*, 122

léi wán 雷丸 omphalia (Omphalia), 201

lèi 泪 tears, 10, 294

lěng 冷 cold, 27, 96, 97, 294

Liver-Settling Wind-Extinguishing
Decoction 镇肝熄风汤 *zhèn gān xī fēng tāng*, 209
liver and gallbladder stand in
interior-exterior relationship 肝与
胆相表里 *gān yǔ dǎn xiāng biǎo lǐ*,
48, 282, 295
liver belongs to wood 肝属木 *gān shǔ mù*, 48, 285, 298
liver blood vacuity 肝血虚 *gān xuè xū*, 150
liver channel damp-heat 肝经湿热 *gān jīng shī rè*, 152
liver depression 肝郁 *gān yù*, 149
liver depression transforming into fire 肝郁化火 *gān yù huà*, 149
liver fire flaming upward 肝火上炎 *gān huǒ shàng yán*, 149, 285
liver governs free coursing 肝主疏泄 *gān zhǔ shū xiè*, 48, 305, 312
liver governs the sinews 肝主筋 *gān zhǔ jīn*, 49, 291
liver is the unyielding viscus 肝为刚脏 *gān wéi gāng zàng*, 50
liver opens at the eyes 肝开窍于目 *gān kāi qiào yú mù*, 50, 298
liver qì invading the spleen 肝气犯脾 *gān qì fàn pí*, 152, 284, 299
liver qì invading the stomach 肝气犯胃 *gān qì fàn wèi*, 152, 284
liver stores blood 肝藏血 *gān cáng xuè*, 49, 285
liver wind stirring internally 肝风内动 *gān fēng nèi dòng*, 150, 282, 285, 298
liver yáng transforming into wind 肝阳化风 *gān yáng huà fēng*, 151, 285
liver... its bloom is in the nails 肝，其华在爪 *gān, qí huá zài zhǎo*, 50, 318
oadstone 磁石 *cí shí* (Magnetitum), 230
ockjaw 破伤风 *pò shāng fēng*, 118
odged 留 *liú*, 161, 166, 296
odged rheum 留饮 *liú yǐn*, 166

long 长 *cháng*, 79, 96, 279
long-rinsing 漂 *piǎo*, 227, 299
long pulse 长脉 *cháng mài*, 96, 279
long voidings of clear urine 小便清长 *xiǎo biàn qīng cháng*, 79, 279, 300
lóng 癃 dribbling urination, 118, 296
lóng bì 癃闭 dribbling urinary block, 119, 296
lóng gǔ 龙骨 dragon bone (Mastodi Ossis Fossilia), 197, 215, 230
lóng yǎn ròu 龙眼肉 longan flesh (Longan Arillus), 211
Longan Arillus 龙眼肉 *lóng yǎn ròu* (longan flesh), 211
longan flesh 龙眼肉 *lóng yǎn ròu* (Longan Arillus), 211
lonicera 金银花 *jīn yín huā* (Lonicerae Flos), 187, 188, 235
Lonicera and Forsythia Powder 银翘散 *yín qiáo sǎn*, 184
Lonicerae Flos 金银花 *jīn yín huā* (lonicera), 187, 188, 235
loosening of the teeth 齿牙松动 *chǐ yá sōng dòng*, 70
loquat leaf 枇杷叶 *pí pá yè* (Eriobotryae Folium), 216
lose, loss 失 *shī*, 88, 304
lotus leaf 荷叶 *hé yè* (Nelumbinis Folium), 203, 204
lotus seed 莲肉 *lián ròu* (Nelumbinis Semen), 214
lotus stamen 莲须 *lián xū* (Nelumbinis Stamen), 215
lòu 漏 spotting, 119, 296
lower 下 *xià*, 38, 310
lower uniting point 下合穴 *xià hé xué*, 38, 310
lozenge 锭 *dìng*, 235
lú 颅 skull, 111, 296
lú gān shí 炉甘石 calamine (Calamina), 228, 230
lú gēn 芦根 phragmites (Phragmitis Rhizoma), 187
lù 露 distillate, 235, 296

Sanguisorbae Radix 地榆 *dì yú*
    (sanguisorba), 204
saposhnikovia 防风 *fáng fēng*
    (Saposhnikoviae Radix), 183–185,
    195, 208
Saposhnikoviae Radix 防风 *fáng fēng*
    (saposhnikovia), 183–185, 195, 208
Sargassum 海藻 *hǎi zǎo* (sargassum),
    201, 227
sargassum 海藻 *hǎi zǎo* (Sargassum),
    201, 227
Sargassum Jade Flask Decoction 海藻玉
    壶汤 *hǎi zǎo yù hú tāng*, 201
scab 疥 *jiè*, 123
scallion-stalk 芤 *kōu*, 94, 294
scallion-stalk pulse 芤脉 *kōu mài*, 94,
    294
scallion white 葱白 *cōng bái* (Allii
    Fistulosi Bulbus), 184
scallion white with root 连须葱白 *lián
    xū cōng bái* (Allii Fistulosi Bulbus
    cum Radice), 183
scant 少 *shǎo*, 70, 79, 90, 303
scant menstruation 月经过少 *yuè jīng
    guò shǎo*, 90, 292, 303, 315
scant phlegm expectorated with
    difficulty 痰少不易咯 *tán shǎo bú
    yì kǎ*, 70, 293, 303
scarring moxibustion 瘢痕灸 *bān hén
    jiǔ*, 249
schizonepeta 荆芥 *jīng jiè*
    (Schizonepetae Herba), 183, 208
Schizonepeta and Saposhnikovia
    Toxin-Vanquishing Powder 荆防败
    毒散 *jīng fáng bài dú sǎn*, 183
Schizonepetae Herba 荆芥 *jīng jiè*
    (schizonepeta), 183, 208
schisandra 五味子 *wǔ wèi zǐ*
    (Schisandrae Fructus), 197, 214,
    216
Schisandra Decoction 五味子汤 *wǔ wèi
    zǐ tāng*, 216
Schisandrae Fructus 五味子 *wǔ wèi zǐ*
    (schisandra), 197, 214, 216

scorch 焦 *jiāo*, 97, 229, 291
scorch-frying 炒焦 *chǎo jiāo*, 229
scorching heat 灼热 *zhuó rè*, 97
Scorpio 全蝎 *quán xiē* (scorpion), 198,
    224
scorpion 全蝎 *quán xiē* (Scorpio), 198,
    224
scrofula 瘰疬 *luǒ lì*, 123, 295, 296
scrofula 瘰 *luǒ*, 123, 296
scrofula 疬 *lì*, 123, 295
Scrofula Internal Dispersion Pill 内消
    瘰疬丸 *nèi xiāo luǒ lì wán*, 201
scrophularia 玄参 *xuán shēn*
    (Scrophulariae Radix), 190, 212
Scrophulariae Radix 玄参 *xuán shēn*
    (scrophularia), 190, 212
scurrying 窜 *cuàn*, 86, 281
scurrying pain around the umbilicus 脐
    周窜痛 *qí zhōu cuàn tòng*, 86, 281,
    300
scutellaria 黄芩 *huáng qín* (Scutellariae
    Radix), 186, 188, 191, 193
Scutellariae Radix 黄芩 *huáng qín*
    (scutellaria), 186, 188, 191, 193
sè 色 color, 9, 302
    complexion, 62, 63, 302
sè 塞 congestion, 70, 302
sè 涩 astringe, astringent (therapeutic
    action), 213–215, 302
    rough (pulse), 93, 302
sè cháng gù tuō 涩肠固脱 astringing the
    intestines and stemming desertion,
    214, 286, 302
sè jīng zhǐ yí 涩精止遗 astringing
    essence and checking (seminal)
    emission and enuresis, 215
sè mài 涩脉 rough pulse, 93, 302
sea 海 *hǎi*, 16, 287
sea of qì 气海 *qì hǎi*, 16, 287
secure, security, securing 固 *gù*, 156,
    213, 286
securing and astriction 固涩法 *gù sè fǎ*,
    213
seminal efflux 滑精 *huá jīng*, 89, 288

zhì zé 治则 principle of treatment, 181

zhì zhēn 滞针 stuck needle, 248

zhōng 中 center, 145, 196, 317
in, 69, 70, 72, 83, 124, 317

zhōng qì bù zú 中气不足 insufficiency of center qì, 145

zhōng qì xià xiàn 中气下陷 center qì fall, 311

zhǒng 肿 swelling, 69, 97, 119, 318

zhòng 中 strike, stroke, 117, 318

zhòng 重 heavy, heaviness, 60, 72, 76, 80, 318

zhòng fēng 中风 wind stroke; wind strike, 117, 318

zhòng tīng 重听 hardness of hearing; hearing impairment, 87

zhòng zhèn ān shén 重镇安神 quieting the spirit with heavy settlers, 207, 277, 316

zhōu 周 generalized, 112, 318

zhōu bì 周痹 generalized impediment, 112, 318

zhǒu 肘 elbow, 14, 318

zhū líng 猪苓 polyporus (Polyporus), 194, 195

zhū shā 朱砂 cinnabar (Cinnabaris), 228, 236

zhú 逐 expel, expelling, 190, 210, 318

zhú hán kāi qiào 逐寒开窍 expelling cold and opening the orifices, 210

zhú rú 竹茹 bamboo shavings (Bumbusae Caulis in Taenia), 192

zhú shuǐ 逐水 expelling water, 190

zhú yū 逐瘀 expelling stasis, 318

zhǔ 主 govern, 43, 318

zhǔ 煮 boiling, 230, 318

zhù 注 pour, 162, 318

zhù 助 assist, assisting, 184, 213, 318

zhù 炷 cone, 243, 250, 318

zhù yáng 助阳 assisting yáng, 213, 318

zhù yáng jiě biǎo 助阳解表 reinforcing yáng and resolving the exterior, 185

zhuǎ 爪 nail, 50, 318

zhuǎn 转 turn, 246, 318

convert, 5, 318 shift, 119, 318

zhuǎn bāo 转胞 shifted bladder, 119, 278, 318

zhuàng 壮 vigorous, 74, 318

zhuàng rè 壮热 vigorous heat [effusion] vigorous fever, 74, 301, 318

zhuàng shù 壮数 number of cones, 250

zhuó 浊 turbid, turbidity, 72, 79, 119, 318

zhuó 着 fixed, 112, 319

zhuó bì 着痹 fixed impediment, 112, 31

zhuó rè 灼热 scorching heat, 97

zī 滋 enrich, enriching, 184, 196, 209, 213, 319
rich, 233, 319

zī yīn 滋阴 enriching yīn, 213, 319

zī yīn jiě biǎo 滋阴解表 enriching yīn and resolving the exterior, 184

zī yīn rùn zào 滋阴润燥 enriching yīn and moistening dryness, 196

zī yīn xī fēng 滋阴息风 enriching yīn and extinguishing wind, 209

zǐ 子 child, 120, 319
pregnant, pregnancy, 319

zǐ 紫 purple, 63, 65, 319

zǐ cǎo 紫草 arnebia/lithospermum (Arnebiae/Lithospermi Radix), 187

zǐ gōng 子宫 uterus, 54

zǐ gōng xià chuí 子宫下垂 prolapse of the uterus, 91

zǐ huā dì dīng 紫花地丁 violet (Violae Herba), 188

zǐ sū 紫苏 perilla (Perillae Folium, Caulis, et Calyx), 192, 205

zǐ sū yè 紫苏叶 perilla leaf (Perillae Folium), 183, 184, 225

zǐ wǎn 紫菀 aster (Asteris Radix), 216

zǐ xuě dān 紫雪丹 Purple Snow Elixir, 210

zì 自 spontaneous, 76, 319

zì hàn 自汗 spontaneous sweating, 76, 287, 319

zì rán tóng 自然铜 pyrite (Pyritum), 23

AUTHORS' BIOGRAPHIES

Nigel Wiseman was born in England on April 21, 1954. He received a Bachelor's degree i Spanish and German interpreting and translation in 1976 from Heriott-Watt University in Edinburgh. He has lived in Táiwān for the last 19 years and taught at China Medical College for many years. He now teaches Chinese medical English in the newly established Department of Traditional Chinese Medicine of Chang Gung University, Táiwān. He is author or coauthor of a number of Chinese medical works including *Fundamentals of Chinese Medicine, Fundamentals of Chinese Acupuncture, An English-Chinese Chinese-English Dictionary of Chinese Medicine*, and *Shāng Hán Lùn* (On Cold Damage) *Translation and Commentaries*. He recently completed his doctorate in Complementary Health and Applied Linguistics at the University of Exeter, England.

Féng Yè (馮曄) was born in Táiwān on November 26, 1967. He graduated from the Chinese Medical School of China Medical College, Táiwān in 1994, and holds R.O.C. licenses in Chinese and Western medicine. He received his Master's degree from the Institute of Chinese Medical Sciences, China Medical College, in 1997. He has co-authore several Chinese medical works including *An English-Chinese Chinese-English Dictionary of Chinese Medicine* and *Shāng Hán Lùn* (On Cold Damage): *Translation and Commentaries*. He is now a resident doctor in the Chinese Internal Medicine Department Chang Gung Memorial Hospital and lectures in diagnostics in the Department of Traditional Chinese Medicine at Chang Gung University's College of Medicine. His speci fields of interest other than general internal medicine include pulse theory, *shāng hán* (col damage), diagnostics, acupuncture, and external injury.

Paradigm Publications
www.paradigm-pubs.com

Wiseman & Féng's

CHINESE MEDICAL CHINESE: GRAMMAR AND VOCABULARY

This is a very sophisticated and highly useful work that provides a sound basis for reading both modern and classical texts for anyone wishing to learn original Chinese medical language. The work assumes readers already have knowledge of how Chinese characters are composed, how they are written by hand, and how they are pronounced.

This book is divided into two parts. The first part describes the basic features of literary Chinese medical language and its relationship to both the classical language and to the modern vernacular of northern China, known as Mandarin. It explains many grammatical constructions commonly encountered in Chinese medical texts, and describes how Chinese medical terms are composed. The second part presents the vocabulary and terminology of Chinese medicine as its component characters.

The lessons are organized by Chinese medical categories and the characters are introduced in sets according to subject matter; for example, terms related to the five phases, terms related to inspection of the tongue, terms related to pulse-taking, or terms related to women's diseases. Each of these sets is followed by a section that presents examples of compound terms formed from characters already introduced. These examples are then followed by drills that self-test these vocabularies.

In all, this text covers basic theories, four examinations, diseases, pathomechanisms and disease patterns, principles and methods of treatment, pharmaceutics, and acupuncture. It includes etymologies of terms, gives component characters in simplified and complex form with their significs, and explains term translations for 1027 characters and 2555 compound terms. The back matter includes answers to the 910 drill questions, appendices containing the names of commonly used medicinals, formulas, and acupuncture points, and a copious index.

CHINESE   MEDICINE   LANGUAGE   SERIES

英文中医词汇入门
英文中醫詞彙入門

Wiseman & Féng's

Introduction to

ENGLISH TERMINOLOGY OF CHINESE MEDICINE

This book serves several basic needs. For the beginning Western student of Chinese medicine, it defines basic concepts. For the learner of Chinese, it furnishes all terms in Chinese characters, both simplified and complex, together with intoned Pīnyīn pronunciation. For Chinese practitioners learning clinical English, it provides English terms with pronunciation in KK transcription. For Táiwān students and practitioners unfamiliar with mainland China's Pīnyīn system, it provides conversion tables for Mandarin Phonetic Symbols (ㄅㄆㄇㄈ). The full index helps readers to locate all terms in the body of the text and furthermore serves as an Chinese-English English-Chinese dictionary.

Features

- Introduces 1129 basic concepts in thematic order.

- Provides both simplified and complex Chinese characters with intoned Pīnyīn for each term.

- Gives English pronunciation for non-native speakers of English.

- Sets nearly 900 questions to test progess, with answers at the end of the book.

- Provides a guide for Pīnyīn pronunciation.

- Includes a Pīnyīn Conversion Table for Mandarin Phonetic Symbols for Táiwān students and practitioners.

- Includes an appendix of 548 basic characters together with examples of terms in which they appear.

- Contains a full index including the names of medicinals and formulas that allows any Chinese term or English equivalent to be accessed.

Other books in the Chinese Medicine Language Series include *Chinese Medical Chinese: Characters* and *Chinese Medical Chinese: Grammar and Vocabulary*.

CHINESE MEDICINE LANGUAGE SERIES